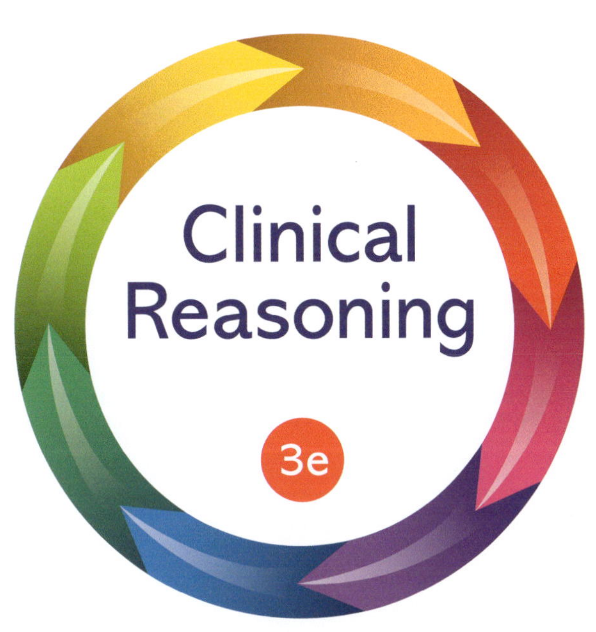
Clinical
Reasoning
3e

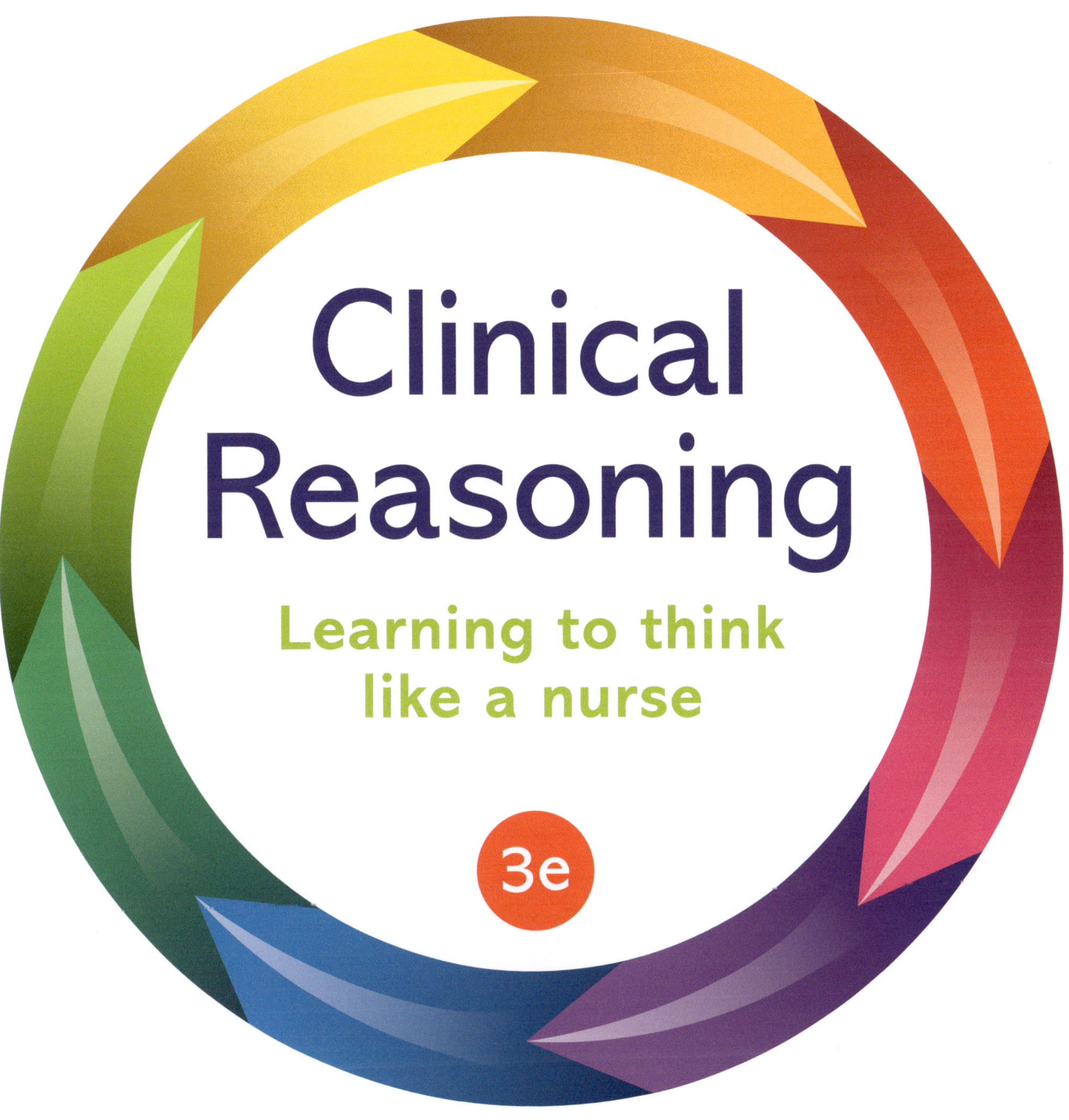

Clinical Reasoning

Learning to think like a nurse

3e

Edited by Tracy Levett-Jones

Pearson Australia
(a division of Pearson Australia Group Pty Ltd)
459–471 Church Street, Level 1, Building B, Richmond, Victoria 3121
PO Box 23360, Melbourne, Victoria 8012

www.pearson.com.au

Pearson respects and honours Aboriginal and Torres Strait Islander Elders past, present and future. We acknowledge the stories, traditions and living cultures of the Traditional Custodians of the lands on which our company is located and where we conduct our business. Pearson is committed to honouring Australian Aboriginal and Torres Strait Islander peoples' unique cultural and spiritual relationships to the land, waters and seas and their rich contribution to society.

Aboriginal and Torres Strait Islander peoples are advised that this text may contain images, voices and names of deceased persons.

Senior Portfolio Manager: Mandy Sheppard
Content Specialist: Anna Carter
Senior Project Manager: Bernadette Chang
Content Producer: Linda Chryssavgis
Senior Digital Producer: Paul Ryan
Senior Rights and Permissions Editor: Madeleine Roberts
Lead Editor/Copy Editor: Sandra Goodall
Proofreader: Marie-Louise Taylor
Indexer: Integra Software Services
Cover and internal design by Lamond Art & Design; internal design elements: Login/Shutterstock, Jonny Drake/Shutterstock
Cover illustration concept courtesy of Tracy Levett-Jones
Typeset by Integra Software Services
Desktop Operator: Jit-Pin Chong

Printed in Australia by Pegasus Media and Logistics

ISBN 9780655703990

1 2 3 4 5 28 27 26 25 24

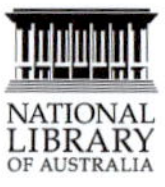

A catalogue record for this work is available from the National Library of Australia

Pearson Australia Group Pty Ltd ABN 40 004 245 943

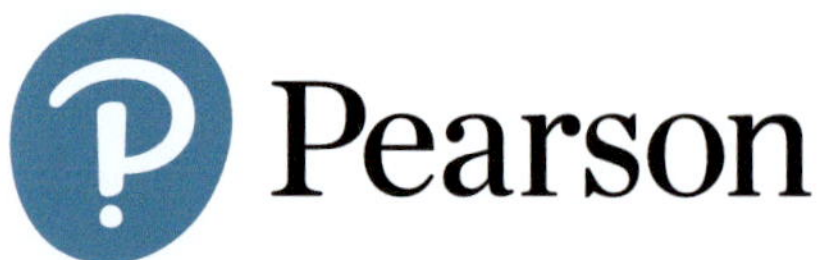

Dedication

This book is dedicated to my son Tyler and my daughter Madeline–inspirational healthcare professionals.

Tracy Levett-Jones

The book to read is not the one that thinks for you
but the one which makes you think.

Harper Lee

Pearson's Commitment to Diversity, Equity, and Inclusion

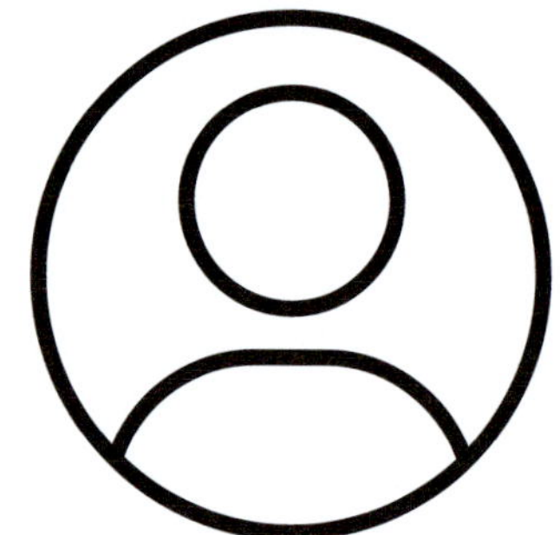

Pearson is dedicated to creating bias-free content that reflects the diversity, depth, and breadth of all learners' lived experiences.

We embrace the many dimensions of diversity, including but not limited to race, ethnicity, gender, sex, sexual orientation, socioeconomic status, ability, age, and religious or political beliefs.

Education is a powerful force for equity and change in our world. It has the potential to deliver opportunities that improve lives and enable economic mobility. As we work with authors to create content for every product and service, we acknowledge our responsibility to demonstrate inclusivity and incorporate diverse scholarship so that everyone can achieve their potential through learning. As the world's leading learning company, we have a duty to help drive change and live up to our purpose to help more people create a better life for themselves and to create a better world.

Our ambition is to purposefully contribute to a world where

- Everyone has an equitable and lifelong opportunity to succeed through learning
- Our educational content accurately reflects the histories and lived experiences of the learners we serve
- Our educational products and services are inclusive and represent the rich diversity of learners
- Our educational content prompts deeper discussions with students and motivates them to expand their own learning (and worldview)

Accessibility

We are also committed to providing products that are fully accessible to all learners. As per Pearson's guidelines for accessible educational web media, we test and retest the capabilities of our products against the highest standards for every release, following the WCAG guidelines in developing new products for copyright year 2022 and beyond.

 You can learn more about Pearson's commitment to accessibility at **https://www.pearson.com/us/accessibility.html**

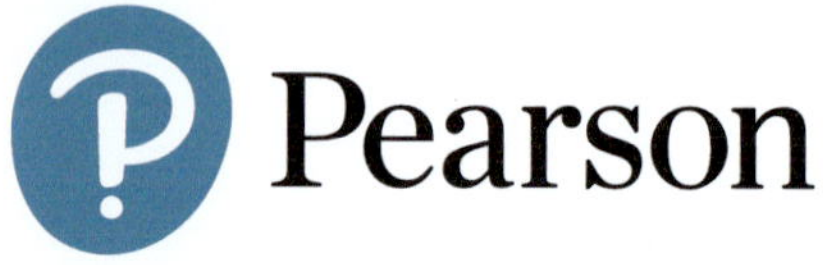

Contact Us

While we work hard to present unbiased, fully accessible content, we want to hear from you about any concerns or needs with this Pearson product so that we can investigate and address them.

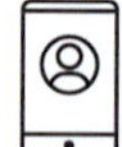 Please contact us with concerns about any potential bias at **https://www.pearson.com/report-bias.html**

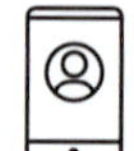 For accessibility-related issues, such as using assistive technology with Pearson products, alternative text requests, or accessibility documentation, email the Pearson Disability Support team at **disability.support@pearson.com**

BRIEF CONTENTS

CONTENTS

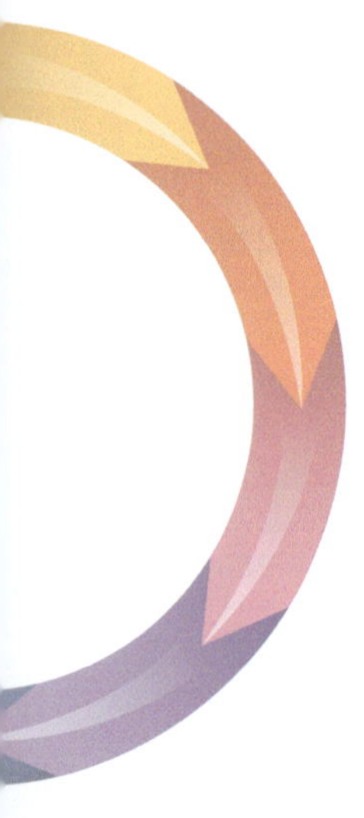

ABOUT THE EDITOR

Tracy Levett-Jones, PHD, RN, MED & WORK, BN, DIPAPPSC (NURSING), is Professor of Nursing Education and Head of School for Nursing and Midwifery at the University of Technology Sydney. She has been the recipient of multiple teaching and research awards, and has led a number of funded research projects designed to improve the quality of teaching and learning for healthcare students, and ultimately improve patient outcomes. Tracy has also authored numerous books, book chapters, journal articles and blogs. Her research interests include clinical reasoning, interprofessional communication, patient safety, cultural competence, belongingness, empathy and simulation. Tracy's doctoral research explored the clinical placement experiences of students in Australia and the United Kingdom.

CONTRIBUTORS

Ms Bernadette Bugeja MN (AD CLIN ED), BN

Clinical Nurse Consultant, Pain Management, Prince of Wales Hospital, Randwick

Mr Vincent Carroll RN, MSc (DEMENTIA CARE), GRADDIP BA BHLTHSC(NURSING), MPHIL CANDIDATE

Parkinson's Clinical Nurse Consultant, Mid-North Coast Local Health District; School of Nursing, Paramedicine and Healthcare Sciences, Faculty of Science and Health, Charles Sturt University

Ms Belinda Causby RN, MCLINN, GCCN (CRITICAL CARE), BN, PHD CANDIDATE

Clinical Nurse Specialist, Intensive Care Services, St Vincent's Hospital, Darlinghurst

Ms Vivienne Chau RN, GRAD CERT TRANSFUSION PRACTICE, GRAD CERT NURSING SCIENCE (APHERESIS), GRAD CERT CANCER NURSING

Clinical Nurse Specialist, Haematology/Oncology/ Apheresis/ Haemovigilance, Concord Repatriation General Hospital

Ms Rochelle Firth RN MN

Nurse Practitioner Neurosurgery, Royal North Shore Hospital, Course Coordinator Master of Nurse Practitioner, School of Nursing and Midwifery, University of Technology Sydney

Lesley Fitzpatrick RN, BSCN (HON), MN (CRIT CARE)

Clinical Nurse Consultant, Royal North Shore Hospital

Ms Jamie Gills RN GRAD DIP AGED CARE

Clinical Nurse Consultant, Orthogeriatrics/Dementia/ Delirium, Aged and Subacute, Central Coast Local Health District

Dr Mark Goodhew RN, MASTERS MH NURSING, PHD

Lecturer, School of Nursing and Midwifery, University of Technology Sydney

Ms Natalie Govind RN, BN (HON), GRAD CERT ICU, PHD CANDIDATE

Lecturer, Faculty of Health, University of Technology Sydney

Associate Professor Stephen Guinea BN, GRAD DIP VOC ED TRAIN, PHD

Associate Dean, Learning, Teaching and Professional Experience, Faculty of Health Sciences, Australian Catholic University

Dr Sharyn Hunter PHD, RN, BSC (HONS), GRAD CERT (AGED CARE), GRAD CERT TERTIARY TEACHING

Honorary Senior Lecturer, School of Nursing and Midwifery, The University of Newcastle

Professor Christine Imms BAPPSC (OT), MSC, PHD, FELLOW OTARA

Apex Australia Chair of Neurodevelopment and Disability, The University of Melbourne

Dr Samantha Jakimowicz PHD, RN, BNURS (HONS1), BCHC

Director Professional Engagement, Australian College of Nursing

Professor Tracy Levett-Jones PHD, RN, MED & WORK, BN, DIPAPPSC (NURSING)

Professor of Nursing Education and Head of School, Nursing and Midwifery, University of Technology Sydney

Associate Professor Joanne Lewis BN, MPallC, PhD

Discipline Lead and Head of Discipline Nursing, School of Nursing Midwifery and Public Health, University of Canberra

Ms Jessica McKirkle BN, GRAD DIP CHILDREN, ADOLESCENT AND FAMILY HEALTH

Lecturer, School of Nursing, Midwifery and Paramedicine, Australian Catholic University

Ms Veronica Mills RN, BN, MHLTH SC

Casual Academic, School of Nursing and Midwifery, CQUniversity, Credentialled Diabetes Nurse Educator

Ms Elizabeth Newman RN MN, MASTER OF NURSING (NURSE PRACTITIONER), GRAD CERT NURS. SCIENCE (APHERESIS), CERT CHEMOTHERAPY, CERT BONE MARROW TRANSPLANT

Nurse Practitioner Haematology, Bone Marrow Transplant & Apheresis, Concord Repatriation General Hospital

Ms Lorinda Palmer RN, BSC, DIP ED, GRAD DIP (NURSING), MN

Casual Academic & Research Associate, School of Nursing and Midwifery, University of Technology Sydney

Professor Deborah Parker RN, BA MSOCSC, PHD

Professor of Nursing Aged Care (Dementia) School of Nursing and Midwifery, University of Technology Sydney

Tyson Perrin RN, BN, GRAD CERTN (CRIT CARE), MADVN

Casual Academic, School of Nursing and Midwifery, University of Technology Sydney

Dr Jacqui Pich RN, PHD

Course Director, Bachelor of Nursing, School of Nursing and Midwifery, University of Technology Sydney

Ms Loretto Quinney RN, RM, CCRN, BAAPPSC, GRAD CERT MNG, PH CANDIDATE

Senior Lecturer, School of Nursing, Midwifery and Paramedicine, Australian Catholic University

Professor Kerry Reid-Searl PHD, RN, RM, BHLTHSC, MCLINED

Emeritus Professor of Nursing, CQUniversity

Dr Tracy Robinson PHD, BA HONS, RN

Adjunct Senior Lecturer, School of Nursing, Midwifery and Indigenous Health, Charles Sturt University

Mr Peter Ross RN
Mental Health Nurse, Mid North Coast Correctional Centre

Dr Rachel Rossiter D.HSC, RN, MN (NP), MCOUNSELLING, BCOUNSELLING, BHLTHSC (NURSING)
Associate Professor of Nursing, School of Nursing, Paramedicine and Healthcare Sciences, Charles Sturt University

Associate Professor Peter Sinclair RN, BN, RENAL CERT, MPHIL, PH
Course Director, Postgraduate Nursing, School of Nursing and Midwifery, University of Technology Sydney

Ms Judith Smith RN, BN, GRAD CERT PERIOP, MA (HONS), PHD CANDIDATE
Lecturer, School of Nursing and Midwifery, University of Technology Sydney

Dr Anna Treloar RN, CMHN, MA, MPHC, PHD
Former Lecturer, School of Nursing and Midwifery, The University of Newcastle

Professor Amanda Wilson RN, BA (HONS), MCA, PHD
Deputy Head of School, School of Nursing and Midwifery, University of Technology Sydney

The Editor and Publisher would also like to thank the contributors from the second edition:

Ms Jacqui Culver RN, BN, MMP
Nurse Practitioner Aged Care (Palliative & Dementia), Hunter New England Health

Ms Frances Dumont RN, MSN, BN, BED
Former Dementia Delirium Clinical Nurse Consultant, Hunter New England Health

Ms Natalie Govind RN, BN (HON), GRAD CERT ICU, PHD CANDIDATE
Lecturer, Faculty of Health, University of Technology Sydney

Dr Stephen Guinea BN, GRAD DIP VOC ED TRAIN, PHD
Associate Dean, Learning, Teaching and Professional Experience, Faculty of Health Sciences, Australian Catholic University

Mr Nathan Haining RN, BN, GRAD CERT CRIT CARE
Clinical Nurse Educator, Neuroscience, Westmead Hospital

Dr Kerry Hoffman RN, BSC, GRAD DIP ED, DIP HEALTH SCI, MN, PHD
Lecturer, School of Nursing and Midwifery, The University of Newcastle

Dr Sharyn Hunter PHD, RN, BSC (HONS), GRAD CERT (AGED CARE), GRAD CERT TERTIARY TEACHING
Honorary Senior Lecturer, School of Nursing and Midwifery, The University of Newcastle

Professor Christine Imms BAPPSC (OT), MSC, PHD FELLOW OTARA
Apex Australia Chair of Neurodevelopment and Disability, The University of Melbourne

Ms Marcia Ingles RN
Clinical Nurse Specialist, Emergency Department, Belmont Hospital

Professor Tracy Levett-Jones PHD, RN, MED & WORK, BN, DIPAPPSC (NURSING)
Professor of Nursing Education and Head of School, Nursing and Midwifery, University of Technology Sydney

Professor Vanessa McDonald PHD, BN, RN, DIP HEALTH SCI
Professor, School of Nursing and Midwifery, The University of Newcastle

Ms Jessica McKirkle BN, GRAD DIP CHILDREN, ADOLESCENT AND FAMILY HEALTH
Lecturer, School of Nursing, Midwifery & Paramedicine, Australian Catholic University

Ms Veronica Mills RN, BN, MHLTH SC
Casual Academic, School of Nursing and Midwifery, CQUniversity, Credentialled Diabetes Nursing Educator

Associate Professor David Newby PHD, GRAD DIP EPI, BPHARM
Acting Discipline Lead, Clinical Pharmacology, School of Medicine and Public Health, The University of Newcastle

Ms Elizabeth Newman RN MN, MASTER OF NURSING (NURSE PRACTITIONER), GRAD CERT NURS. SCIENCE (APHERESIS), CERT CHEMOTHERAPY, CERT BONE MARROW TRANSPLANT
Nurse Practitioner Haematology, Bone Marrow Transplant & Apheresis, Concord Repatriation General Hospital

Ms Lorinda Palmer MN, RN, BSC, DIP ED, GRAD DIP (NURSING), MN
Casual Academic and Research Associate, School of Nursing and Midwifery, University of Technology Sydney

Ms Caroline Phelan RN, MPH, BN, PHD CANDIDATE
Clinical Nurse Consultant Pain Management, Hunter Integrated Pain Service

Dr Victoria Pitt RN, PHD, MNUR (RESEARCH), GRAD DIP NURS (PAL. CARE), GRAD CERT TERTIARY TEACHING, DIP APSC (NURSING)
Bachelor of Nursing Program Convenor, School of Nursing and Midwifery, The University of Newcastle

Ms Loretto Quinney RN, RM, CCRN, BAAPPSC, GRAD CERT MNG, PHD CANDIDATE
Senior Lecturer, School of Nursing and Midwifery and Paramedicine, Australian Catholic University

Professor Kerry Reid-Searl PHD, RN, RM, BHLTHSC, MCLINED
Emeritus Professor of Nursing, CQUniversity

Mr Peter Ross RN
Mental Health Nurse, Mid North Coast Correctional Centre

Dr Rachel Rossiter D.HSC, RN, MN (NP), MCOUNSELLING, BCOUNSELLING, BHLTHSC
Associate Professor of Nursing, Paramedicine and Healthcare Sciences, Charles Sturt University

Associate ProfessorPeter Sinclair RN, BN, RENAL CERT, MPHIL, PH
Course Director, Postgraduate Nursing, School of Nursing and Midwifery, University of Technology Sydney

Professor Teresa Stone PHD, RN, RMN, BA, M HEALTH MANAGEMENT, GRAD CERT TERTIARY TEACHING
Professor, International Nursing, Faculty of Health Sciences, Yamaguchi University

Dr Anna Treloar RN, CMHN, MA, MPHC, PHD
Former Lecturer, School of Nursing and Midwifery, The University of Newcastle

Associate Professor Pamela van der Riet PHD, RN, MED, BA, DIP ED (NURSING), ICU/CCU CERT
Associate Professor, School of Nursing and Midwifery, The University of Newcastle

Ms Bree Walker RN, BN
Nurse Educator, Paediatrics, Rockhampton Hospital

Dr Amanda Wilson RN, BA (HONS), MCA, PHD
Deputy Head of School, School of Nursing and Midwifery, University of Technology Sydney

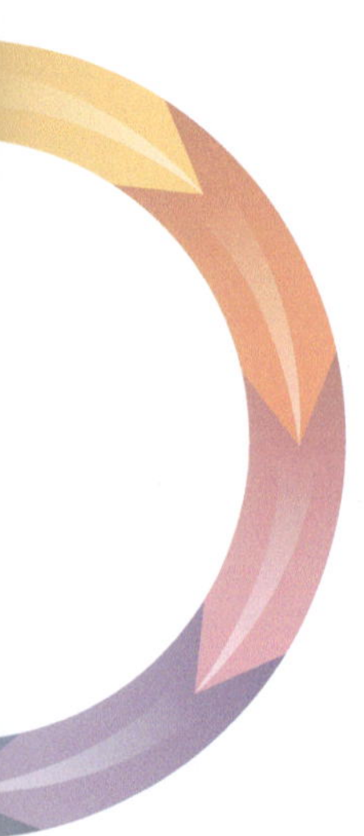

PREFACE

FOR STUDENTS

> *The most important practical lesson that can be given to nurses is to teach them what to observe–how to observe–what symptoms indicate improvement–what the reverse–which are of importance–which are none–which are the evidence of neglect–and of what kind of neglect.*
>
> (Florence Nightingale, 1860, p. 105)

Competent nursing practice requires not only knowledge and skills but also sophisticated thinking abilities. Safe and effective nurses use disciplined, systematic and logical thought processes to guide their practice and inform their decision making. Their clinical reasoning ability is a key factor in the provision of quality care and the prevention of adverse patient outcomes.

In order to become a safe and effective nurse, it is essential to learn the process and steps of clinical reasoning. Students need to understand the rules that determine how cues influence clinical decisions and the connections between cues, decisions and outcomes. Becoming skilled in clinical reasoning requires practice, determination and active engagement in deliberate learning activities; it also requires reflection on activities designed to improve performance.

This edition of *Clinical Reasoning* includes 17 authentic, engaging and meaningful chapters that will guide you through the clinical reasoning process while challenging you to think critically and creatively about the nursing care you provide. Each chapter promotes deep learning and provides opportunities for you to rehearse how you will respond to emergent clinical situations in ways that are both person-centred and clinically astute.

A key feature of this text is its clinical relevance; the chapters have been written collaboratively with expert clinicians to ensure the focus and content are current, accurate and authentic. To ensure alignment with contemporary healthcare priorities, the chapters have been updated and many have been expanded for this edition.

The scenarios included in each chapter have been adapted from real clinical situations that occurred in healthcare and community settings. The clinical conditions that feature in this text are framed by Australia's National Health Priorities, and the patients/clients profiled are of different ages and from diverse backgrounds. Each chapter emphasises patient safety and quality care; and there are references to the *Patient Safety Competency Framework* (2017), the National Safety and Quality Health Service (NSQHS) Standards (2021), and the Nursing and Midwifery Board of Australia (NMBA) *Registered Nurse Standards for Practice* (2016).

We hope you enjoy learning about clinical reasoning and that this textbook helps you on your journey to becoming a safe, person-centred and competent nurse.

HOW TO USE THIS TEXT

While there is no one way to read this text, here are some suggested approaches. Start with Chapter 1—it will help you to understand the importance of clinical reasoning and introduce you to the process. Chapter 2 is an introductory chapter that takes you through the clinical reasoning process by juxtaposing two scenarios: the first demonstrates what can happen when clinical reasoning is not used and the second 'rewinds' and illustrates how effective clinical reasoning skills can make a significant difference to patient outcomes. With the foundation skills from Chapter 1 and the application skills from Chapter 2, you will be prepared for the other chapters. Scan the list of contents and select the topics that interest you the most, that you are currently studying or that you have encountered in your clinical practice. Your lecturers may also require you to read particular chapters as part of your course work.

While many of the chapters illustrate how effective clinical reasoning skills can help you recognise and manage patient deterioration early and, in effect, 'rescue' the patient, Chapter 17 considers the ethical implications of withholding potentially life-saving treatments when an attempt to 'rescue' may not be in the person's best interests or in accord with their wishes. These are some of the most difficult clinical decisions that have to be made, and require effective clinical and moral reasoning skills.

LEARNING OUTCOMES
Completion of the activities in thi
- explain why an understanding c essential to competent practice (
- explain the nurse's role in the m
- identify potential clinical manife the collection and interpretation

PEDAGOGICAL FEATURES

Learning outcomes are listed at the beginning of the chapter, and a sequential, step-through approach is used to tell an 'unfolding story'.

Key concepts are integrated throughout the book and include person-centred care, holistic practice, empathy, diversity, therapeutic communication, intra- and interprofessional communication, cultural competence, pathophysiology and safe medication practices.

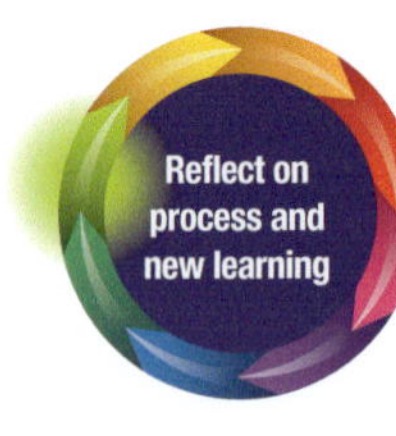

Advanced organisers are provided to enhance understanding and recall of the clinical reasoning cycle.

Questions (multiple-choice, true or false, rank and sort, and short-answer) provide multiple opportunities to test your knowledge, make mistakes and learn from the process.

Answers to the questions are provided on the *Clinical Reasoning* website (www.pearson.com/en-au/9780655703990).

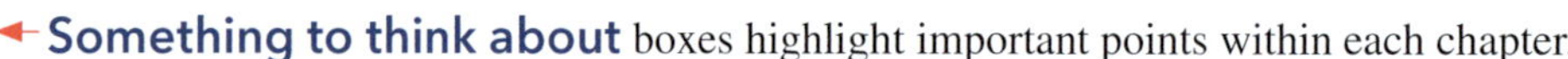

Something to think about boxes highlight important points within each chapter.

Reflective thinking is the final stage of the clinical reasoning cycle and, in order for you to maximise your learning, guided reflection questions are provided at the end of each scenario. Answers to these questions are not provided, as their purpose is to help you think critically and creatively about what you have learned and, most importantly, how your learning will inform and translate to your future practice.

It appears on face value that Giuseppe is in a positive balance. Do you think this is an accurate reflection of his fluid status? Why?

Margin notes provide helpful hints, advice and links to relevant resources.

Suggested readings are provided at the beginning of each chapter to enable preparation for the learning activities.

Further reading lists are provided at the end of each chapter to build on and extend your knowledge about topics of interest.

Nursing and Midwifery Board of
Standards for Practice Reid-Searl e
Although a commonly used form of su
neither legal nor professional. Superv
medication administration at all times (

A **glossary** of terms is provided on page 320.

Nursing and Midwifery Board of Australia (NMBA) Registered Nurse Standards for Practice boxes appear in the chapters where applicable to demonstrate relevant Nursing Standards for Practice, thereby aligning the content to contemporary professional practice in Australia. For up-to-date information, standards and guidelines, visit www.nursingmidwiferyboard.gov.au

Patient Safety Competency Framew
Domain 9 – Medication S
The PSCF specifies that nurses studen
information when administering medi

Patient Safety Competency Framework (PSCF) boxes appear in the chapters where applicable to demonstrate how concepts relate back to the skills and knowledge that underpin patient safety.

National Safety and Quality Health S
Communicating for safety
The importance of effective communica
NSQHS Standards (ACSQHC, 2021), w
must facilitate structured and effective c

National Safety and Quality Health Service (NSQHS) Standards boxes appear in the chapters where applicable to demonstrate how concepts relate back to patient safety standards. Visit www.safetyandquality.gov.au/standards for access to the full standards.

FOR EDUCATORS

Nursing programs must enable the development of clinical reasoning, problem solving and critical thinking.

(World Health Organization, 2009)

This text is premised on the understanding that a requisite level of clinical reasoning skills is imperative for safe and effective nursing practice. This requires educators to model, teach and assess students' developing clinical reasoning skills in both academic and clinical settings. The scenarios in this book have been developed to encourage the acquisition of both content knowledge (domain-specific) and process knowledge (clinical reasoning ability). The constructivist approach that informs each chapter will allow both undergraduate and postgraduate students to construct knowledge by being actively engaged in learning that is situated, experiential and authentic. The unfolding clinical stories provide meaningful opportunities for reiterative learning which leads to deeper levels of processing, thus improving retention and recall of information. The consistent structure of the scenarios allows for cognitive rehearsal of the clinical reasoning process to enable students to integrate this cognitive skill into their repertoire of clinical behaviours.

The scenarios can be used in multiple ways: as stimulus materials prior to or during tutorial activities or online learning; for self-directed learning, assignments and exam preparation; or for continuing professional development. Additionally, the scenarios can be used as a framework for the development of simulation scenarios using manikins, standardised patients/actors or a range of other modalities.

The reflective thinking activities can be used to design assignment and exam questions, for tutorial discussion or to structure debriefing following simulation sessions or clinical placements. They can also be extended and contextualised by adding specific questions that align with your course objectives.

Feedback from students about *Clinical Reasoning* has been consistently positive. For example:

- *Each chapter made me feel like an investigator trying to put all the clues together to solve the patient problem.*
- *The scenarios showed me how I jump to conclusions before considering the information given; I learnt that some things aren't always what they seem.*
- *The scenarios involved constant thinking and decision making and I found them to be a great tool for learning what could go wrong when a patient's nursing diagnosis is incorrect.*
- *Going step by step through the clinical reasoning cycle was a good way to learn. I found it made me research a lot of things I didn't know and look into conditions I was unfamiliar with.*

In writing this textbook for nursing students, our aim has been to have a positive impact on patient safety and quality care. We hope that you find the scenarios engaging, meaningful and beneficial in your teaching of clinical reasoning.

Tracy Levett-Jones and the 'Thinking like a nurse' writing team

REFERENCES

Florence Nightingale. (1860). *Notes on Nursing: What It Is and What It Is Not*. New York: D. Appleton and Co. Reprint 1969. New York: Dover Publications, Inc.

World Health Organization. (2009). *Global Standards for the Initial Education of Professional Nurses and Midwives.* Geneva: WHO. https://apps.who.int/iris/handle/10665/44100

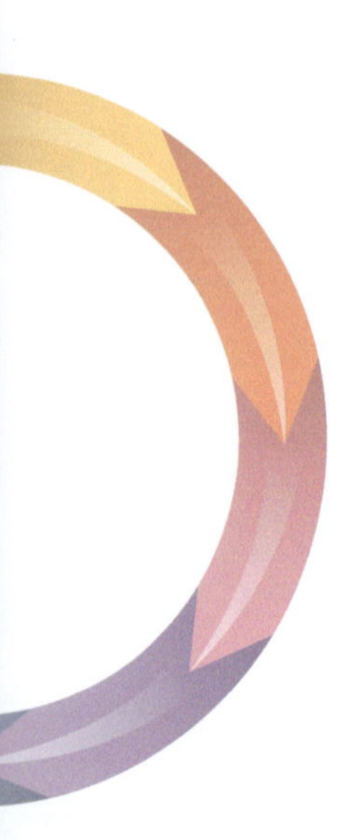

ACKNOWLEDGEMENTS

I would like to acknowledge and offer sincere thanks to my wonderful writing team. Their commitment to student learning, patient safety and person-centred care informs every chapter and has resulted in a book that will inspire, motivate and engage nursing students. I would also like to thank the expert clinicians and academics who reviewed the book for accuracy and clinical relevance. Finally, thank you to the editorial and production team at Pearson including: Mandy Sheppard, Senior Portfolio Manager; Anna Carter, Development Editor; Linda Chryssavgis, Content Producer; Madeleine Roberts, Senior Rights and Permissions Editor; and Sandra Goodall, Lead Editor/Copy Editor.

REVIEWERS

Kate Barnewall, Griffith University
Jacqueline Bloomfield, The University of Sydney
Didy Button, Flinders University
Valda Frommolt, Griffith University
Benjamin Hay, Notre Dame University
Carly Jans, University of Wollongong
Tanya Langtree, James Cook University
Sam Lapkin, University of Wollongong
Lee Lethbridge, The University of Newcastle
Rebekkah Middleton, University of Wollongong
Kolleen Miller-Rosser, Southern Cross University
Lee O'Malley, UniSQ
Sean Parker, La Trobe University
Floridah Rolf, UniSQ
Jane Walker, Deakin University
Amanda Wilson, University of Technology Sydney
Lisa Wirihana, CQUniversity

Chapter 1

Clinical reasoning: What it is and why it matters

TRACY LEVETT-JONES and JUDITH SMITH

LEARNING OUTCOMES

Completion of the activities in this chapter will enable you to:

- discuss what 'thinking like a nurse' means
- explain why nursing students need to learn about clinical reasoning
- outline the clinical reasoning process
- explain the relationship between clinical reasoning and critical thinking
- discuss how clinical reasoning errors can adversely affect patient outcomes
- explain how stigmatising, stereotyping, preconceptions and assumptions can negatively impact clinical reasoning
- explore and discuss different types of clinical reasoning errors.

Nurses are the caregivers most directly involved with patients 24/7, responsible for monitoring and assessing clinical changes in patients, intervening when necessary, and communicating changes in status to ensure appropriate intervention and coordination of care. (Duffield et al., 2007)

INTRODUCTION

In this introductory chapter, we explore what 'thinking like a nurse' means. We discuss the importance of clinical reasoning, outline the clinical reasoning process and illustrate how clinical errors are linked to poor reasoning skills. This chapter creates a foundation for the ones that follow and a backdrop to a series of authentic and clinically relevant clinical scenarios.

Learning to 'think like a nurse' is challenging and requires commitment, practice and multiple opportunities for application of learning. However, the benefits are significant for you, as a curious, competent and intelligent nurse, and for the people who will be the recipients of your care. Simply stated, effective clinical reasoning skills will improve the quality of your patient care, prevent adverse patient outcomes and enhance your work satisfaction.

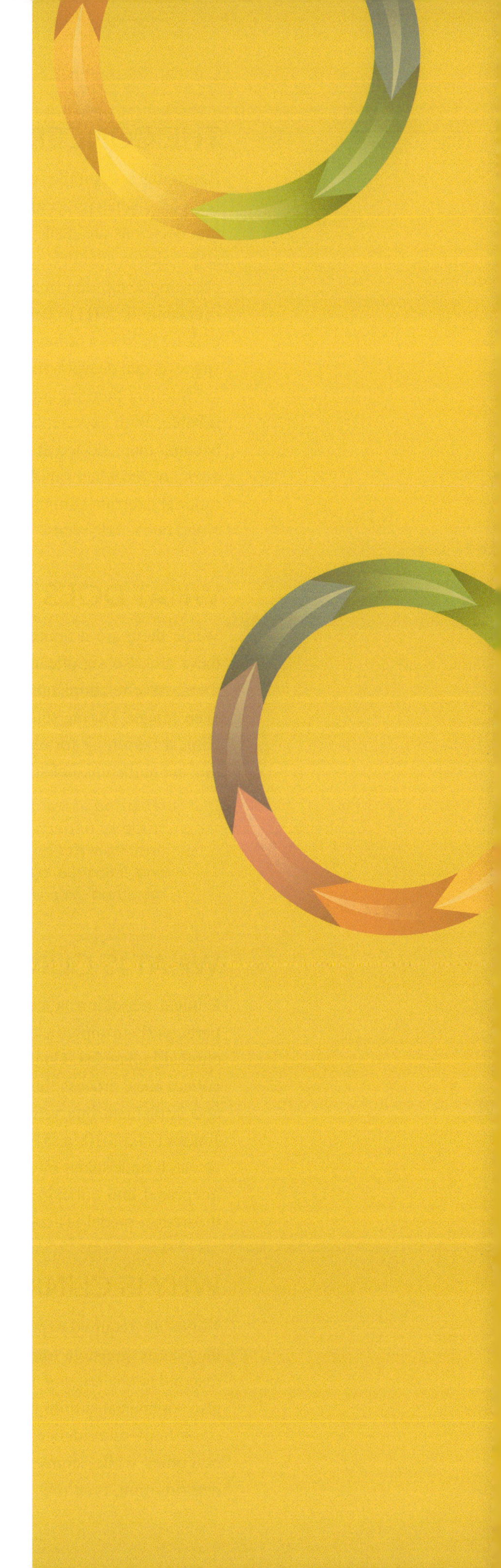

THE CONCEPT OF REASONING

Reasoning is a complex concept that is typically used to describe thinking skills. A number of theories have been used when referring to the cognitive processes that precede decision making. Some theories suggest that decisions are made either rationally or intuitively. The rational decision-making approach includes steps such as identifying the problem, generating alternative solutions, evaluating alternative solutions, choosing a solution, making and implementing a decision, and evaluating the decision's effectiveness (Schoenfeld, 2011). This is similar to the information-processing theory that proposes that decision making follows a rational and logical process (Simmons, 2010). Conversely, the intuitive-humanist model suggests that decision making is often informed by intuition (Johansen & O'Brien, 2016).

Intuitive thinking processes are very fast whereas rational processes are slower, deliberate and more reliable. With experience, healthcare professionals build a repertoire of experiences that allow them to become more skilled at intuitive processing. However, it is important to remember that most reasoning errors occur when rapid intuitive processing is used to make decisions without sufficient thought and rational override (Simmons, 2010), and particularly when preconceptions, assumptions and stereotypes cloud one's judgments.

WHAT DOES 'THINKING LIKE A NURSE' MEAN?

While there are a number of similarities in the way nurses and other healthcare professionals think, there are also significant differences. Unlike many healthcare professionals who 'treat' and 'retreat', therapeutic relationships between nurses and the patients they care for can extend over hours, days or even longer. During this time, nurses maintain constant vigilance and engage in multiple episodes of clinical reasoning for each person, responding to the complex nature of the illness experience in ways that are authentic, holistic and person-centred.

> *'Thinking like a nurse' is a form of engaged moral reasoning. Educational practices must help students engage with patients with a deep concern for their well being. Clinical reasoning must arise from this engaged, concerned stance, always in relation to a particular patient and situation and informed by generalised knowledge and rational processes, but never as an objective, detached exercise.* (Tanner, 2006, p. 209)

WHAT IS CLINICAL REASONING?

Clinical reasoning is a logical, systematic and cyclical process that guides clinical decision making, particularly in unpredictable, emergent and non-routine situations, and that leads to accurate and informed clinical judgments. Clinical reasoning is defined as 'the process by which nurses (and other clinicians) collect cues, process the information, come to an understanding of a patient problem or situation, plan and implement interventions, evaluate outcomes, and reflect on and learn from the process' (Levett-Jones et al., 2010, p. 516). Over the last decade, the clinical reasoning cycle (Figure 1.1), drawn from research undertaken by Levett-Jones et al. (2010) and Hoffman, Aitken and Duffield (2009), has been integrated into nursing, medical and allied health curricula across the world and found to be a sound theoretical model (Theobald & Ramsbotham, 2019; Vierula et al., 2020).

WHY IS CLINICAL REASONING IMPORTANT?

Nurses are required to care for and make decisions about complex patients with diverse health needs. As they are responsible for a significant proportion of the clinical judgments in healthcare, their ability to respond to challenging and dynamic situations requires not only psychomotor skills and knowledge but also sophisticated thinking abilities.

A body of evidence has identified that clinical reasoning skills have a positive impact on patient outcomes while, conversely, nurses with poor clinical reasoning skills often fail to detect patient deterioration, resulting in a 'failure to rescue' (Cooper et al., 2011). Clinical reasoning errors have

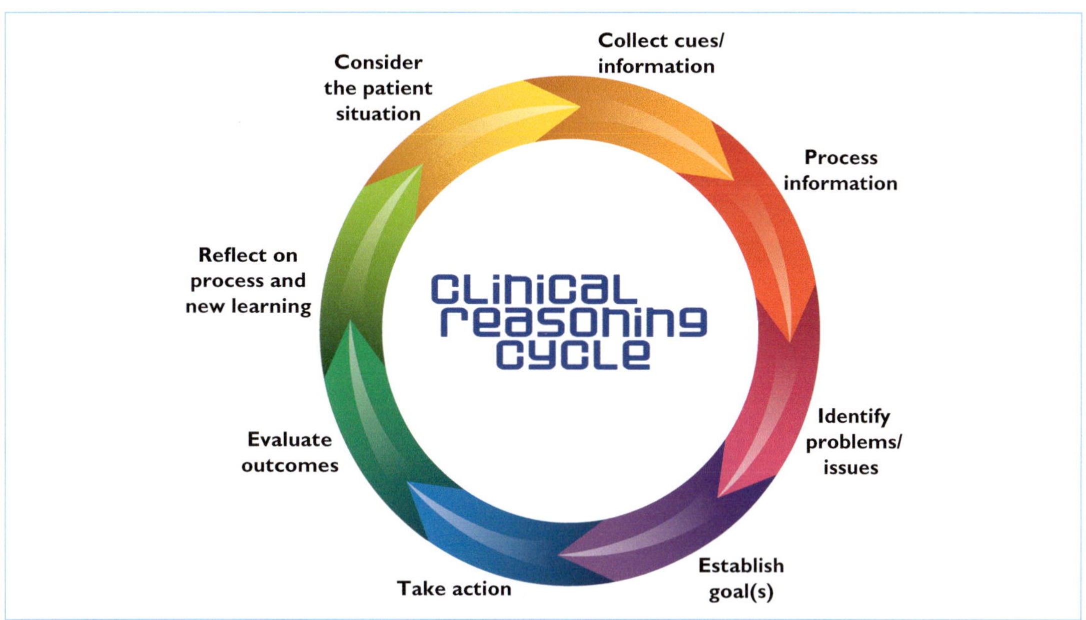

Figure 1.1
The clinical reasoning cycle

Source: T. Levett-Jones, K. Hoffman, Y. Dempsey, S. Jeong, D. Noble, C. Norton, J. Roche, & N. Hickey (2010). The 'five rights' of clinical reasoning: An educational model to enhance nursing students' ability to identify and manage clinically 'at risk' patients. *Nurse Education Today, 30*(6), 515–520.

been implicated as a factor in most adverse patient outcomes (Institute of Medicine, 2010). The reasons for this are multidimensional and include the tendency to make errors in time-sensitive situations where there is a large amount of complex data to process, and difficulties in distinguishing between a clinical problem that needs immediate attention and one that is less acute (Hoffman, Aitken & Duffield, 2009).

THE CLINICAL REASONING PROCESS

A diagram showing the clinical reasoning cycle and describing the nursing actions that occur during each stage is provided in Figure 1.2. The cycle begins at 1200 hours and moves in a clockwise direction through eight stages: *look, collect, process, diagnose, plan, act, evaluate* and *reflect*. Although each stage is presented as a separate and distinct element in this diagram, in reality clinical reasoning is a dynamic process and nurses often combine one or more stages or move back and forth between them before reaching a diagnosis, taking action and evaluating outcomes. Table 1.1 provides an example of a nurse's clinical reasoning while caring for a man following surgery for an abdominal aortic aneurysm.

Stages of the clinical reasoning cycle

Patient Safety Competency Framework (PSCF)

Domain 5–Clinical reasoning

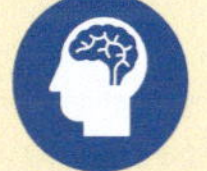

The PSCF specifies that nurses must demonstrate the ability to accurately assess, interpret and respond to individual patient data in a systematic and timely way.

Source: *The Patient Safety Competency Framework for Nursing Students*, https://patientsafetyfornursingstudents.org

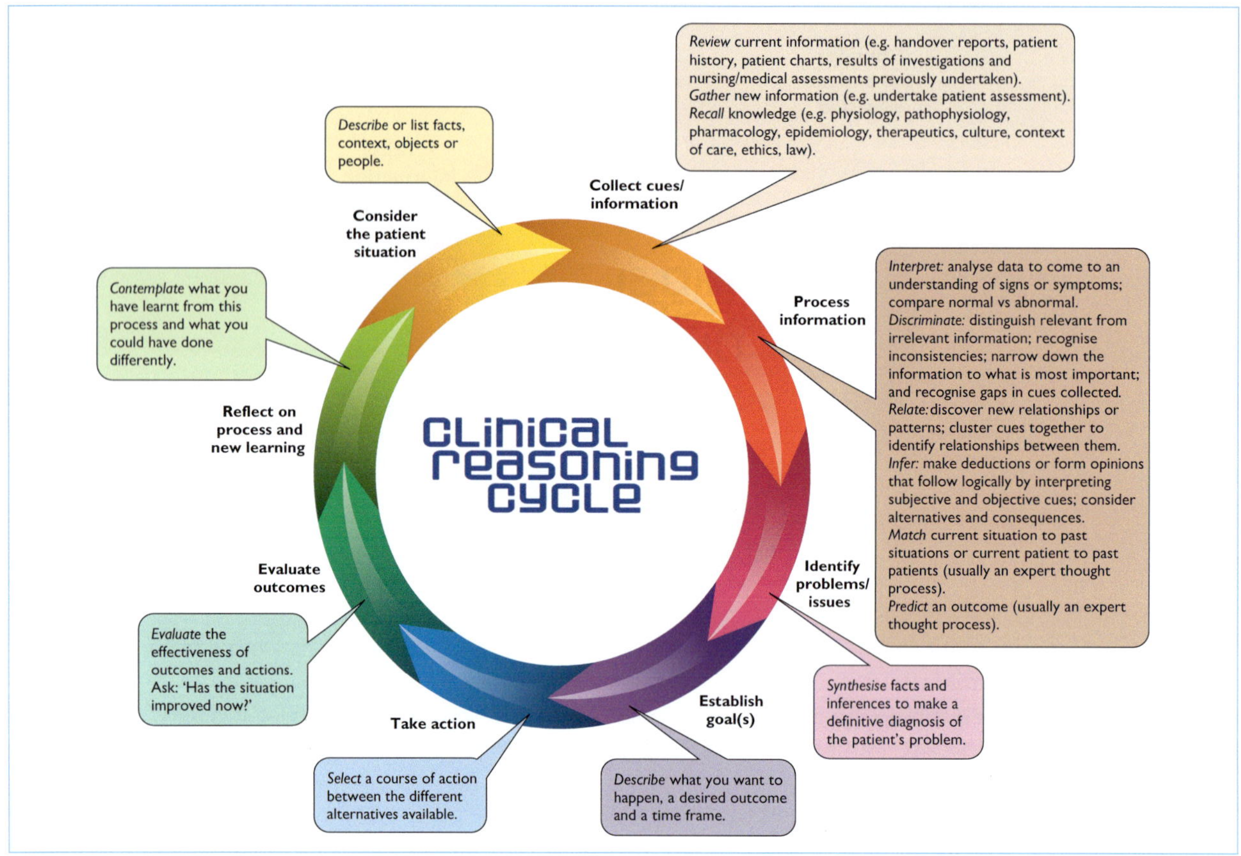

Figure 1.2
The clinical reasoning process with descriptors

Source: Adapted from T. Levett-Jones, K. Hoffman, Y. Dempsey, S. Jeong, D. Noble, C. Norton, J. Roche, & N. Hickey (2010). The 'five rights' of clinical reasoning: An educational model to enhance nursing students' ability to identify and manage clinically 'at risk' patients. *Nurse Education Today, 30*(6), 515–520.

Table 1.1 *Phases of the clinical reasoning cycle with examples*

Process	Description	Example of a nurse's thinking
Consider the patient situation	**Describe** person and context, notice salient features and anticipate emergent issues.	Mr Smith is a 60-year-old man admitted to ICU yesterday following surgery for an abdominal aortic aneurysm (AAA).
Collect cues/ information	**Review** current information (e.g. handover reports, patient history, patient charts, results of investigations and nursing/ medical assessments previously undertaken).	Mr Smith has a history of hypertension and he takes beta-blockers. His BP was 140/80 mmHg an hour ago.
	Gather new information (e.g. undertake patient assessment).	Mr Smith's vital signs are: T 37.6°C, PR 116, RR 20, BP 110/60 mmHg. His urine output is averaging 20 mL/hr. He has an epidural running @ 10 mL/hr.
	Recall knowledge (e.g. physiology, pathophysiology, pharmacology, epidemiology, therapeutics, culture, context of care, ethics, law).	BP and PR are influenced by fluid status. Epidurals can lower the BP because they can cause vasodilation.

Table 1.1 *Phases of the clinical reasoning cycle with examples (continued)*

Process	Description	Example of a nurse's thinking
Process information	**Interpret:** analyse cues to come to an understanding of signs or symptoms. Compare normal vs abnormal.	Mr Smith's BP is low, especially for a person with a history of hypertension. He is tachycardic and oliguric.
	Discriminate: distinguish relevant from irrelevant information; recognise inconsistencies; narrow down information to what is most important; and recognise gaps in cues collected.	Mr Smith is slightly febrile. However, I'm more concerned about his hypotension, tachycardia and oliguria.
	Relate: discover new relationships or patterns; cluster cues together to identify relationships between them.	Although Mr Smith's hypotension, tachycardia and oliguria could be signs of impending shock, his BP decreased soon after his epidural rate was increased.
	Infer: make deductions or form opinions that follow logically by interpreting subjective and objective cues; consider alternatives and consequences.	Mr Smith's BP is probably low because of vasodilation caused by his epidural and blood loss during surgery.
	Match current situation to past situations or current patient to past patients (usually an expert thought process).	AAAs are often hypotensive post-op.
	Predict an outcome (usually an expert thought process).	If I don't give Mr Smith a fluid challenge, he could develop acute kidney injury or go into shock.
Identify the problem/issue	**Synthesise** facts and inferences to make a definitive nursing diagnosis.	Mr Smith has reduced cardiac output related to decreased intravascular volume and vasodilation evidenced by hypotension, tachycardia and oliguria.
Establish goals	**Describe** what you want to happen, a desired outcome and a time frame.	To improve Mr Smith's cardiac output, haemodynamic status and urine output over the next 1–2 hours.
Take action	**Select** a course of action between the different alternatives available.	I will phone the medical officer (using ISBAR) to request an order for a fluid challenge, increased IV rate and metaraminol if needed.
Evaluate	**Evaluate** the effectiveness of outcomes and actions. Ask: 'Has the situation improved now?'	Mr Smith's BP has now improved and his urine output is averaging > 30 mL/hr. I'll continue to monitor him as he may need another fluid challenge or metaraminol later.
Reflect on process and new learning	**Contemplate** what you have learnt from this process and what you could have done differently.	I now understand . . . I should have . . . Next time I will . . .

Sources: K. Hoffman (2007). A comparison of decision-making by 'expert' and 'novice' nurses in the clinical setting, monitoring patient haemodynamic status post abdominal aortic aneurysm surgery [Unpublished PhD thesis]. University of Technology Sydney; and T. Levett-Jones, K. Hoffman, Y. Dempsey, S. Jeong, D. Noble, C. Norton, J. Roche, & N. Hickey (2010). The 'five rights' of clinical reasoning: An educational model to enhance nursing students' ability to identify and manage clinically 'at risk' patients. *Nurse Education Today*, *30*(6), 515–520.

1. Consider the patient situation

During the first stage of the clinical reasoning cycle, the nurse 'anticipates' potential issues, begins to gain an initial impression of the patient and identifies salient features related to the situation. This first impression, which is sometimes referred to as 'noticing', is critical but can be negatively influenced by the nurse's preconceptions, assumptions and biases (see Table 1.2 later in this chapter).

2. Collect cues/information

The importance of the cue collection stage of the clinical reasoning cycle cannot be underestimated, as early subtle cues when missed can lead to adverse patient outcomes (Levett-Jones et al., 2010). During this stage, the nurse begins to collect relevant information about the patient. He or she reviews the information that is currently available, including the handover report, the patient's medical and social history, clinical documentation, electronic medical records, and other available information.

The nurse then identifies any additional information that is required, such as vital signs and/or a focused health assessment, and focuses on collecting specific cues relevant to the person's condition at this point in time. Importantly, it is during this stage that the nurse elicits the patient's and family's concerns and understanding of the situation.

Lastly, the nurse recalls knowledge related to the patient's particular situation. A breadth and depth of knowledge is therefore imperative for accurate clinical reasoning. Unless a nurse has a deep understanding of the applied sciences, especially pathophysiology, the ability to make sense of and correctly interpret cues will be impacted.

3. Process information

In the third stage of the clinical reasoning cycle, the nurse interprets the cues that have been collected and identifies significant aberrations from normal. Cues are grouped into meaningful clusters, clinical patterns are identified, inferences are made and hypotheses are generated. During this stage, experienced nurses call upon their wide repertoire of previous clinical experiences matching the salient features of the patient's presentation with other similar situations. They are also able to 'think ahead', anticipating potential outcomes and complications depending on the particular course of action (or inaction).

4. Identify problems/issues

> *Improving the diagnostic process is not only possible, but it also represents a moral, professional, and public health imperative.* (Institute of Medicine, 2010)

The fourth stage of the cycle is where the nurse synthesises all of the information that has been collected and processed in order to identify the most appropriate nursing diagnoses. A three-part 'actual' diagnosis or a two-part 'risk' diagnosis may be formulated. The accuracy of this step is critical as the nursing diagnosis is used to determine appropriate goals of care and subsequent nursing actions. The following examples are adapted from Berman et al. (2020).

Nursing diagnosis

1. A nursing **diagnosis** is a problem that becomes apparent following a thorough and systematic interpretation of subjective and objective data. An actual nursing diagnosis consists of the person's **problem**, the related **aetiology** (causal relationship between a problem and its related or risk factors), and supporting **evidence/**cues.

   For example: *Dehydration* related to *post-operative nausea* and *vomiting* evidenced by *dry mucous membranes, oliguria, poor skin turgor, hypotension* and *tachycardia.*
2. A **risk nursing diagnosis** is a clinical judgment about a potential problem where the presence of **risk factors** indicates that a problem may develop unless nurses intervene appropriately. A risk diagnosis is written in two parts and does not include signs and symptoms.

   For example: *Risk of infection* related to *skin tear* and *type 2 diabetes.*

5. Establish goals

The fifth stage of the cycle is where the nurse clarifies and prioritises the goals of care depending on urgency. Goals must be SMART (**S**pecific, **M**easureable, **A**chievable, **R**ealistic and **T**imely) and designed to address the nursing diagnoses previously identified. Without SMART goals, the nurse cannot determine the efficacy of their actions.

6. Take action

In this stage the nurse selects the most appropriate course of action to achieve the goals of care and address the nursing diagnoses. The nurse also decides who is best placed to undertake the interventions, and who should be notified and when. During this stage, members of the healthcare team may be consulted and collaborative decision making undertaken.

7. Evaluate outcomes

This stage requires the nurse to re-examine objective and subjective data (patient cues) in order to evaluate how effective the nursing interventions have been, and whether the patient's problem has been addressed. If the evaluation identifies that the patient's condition has not improved, the nurse reconsiders the patient's situation and seeks to identify a more appropriate course of action. There may be a need for further consultation and/or to begin the clinical reasoning process again.

8. Reflect on process and new learning

Effective clinical reasoning requires both cognitive and metacognitive (thinking about one's thinking) skills in order to develop the ability to 'think like a nurse'. Thus, the final step of the clinical reasoning cycle involves reflection. This requires nurses to critically review their practice with a view to refinement, improvement or change. Reflection is intrinsic to learning. It is a deliberate, orderly and structured intellectual activity that allows nurses to process their experience and explore their understanding of what they did, why they did it, and the impact it had on themselves and others (Boud, 2015).

Nurses reflect *in* and *on* practice by asking themselves questions such as:

- What happened and why?
- What was done well?
- What could have been done better?
- What should be done differently if presented with the same or similar situation?
- What has been learnt that can be used when caring for other patients in the same or similar situations?
- What is needed to improve future practice, for example more knowledge about a specific condition or more practice in particular skills?

CLINICAL REASONING AND CRITICAL THINKING

> *As a client's status changes, the nurse must recognise, interpret and integrate new information, and make decisions about the course of action to follow. For satisfactory client outcomes clinical reasoning goes hand in hand with critical thinking.* (Martin, 2002, p. 245)

Clinical reasoning is the practical application of critical thinking skills to clinical situations (Victor-Chmil, 2013). Clinical reasoning is dependent on a critical thinking 'disposition'. Critical thinking is a complex collection of cognitive skills and effective habits of the mind, and has been described as the process of analysing and assessing thinking with a view to improving it (Paul & Elder, 2007). To think like a nurse requires you to learn the knowledge, ideas, skills, concepts and theories of nursing, and develop your intellectual capacities to become a disciplined, self-directed, critical thinker capable of clinical reasoning (Paul & Elder).

Nurses who are critical thinkers strive to be clear, accurate, precise, logical and fair when they listen, speak, read and write (Paul & Elder, 2007). Critical thinkers think deeply and broadly, eliminating irrelevant, inconsistent and illogical thoughts as they reason about patient care. The quality of their thinking improves over time and through reflection. Below is a list of attributes nurses need in order to develop their critical thinking and clinical reasoning skills (Rubenfeld & Scheffer, 2006, pp. 16–24).

- **A holistic and contextual perspective**—consideration of the whole person, taking into account the entire situation, including relationships, background and environment
- **Creativity**—the ability and desire to generate, discover or restructure ideas, and to imagine alternatives
- **Inquisitiveness**—a thoughtful, questioning and curious approach, and an eagerness to explore possibilities and alternatives
- **Perseverance**—a dedication to the pursuit of knowledge despite any obstacles that are encountered
- **Intuition**—insightful patterns of knowing, brought about by previous experiences and pattern recognition
- **Flexibility**—the capacity to adapt, modify or change thoughts, ideas and behaviours
- **Integrity**—seeking the truth through sincere, honest processes, even if the results are contrary to one's assumptions or beliefs
- **Reflexivity**—contemplation of assumptions, thinking and behaviours for the purpose of deeper understanding and self-evaluation
- **Confidence**—a firm belief in one's reasoning abilities
- **Open-mindedness**—receptiveness to different views and sensitivity to one's biases, prejudices, preconceptions and assumptions.

QUESTIONING ASSUMPTIONS AND UNDERSTANDING ERRORS

Nurses are human and we make the same kinds of thinking errors in our practice as we do in our day-to-day lives. Sometimes we overlook or misinterpret the significance of an important cue, or we jump to conclusions or fail to take into account alternative possibilities or options. Additionally, preconceptions, assumptions, biases, stereotypes and stigmatism can negatively influence our clinical reasoning and in some cases even prevent clinical reasoning from occurring. We may be unaware of the assumptions and prejudices that we hold as they are often long-standing and deeply embedded. For this reason, nurses must develop humility, insight and self-awareness by deliberately reflecting on their biases and preconceptions. Failure to do so can undermine the accuracy of clinical reasoning and consequently patient safety. Nurses can help avoid clinical reasoning errors by being humble, mindful and reflective, and by using the multitude of decision-support resources available to help them make a decision. They can also maintain a healthy scepticism and make it a habit to ask: 'What is influencing my thinking about this patient?', 'Could my interpretation be flawed?' and 'What other nursing diagnosis is possible in this situation?'.

Table 1.2 provides a list of clinical reasoning errors, many of which arise because of flawed assumptions and beliefs. These errors are then illustrated in the narratives that follow.

Examples of clinical reasoning errors

The clinical reasoning errors listed in Table 1.2 are illustrated with authentic clinical narratives. As you read these narratives, it will become evident that even experienced, committed and well-intentioned healthcare professionals can make errors if they allow their thinking process to be clouded by assumptions, preconceptions and stereotypes. Environmental and situational factors such as noise, fatigue, stress, multitasking and interruptions can also impede rational thinking processes. As you read these examples, it is important to reflect on your own biases and prejudices, and any personal or contextual factors that negatively influence your thinking, as this will enhance your self-awareness, emotional intelligence and clinical reasoning ability.

Table 1.2 *Clinical reasoning errors*

Error	Definition
Anchoring	The tendency to lock onto salient features in the patient's presentation too early in the clinical reasoning process, and failing to adjust this initial impression in the light of later information. This error is compounded by confirmation bias.
Ascertainment bias	When a nurse's thinking is shaped by prior assumptions and preconceptions; for example, ageism, stigmatism and stereotyping.
Confirmation bias	The tendency to look for confirming evidence to support a nursing diagnosis rather than look for disconfirming evidence to refute it, despite the latter often being more persuasive and definitive.
Diagnostic momentum	Once labels are attached to patients, they tend to become stickier and stickier. What started as a possibility gathers increasing momentum until it becomes definite and other possibilities are excluded.
Fundamental attribution error	The tendency to be judgmental and to blame patients for their illnesses (dispositional causes) rather than examine the circumstances (situational factors) that may have been responsible. Patients with a mental illness, and from minority or marginalised groups, are at particular risk of this error.
Overconfidence bias	A tendency to believe we know more than we do. Overconfidence bias reflects a tendency to act on incomplete information, intuition or hunches. Too much faith is placed on opinion instead of carefully collected cues. This error may be augmented by anchoring.
Premature closure	The tendency to accept a nursing diagnosis without sufficient evidence and before it has been fully verified. This error accounts for a high proportion of inaccurate or incomplete nursing diagnoses.
Psych-out error	People with a mental illness are particularly vulnerable to clinical reasoning errors, and co-morbid conditions may be overlooked or minimalised. A variant of this error occurs when medical conditions (such as hypoxia, delirium, electrolyte imbalance and head injuries) are misdiagnosed as psychiatric conditions.
Unpacking principle	Failure to collect and unpack all of the relevant cues and consider differential diagnoses may result in significant possibilities being missed.

Source: Adapted from P. Croskerry (2003). The importance of cognitive errors in diagnosis and strategies to minimize them. *Academic Medicine, 78*(8), 1–6.

Anchoring

Working as a nurse educator, I had been paged to come to PACU (post-anaesthetic care unit). Two RNs were seeking advice about the management of a patient (Mrs L) who had had a left hip replacement and was in severe pain, very distressed and calling out loudly and incoherently. The anaesthetist had been notified but was in theatre with another patient. Mrs L had been given morphine by the anaesthetist before being transferred to recovery. As ordered, she was given three further bolus doses of morphine at 3-minute intervals but with minimal effect. The nurses were encouraging her to use her PCA button but she was not coherent enough to comply. I tried to do a thorough pain assessment but was hampered in my attempts as the patient was unable to reply to my questions. I did an assessment of the wound and found that the dressing was dry and intact and the bellovac draining a small amount. There was a small amount of urine in the catheter bag. I examined the area surrounding the wound, convinced that there must be a surgical problem. But it appeared normal and I could see no obvious reason for the pain.

Time was passing without any improvement and we were all becoming anxious and concerned about Mrs L's distress and pain. I was about to phone the anaesthetist again but decided to check her wound one more time. In the process, I briefly noticed that Mrs L's catheter had not been taped to her leg and was actually lying under her thigh. Lifting it over her leg I saw that it had also been kinked. As I untwisted it, urine began to quickly flow. Within minutes there was close to 1600 mL in the catheter bag and Mrs L had drifted off into a morphine-induced state. Her resps were now 6 and oxygen sats 85 per cent. We increased the oxygen to 10 L per minute with little effect and phoned the anaesthetist for an order of naloxone as she had become narcotised. Had I not anchored onto the belief that Mrs L's pain must be coming from the surgical site I would have done a more comprehensive assessment, identified the cause of her pain, not administered as much morphine, and prevented respiratory depression from occurring. Checking that catheters are draining properly and not kinked or blocked became part of my routine post-operative patient assessment following this experience.

Distinguished Professor Tracy Levett-Jones
University of Technology Sydney

Ascertainment bias

While employed as a mental health nurse in a general practice, I assessed a 65-year-old woman, Alice (pseudonym), who was referred by her general practitioner (GP) as he was concerned about her mental state. Alice had been diagnosed three years prior with the degenerative neurological condition, amyotrophic lateral sclerosis (ALS). She was divorced, lived alone in a council flat in a small seaside village and had limited contact with her daughter and grandchildren who lived six hours away. Alice had a prior history that included childhood sexual abuse, a previous suicide attempt (in the context of domestic violence) and two episodes of major depression which had responded well to psychotropic medication and supportive psychotherapy.

Although Alice had significant physical symptoms that affected her mobility at times, she described having managed well until four months ago when her relationship with her daughter had deteriorated severely. The abandonment had increased her sense of isolation and this estrangement appeared to have been a trigger for a relapse into major depression, with decreased motivation, tearfulness, disordered sleep, loss of appetite and a heightened sense of hopelessness and suicidal ideation. Further discussion revealed that her GP had initiated a neurological review, which revealed minimal deterioration in physical functioning, and an aged care assessment (ACAT) with a view to increasing the level of support services available to Alice.

After consultation with Alice's GP, it was agreed that a psychiatrist review was warranted and I prepared a comprehensive referral to the mental health services. At the time, I was working part-time with the Community Mental Health Team and thus was present at the intake meeting where all referrals were reviewed as part of a multi-disciplinary team process. The nurse from the Acute Care Service responsible for presenting the referrals to the team commenced reading the referral. Before he had finished, he commented, 'This is a waste of time; of course the woman's depressed, who wouldn't be with a degenerative illness; besides, she's old.' Another team member responded, 'Tell the GP to refer her to palliative care.'

Sadly for Alice, the mental health service declined a psychiatrist review; the Mental Health Service for Older Persons likewise declined a review and recommended instead that the application process for placement in an aged care facility be started. Alice's 'real' issues were not addressed because of the ageism and preconceptions of the mental health team.

Associate Professor Rachel Rossiter
Charles Sturt University

Diagnostic momentum and confirmation bias

At handover on the second week of my third-year placement in an emergency department I learnt that one patient I was to assist in caring for was a young man of 16 with queried hepatitis A. It was at this point my clinical reasoning errors began. The 'bandwagon effect' known as diagnostic momentum took over and I found myself treating this young man as if his diagnosis had been confirmed. This was compounded by confirmation bias when he indicated that his abdominal pain was located at the site of his liver. As it turned out, the young man had gastroenteritis. The one strength I took out of this episode was my capacity to review current information, gather cues and recall knowledge to form a nursing diagnosis, even though in this case it was erroneous. Of course, my weakness was jumping to conclusions before all the information and cues were gathered. My thinking in this episode was affected by my desire to sound 'clever' to my mentor and the other nurses, so as to establish a little bit of 'credibility' in the ED. I have come to realise now that the only way to have 'credibility' is to be more critical in my thinking. My strategies for addressing the weaknesses exhibited in this episode are to continue to gather cues, use current information and the recall of knowledge prior to forming a nursing diagnosis.

Source: Adapted from Levett-Jones et al. (2010) Learning to think like a nurse, *Handover for Nurses, 3*(1): 15–20.

Fundamental attribution error

This incident occurred when I was a newly registered nurse working on a medical ward. The patient was an elderly man (70+ years) who was admitted for a stroke and had mild hemiparesis. The man appeared to be extremely resistive to our efforts to help him become as independent as possible. He wanted a great deal of assistance with his activities of daily living–more than would normally be required for his level of disability. He required constant encouragement to participate in any sort of physical activity, no matter how minimal. The man was eventually transferred to a rehabilitation unit. Some weeks later he returned to our ward as he would 'not participate' in his rehabilitation program. The handover reported that he had 'failed rehab'. I judged him on his previous behaviour and (based on the information from the rehab staff) I assumed he was just lazy. On his return to my ward he continued to constantly want assistance but I insisted (often strenuously and, on reflection, harshly) that he walk and participate in his own care. Around this time, he also started to mention pain which hadn't really featured till then. He was investigated and was found to have widespread bony metastasis from an unknown primary cancer. He died three weeks later. I was astounded and felt very guilty as I had judged this man, making assumptions that were later proven to be erroneous. I did, however, ensure that this man received the very best care for the last three weeks of his life.

Doctor Jennifer Dempsey
Former Senior Lecturer at The University of Newcastle

Overconfidence bias and unpacking principle

A 52-year-old male, John (pseudonym), was brought into the emergency department by the police and the local mental health team. John was in breach of his community treatment order. On presentation, John had slurred speech, was unable to stand or walk unassisted and was very aggressive. A code black was called after the triage nurse was punched and the attending nurse was bitten whilst obtaining a blood pressure. The emergency medical officer and two security personnel responded, with John being restrained. I had been asked to obtain a patient history. However, upon presentation, I had already labelled John as an alcoholic who was homeless and suffering from some sort of mental illness. I didn't see the purpose of taking a full patient history and thought that we just needed to sober him up and then release him back to the mental health team. The clinical reasoning errors that influenced my attitude and thinking included overconfidence bias and unpacking principle: I did not believe this patient had any real medical issues due to my labelling him as an alcoholic. Due to my assumptions, I did not collect a thorough history or assessment of this patient and disregarded the real medical and social problems that he was presenting with. John was homeless and had been for the past six years since his wife, daughter and two grandchildren had been killed in a car accident; he was simply unable to function anymore. Three years ago, John had come to the attention of the mental health team and he was diagnosed with an anxiety disorder, delusions, paranoia and panic attacks. He was also misusing alcohol and drugs, however, he had been clean and sober for the past 18 months. It was later established that, on presentation, John had a blood alcohol reading of zero. He was diagnosed with severe dehydration and a mild cerebrovascular haemorrhage. I was fortunate to have been supervised throughout this experience so my personal judgments did not endanger this patient. However, this has been an invaluable experience for me as I have learnt that you need to treat every patient individually without judgment, and that a thorough history is essential to understand what may be impacting on the patient's health status. I will endeavour to remember this in the future and not allow my biases to cloud my thinking.

Source: Adapted from Levett-Jones et al. (2010) Learning to think like a nurse, *Handover for Nurses, 3*(1):15–20.

Premature closure

This incident occurred while I was working as a registered nurse in an emergency department (ED). I was looking after a 7-year-old boy named Jamie (pseudonym). Jamie had been playing with his older brothers in the park when he fell, landing heavily on his right arm. On arrival into the ED, Jamie appeared very distressed: he was crying, pale and clutching his right arm. Jamie stated that his arm hurt 'really bad' and when asked to point to the pain, he indicated the whole forearm and elbow. On initial inspection, there was an obvious deformity to his right wrist. An X-ray of Jamie's wrist confirmed a transverse fracture of his distal radius. As it was not displaced, the doctor decided management of his fracture would include pain relief and a plaster backslab to his wrist. Jamie was given intranasal fentanyl with good pain relief and was able to tolerate the application of the backslab.Jamie's presentation appeared to be a straightforward case of a fractured distal radius. Therefore, we were surprised when approximately 30 minutes after the administration of the fentanyl and the application of the backslab, Jamie became very unsettled and inconsolable stating the pain was 'really, really bad'. He continued clutching his arm and was rocking back and forth in the bed, and would not let his mother comfort him. Jamie was given oral paracetamol for the pain. Neurovascular observations were conducted and were normal. Jamie's mum stated that this behaviour was unlike Jamie. The doctor determined that Jamie was overtired and stressed from the 'ordeal' and it would be best to discharge him home to rest. From my previous experience of caring for children with a distal radius fracture, this management seemed appropriate, even though his pain response was inconsistent with what would normally be expected. Later that evening, Jamie and his mother re-presented to the ED. Jamie had not been able to settle at home; his mother had given him a further dose of paracetamol as well as ibuprofen with no effect. Jamie was now complaining of pins and needles in his fingers. Jamie appeared pale and was tachycardic and diaphoretic. Following a review by the orthopaedic registrar, Jamie was sent for further X-rays where it was discovered that, in addition to the fractured distal radius, he had a fracture in his right olecranon which was impinging on his ulnar nerve and required immediate surgical repair. Failing to note the second fracture is an example of premature closure. Although the evidence (X-ray) supported the diagnosis of a fractured radius, it did not account for the excessive pain and lack of response to analgesia. 'When the diagnosis is made the thinking stops' (Croskerry, 2003). After the initial diagnosis, a reasonable alternative for Jamie's ongoing pain and symptoms was not sought and, instead, Jamie was considered to be 'overtired and stressed'. This was an example of ascertainment bias and was based on the flawed belief that children can be overly demonstrative in hospital environments.

Judy Smith
Lecturer, University of Technology Sydney

Psych-out error

Jill (pseudonym), a 44-year-old woman previously diagnosed with schizophrenia, was admitted to ICU in a catatonic state. Catatonia is linked to schizophrenia and is also associated with depression, anxiety, and severe stress. It can also occur as an atypical reaction to antipsychotic medications. My mentor and I found that Jill was tachycardic, diaphoretic, tachypneic and febrile. These observations were only moderately outside normal limits and, at the time, I believed that they were most likely due to anxiety consistent with Jill's mental illness. I admit that, from the start, I had made the clinical reasoning error described as psych-out error by seeing her as primarily mentally ill. I had assumed that her previous admissions and psychological state were the most likely causes of her present physiological condition. I searched her file for supporting evidence but instead my attention was drawn to the fact that she had recently commenced the antipsychotic drug clozapine. After reviewing Jill's condition, the doctors decided that she required specialist care and transferred her to a larger hospital. On reviewing evidence-based literature, I identified the adverse effects of clozapine. I could now appreciate that her condition was far more serious than I had first thought, with a possibility of neuroleptic malignant syndrome (NMS). NMS is a severe, potentially life-threatening response to antipsychotic therapy. The most obvious symptoms include muscle rigidity, tachycardia, tachypnoea, diaphoresis and fever. Jill's symptoms were consistent with all of the described signs, including her elevated temperature. On analysing my thinking, I recognised that, as a third-year student, my views were impacted by my lack of knowledge and experience which led to several naïve and biased judgments.

Source: Adapted from Levett-Jones et al. (2010) Learning to think like a nurse, *Handover for Nurses, 3*(1): 15–20.

CONCLUSION

This chapter has outlined the clinical reasoning process and emphasised that clinical reasoning skills are imperative for safe and effective nursing practice. The unfolding stories throughout the remainder of this text will capture your clinical imagination and provide opportunities for cognitive rehearsal of the clinical reasoning process. Repeated exposure to these meaningful clinical scenarios will enhance your acquisition of in-depth, clinically relevant knowledge and storage in your long-term memory; and, as you become immersed in these authentic stories, you will develop memory schemes for responding appropriately to diverse clinical problems.

Nursing and Midwifery Board of Australia (NMBA) *Registered Nurse Standards for Practice* The NMBA's *Registered Nurse Standards for Practice* (2016) state that registered nurses must use a variety of thinking strategies and the best available evidence in making decisions and providing safe, quality nursing practice within person-centred and evidence-based frameworks.

REFERENCES

Berman, A., Snyder, S., Levett-Jones, T., Dwyer, T., Hales, M., Harvey, N., . . . Stanley, D. (2020). *Kozier and Erb's Fundamentals of Nursing* (5th edn). Sydney: Pearson.

Boud, D. (2015). Feedback: Ensuring that it leads to enhanced learning. *The Clinical Teacher*, *12*(1), 3–7.

Cooper, S., Buykx, P., McConnell-Henry, T., Kinsman, L. & McDermott, S. (2011). Simulation: Can it eliminate failure to rescue? *Nursing Times*, *107*(3).

Croskerry, P. (2003). The importance of cognitive errors in diagnosis and strategies to minimize them. *Academic Medicine*, *78*(8), 1–6.

Duffield, C., Roche, M., O'Brien-Pallas, L., Diers, D., Alsbett, C., King, M., . . . Hall, J. (2007). *Gluing It Together: Nurses, Their Work Environment and Patient Safety*. University of Sydney, NSW.

Hoffman, K., Aitken, L. & Duffield, C. (2009). A comparison of novice and expert nurses' cue collection during clinical decision making: Verbal Protocol Analysis. *International Journal of Nursing Studies*, *46*(10), 1335–44.

Institute of Medicine. (2010). *The Future of Nursing: Focus on Education*. Retrieved from: www.nursingworld.org/MainMenuCategories/ThePracticeofProfessionalNursing/workforce/IOM-Future-of-Nursing-Report-1

Johansen, M. L. & O'Brien, J. L. (2016). Decision making in nursing practice: A concept analysis. *Nursing Forum*, *51*(1), 40–48.

Levett-Jones, T., Dwyer, T., Reid-Searl, K., Heaton, L., Flenady, T., Applegarth, J., Guinea, S. & Andersen, P. (2017). *The Patient Safety Competency Framework (PSCF) for Nursing Students*. Sydney, NSW. Retrieved from: http://psframework.wpengine.com/wp-content/uploads/2018/01/PSCF_Brochure_UTS-version_FA2-Screen.pdf

Levett-Jones, T., Hoffman, K., Dempsey, Y., Jeong, S., Noble, D., Norton, C., . . . Hickey, N. (2010). The 'five rights' of clinical reasoning: An educational model to enhance nursing students' ability to identify and manage clinically 'at risk' patients. *Nurse Education Today*, *30*(6), 515–20.

Martin, C. (2002). The theory of critical thinking. *Nursing Education Perspectives*, *23*(5), 241–47.

Nursing and Midwifery Board of Australia (NMBA). (2016). *Registered Nurse Standards for Practice*. Retrieved from: www.nursingmidwiferyboard.gov.au/Codes-Guidelines-Statements/Professional-standards.aspx

Paul, R. & Elder, L. (2007). *The Thinker's Guide for Students on How to Study and Learn a Discipline*. Dillon Beach, USA: Foundation for Critical Thinking Press.

Rubenfeld, M. & Scheffer, B. (2006). *Critical Thinking Tactics for Nurses*. Boston: Jones and Bartlett.

Schoenfeld, A. H. (2011). *How We Think: A Theory of Goal-Oriented Decision Making and Its Educational Applications*. New York, NY: Routledge.

Simmons, B. (2010). Clinical reasoning: Concept analysis. *Journal of Advanced Nursing*, *66*(5), 1151–58.

Tanner, C. (2006). Thinking like a nurse: A research-based model of clinical judgement in nursing. *Journal of Nursing Education*, *45*(6), 204–11.

Theobald, K. A. & Ramsbotham, J. (2019). Inquiry-based learning and clinical reasoning scaffolds: An action research project to support undergraduate students' learning to 'think like a nurse'. *Nurse Education in Practice*, *38*(7), 59–65.

Victor-Chmil, J. (2013) Critical thinking versus clinical reasoning versus clinical judgment: Differential diagnosis. *Nurse Educator*, *38*(1), 34–36.

Vierula, J., Hupli, M., Talman, K. & Haavisto, E. (2020). Identifying reasoning skills for the selection of undergraduate nursing students: A focus group study. *Contemporary Nurse*, *56*(2): 120–31.

Chapter 2

Caring for a person experiencing an adverse drug reaction

TRACY LEVETT-JONES and JUDITH SMITH

LEARNING OUTCOMES

Completion of the activities in this chapter will enable you to:

- explain why an understanding of medication safety and person-centred care is essential to competent practice (**recall** and **application**)
- explain the nurse's role in the medication team (**recall** and **application**)
- identify potential indications of an adverse drug reaction that will guide the collection and interpretation of appropriate cues (**gather, review, interpret, discriminate, relate** and **infer**)
- identify potential risk factors for medication safety and from medication errors (**match** and **predict**)
- review clinical information to identify the main nursing diagnoses for a patient experiencing an adverse drug reaction (**synthesise**)
- describe the priorities of care for a patient experiencing an adverse drug reaction (**goal setting** and **taking action**)
- identify clinical criteria for determining the effectiveness of nursing actions taken to manage an adverse drug reaction (**evaluate**)
- apply what you have learnt about medication safety to new clinical situations with different patients (**reflection** and **translation**).

INTRODUCTION

Medication errors result from multiple factors. However, nursing students (and occasionally more senior nurses) sometimes assume that if they learn about pharmacology and the 'six rights', and practise the technical aspects of medication administration, medication safety will be assured. In reality, there are many contextual and interpersonal factors that impact on safe medication practices. These include knowledge and skill deficits, poor communication with patients and their families, ineffective communication and coordination of care between members of the healthcare team, work pressures and distractions, and medication administration errors (World Health Organization, 2016). Additionally, each person who is the recipient of care will respond in an individual way to the medications prescribed and will need to be monitored for these responses. Clinical reasoning skills allow nurses to manage the many interconnected and complex factors that influence medication safety.

This chapter was written to introduce you to the clinical reasoning process. Two scenarios related to medication safety are juxtaposed to illustrate how clinical reasoning can make a significant difference to patient outcomes. The first scenario describes what actually occurred in the care of Mr Giuseppe Esposito. In the second scenario, we 'rewind' and illustrate what might have happened had the first-year nursing student caring for Mr Esposito demonstrated effective clinical reasoning skills. These scenarios are typical of those played out in Australian hospitals every day. They illustrate how clinical reasoning can make a difference to patient safety and why effective clinical assessment and communication skills are key components of medication safety. Importantly, these scenarios will help you to understand your role and the difference you can make, even as a beginning nursing student or graduate nurse, to your patients' clinical outcomes.

KEY CONCEPTS

adverse drug event
medication error
medication safety

SUGGESTED READINGS

A. Berman, S. Snyder, T. Levett-Jones, T. Burton & N. Harvey (Eds). (2020). *Skills in Clinical Nursing* (2nd Australian edn). Sydney: Pearson.
Unit 6: Medication administration

T. Levett-Jones (Ed.) (2020). *Critical Conversations for Patient Safety: An Essential Guide for Health Professionals.* Sydney: Pearson.
Chapter 10: Communicating to promote medication safety

SCENARIO 2.1 What did happen...

SETTING THE SCENE

One of the causes of medication errors is inconsistent and inaccurate use of medication abbreviations. Access this link for the approved terms for use in Australian hospitals: https://www.safetyandquality.gov.au/our-work/medication-safety/safer-naming-and-labelling-medicines/recommendations-terminology-abbreviations-and-symbols-used-medicines-documentation

Mr Giuseppe Esposito, 81 years, was admitted to the medical ward of Griffith Community Hospital with dehydration as a result of suspected gastroenteritis. He'd had vomiting and diarrhoea for two days prior to admission. Intravenous (IV) fluids were commenced and his diarrhoea and vomiting began to improve the following day, although some nausea persisted. Mr Esposito's IV was not re-sited when it 'tissued' later that evening.

On the second day following Mr Esposito's admission, Madeline Rose, a first-year nursing student, was to administer his usual oral medications (frusemide 80 mg, atorvastatin 20 mg and enalapril 20 mg) at 0800 hours.

At first, Madeline was supervised by a registered nurse (RN), but when another nurse called for assistance the RN left to attend to a patient in a nearby bed, saying to Madeline, 'Keep going—I'll watch what you are doing from over here.'

Reid-Searl et al. (2010) refer to the RN's behaviour in this scenario as 'being near'. Although a commonly used form of supervision during medication administration, it is neither legal nor professional. Nursing students are to be directly supervised by an RN when administering medications and the medication chart must be co-signed by the supervising RN.

Madeline was new to the ward and felt quite intimidated by the RN who was mentoring her, so she continued to administer the medications following the 'six rights' of medication administration (right patient, right drug, right dose, right time, right route and right documentation) as she had been taught at university. Madeline had heard of each of the medications but did not know very much about them. She did not refer to a drug reference as she was conscious that the RN was busy and wanted to get on with the medication round for her other patients.

Later that morning, the RN told Madeline that the bed was needed and asked her to quickly shower Mr Esposito, take his vital signs and get him ready for discharge. Madeline entered Mr Esposito's room and explained that his daughter would be in to pick him up soon but that she was going to take him to have a shower first. As Mr Esposito got out of bed he staggered a little and said, 'I'm a bit wobbly today.' He quickly regained his balance and Madeline reassured him that she would put a shower chair in the bathroom for him. She was concerned as time was getting away, so she settled Mr Esposito in the shower then left to pack up his belongings. When Madeline returned, she found him leaning forward in the chair with his head down. Mr Esposito reassured her by saying, 'Don't you worry, love, it's just the hot water... it made me a bit giddy.' Madeline helped him dress, then walked with him back to his room and sat him in the chair next to his bed to wait for his daughter.

Madeline returned a few minutes later with an electronic blood pressure machine and took Mr Esposito's temperature, pulse, respiration and blood pressure, as she had been instructed. His vital signs were: T 36.6ºC, PR 96, RR 20, BP 110/60 mmHg. Madeline then documented the observations in Mr Esposito's chart.

Would these results be considered 'normal' for Mr Esposito?

The RN was busy when Mr Esposito's daughter arrived, so she asked Madeline to give him his discharge papers and take him to the car in a wheelchair.

Mr Esposito's daughter took her father home. She would have preferred that he spend a few days with her in town but he refused, saying he wanted to get back to the farm as his dog would be fretting without him. She made him a sandwich and a cup of tea, ensured he was comfortable and left, saying she would be back in a couple of hours after she had finished with some things at work. Mr Esposito, relieved to be home and feeling very tired, fell asleep in his recliner chair. He woke up an hour later needing to go to the bathroom. He began to walk to the bathroom but felt lightheaded and very dizzy. Later, he couldn't recall whether he had lost his footing or fainted, but when he regained consciousness he had a lot of pain in his right forearm, wrist and chest. He also had a laceration to his forehead. Shortly after, his daughter found him lying on the floor and immediately called an ambulance.

Mr Esposito was taken to the emergency department and, following X-rays, was diagnosed with a Colles' fracture, three fractured ribs and a concussion. The admitting medical officer attributed Mr Esposito's collapse to postural hypotension caused by dehydration and an adverse drug reaction.

Mr Esposito was discharged to his daughter's home seven days later, but it took many months for his fractures to heal and for him to regain his independence, confidence, strength and sense of wellbeing.

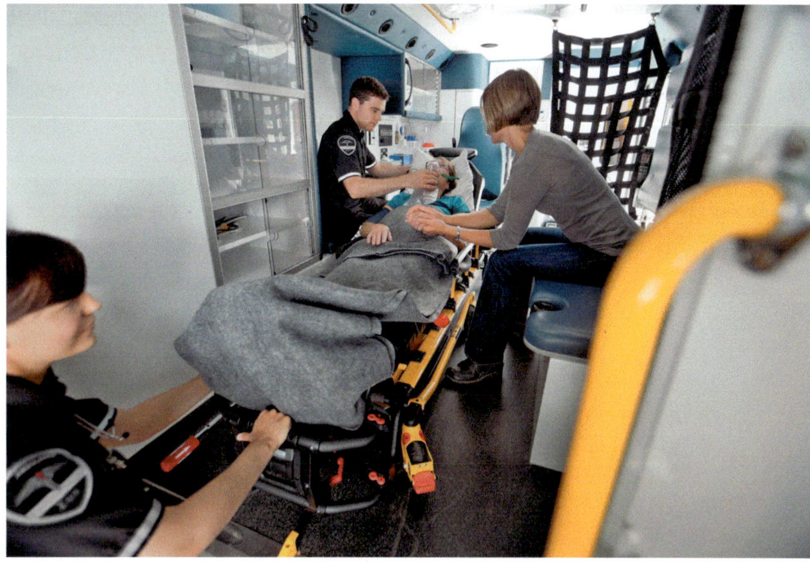

Mr Esposito returns to hospital via ambulance © Tyler Olson | 123RF

Epidemiology of medication errors

Medication administration is a complex process involving counting, calculating, measuring, mixing and ensuring that the right person receives the right medicine, in the right dose, at the right time, by the right route and for the right reason (Manias, 2020). The complexity of the medication administration process is compounded by polypharmacy, patient acuity, interruptions, use of electronic technologies, facility design and time constraints (World Health Organization, 2016). The unpredictable and dynamic nature of the clinical environment further adds to this complexity.

Medication administration errors can be clinical, such as giving the wrong drug or dose, by the wrong route, to the wrong patient or at the wrong time (Westbrook et al., 2015). However, errors can also be procedural and include failure to adhere to established practices, standards or policies in any aspect of the medication administration process, for example, failure to check a patient's identification, read the medication label/expiry date or accurately document medication administration (Westbrook et al.).

Medication errors are the second most common type of incident reported in Australian hospitals (Johnson & Young, 2011), and the World Health Organization (2016) estimates that more than 50 per cent of all medications are prescribed, dispensed, administered or used inappropriately. However, it is likely that this is an underestimate as many errors are not reported (Johnson & Young).

Nurses are the last line of defence in protecting patients against medication errors.

Approximately two to three per cent of all Australian hospital admissions are related to medications. This suggests at least 230,000 admissions annually are caused by patients taking too much or too little of a particular medicine, or taking the wrong medicine—with an estimated annual cost of at least $1.2 billion (Australian Commission on Safety and Quality in Health Care, 2017).

An adverse drug reaction is a harmful and unintended response to a medication or combination of medications given in normal doses that requires treatment and/or a decreased dose.

Reflection

Q1 In this scenario, Madeline did every task she had been asked to do by the RN. Should anything else have been expected of her?

Q2 What interpersonal and situational factors influenced how this scenario unfolded?

Q3 How might the outcome for Mr Esposito have been different had Madeline had a requisite level of clinical reasoning skills?

Q4 What aspects of this adverse drug reaction were preventable?

Q5 Should this adverse drug reaction be documented and reported? If so, where, by whom, to whom and why?

National Safety and Quality Health Service (NSQHS) Standards

Medication safety standard

The NSQHS Standards specify that each health service organisation must have processes for documenting adverse drug reactions in the healthcare record and in an organisation-wide incident reporting system (ACSQHC, 2021).

Access Young-Min Lee's story in this online module to learn about open disclosure following medical errors: https://patientsafetyfornursingstudents.org/resources/medication-safety

Q6 The medical officer and nurse discussed whether Mr Esposito and his daughter should be told that he had experienced an adverse drug reaction. The nurse thought they should be told but the doctor disagreed, saying that telling Mr Esposito and his daughter would make them worry needlessly. What do you think and why?

Sometimes healthcare professionals adopt an overly simplistic approach to clinical errors such as adverse drug reactions by blaming the person who administered, prescribed or dispensed the medication. However, this does not take into account the multiple contextual and system-wide factors that create the conditions in which errors can occur.

It is helpful to use James Reason's 'Swiss Cheese Model' (2000) when reviewing the causes of adverse drug reactions such as the one described in Scenario 2.1. In Reason's model of system failure, every step in a process has the potential for failure, to varying degrees. The ideal system is like a stack of Swiss cheese slices. In this analogy, each hole is an opportunity for a process to fail and each slice is a 'defensive layer' in the process. An error may allow a problem to pass through a hole in one layer but in the next layer the holes are in different places and the problem should be caught. The fewer the holes, the more likely it is that an error will be caught or stopped.

Q7 Reflect on Scenario 2.1 and label Figure 2.1 with some of the errors that occurred and led to Mr Esposito's adverse drug reaction.

PERSON-CENTRED CARE

Person-centred health professionals are ethical, open-minded, empathetic, respectful and self-aware with a profound sense of moral agency (Levett-Jones et al., 2020). Person-centred care means seeing the *person,* not just the patient or their disease. Integral to person-centred care is the nurse's understanding of the patient's beliefs and values, and respect for and appreciation of the patient's life history. Person-centred care is a holistic approach to healthcare that is grounded in a philosophy of personhood. Although there

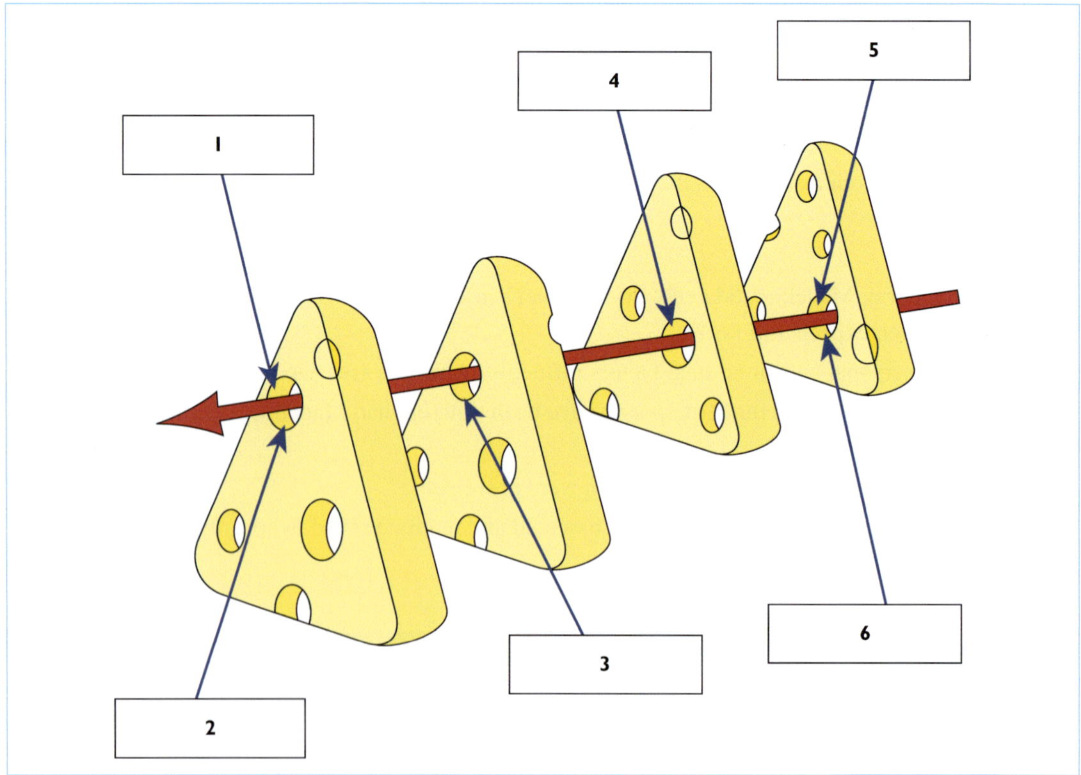

Figure 2.1 *Adverse drug reaction—Reason's Swiss Cheese Model*

Source: Based on J. Reason. (2000). Human error: Models and management. *British Medical Journal, 320*, 768–70.

are varying definitions of person-centred care, each promotes self-determination, empowerment and a commitment to providing healthcare that is responsive to the needs and preferences of the individual (Rossiter, Scott & Walton, 2020). Key dimensions of person-centered care include respect, emotional support, physical comfort, information and communication, as well as care coordination that involves the patient, carers and family (ACSQHC, 2019).

Something to think about . . .

Person-centred care and effective communication help nurses to develop an understanding of the patient as a person and to work collaboratively in a therapeutic relationship (Rossiter, Scott & Walton, 2020). Nurses who communicate effectively with their patients are better able to collect and validate assessment data, initiate appropriate nursing actions, evaluate the effectiveness of outcomes and prevent unsafe practice.

SCENARIO 2.2 What might have happened . . .

CHANGING THE SCENE

Let's imagine that we could rewind Scenario 2.1 and this time we'll see how Mr Esposito's outcomes are influenced by the use of clinical reasoning skills and person-centred care.

Mr Giuseppe Esposito, 81 years, was admitted to the medical ward of Griffith Community Hospital with dehydration as a result of suspected gastroenteritis. He had been vomiting and had diarrhoea for two days prior to admission. Intravenous fluids were commenced and his diarrhoea began to improve the following day, although some nausea persisted. Mr Esposito's IV was not re-sited when it 'tissued' later that evening.

> 'Words are, of course, the most powerful drug used by mankind' (Rudyard Kipling, 1923).

Madeline Rose, a nursing student, was caring for Mr Esposito following his admission and spent time talking to him and his daughter, Bella. He asked Madeline to call him Giuseppe and, as she got to know him, he began to tell her about his past.

> Cultural awareness: How might Giuseppe's personal history, culture and life experiences influence the way he interacts in healthcare environments?

Giuseppe had lived alone on his five-hectare farm in Yenda, approximately 10 kilometres from Griffith in New South Wales, since his wife Fiore's death a year ago. He arrived in Australia in 1944 from a village near the town of Verona. Like many of his fellow Italians, he came to Australia in search of *benessere* (prosperity). He worked as a labourer on road construction in order to buy and pay off his farm. It was a tough existence made worse by the racist taunts and other displays of vilification that he and many of the other Italian farmers endured. To this day, Giuseppe is embarrassed by his accent and he often feels like an 'outsider'.

Giuseppe and Fiore had three sons and one daughter, Bella. His sons now live in Sydney and Bella lives in Griffith. Giuseppe loves to spend time with his daughter and grandsons, but they have busy lives and he sees them only once or twice a week. Bella worries about him and wishes he lived closer to town, but he has refused to move. For most of Giuseppe's life his health has been reasonably good, although he has had some arrhythmias and hypertension over the past few years. Lately, Bella has been concerned that Giuseppe isn't taking care of himself properly and she thinks he is becoming a little forgetful. She believes that his gastroenteritis is a result of eating a chicken dish that had been in his refrigerator for more than a week.

> Researchers have identified a significant association between interruptions during medication preparation and administration, and medication errors (Shahbaz et al., 2020).

At 0800 hours, two days following Giuseppe's admission, Madeline was asked to administer his usual oral medications (frusemide 80 mg, atorvastatin 20 mg and enalapril 20 mg). It was a busy shift and the RN supervising Madeline was interrupted with a request to attend to another patient. She said, 'Keep going—I'll watch what you are doing from over here.'

Madeline, although new to the ward and feeling quite intimidated, was conscious that what the RN was asking her to do contravened university and healthcare policies, and was outside of her scope of practice. She replied, 'I'm sorry but I am not allowed to administer medications without direct supervision by a registered nurse.' The RN looked surprised but said, 'Oh… okay, I'll be there in a tick.'

Nursing and Midwifery Board of Australia (NMBA) *Registered Nurse Standards for Practice* The NMBA standards for practice (2016) specify that registered nurses must comply with legislation, regulations, policies, guidelines and other standards or requirements relevant to the context of practice.

While she waited, Madeline checked whether Giuseppe had any allergies and that there was a valid order for the medications. She also reviewed the *Australian Medicines Handbook* (Rossi, 2021) to find out more about the medications she was administering.

Patient Safety Competency Framework (PSCF)

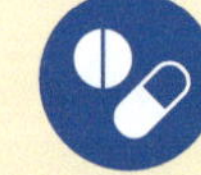

Domain 9—Medication safety

The PSCF specifies that nursing students must use evidence-based sources of information when administering medications.

Source: *The Patient Safety Competency Framework for Nursing Students*, https://patientsafetyfornursingstudents.org

Medication safety is enhanced when patients are actively engaged in the medication management process, this includes an active dialogue between the patient and the nurse (Manias et al., 2015).

Once the RN returned, Madeline administered the medications following the 'six rights' (right patient, right drug, right dose, right time, right route and right documentation). She also asked Giuseppe to check his medications as she gave them to him, saying, 'I'm giving you your Lipitor, Lasix and Renitec, is that right? Do you know what they're for, Giuseppe?' He nodded and replied, 'Yes, yes, they're for my ticker and my water.'

Q1 What other 'rights' are essential to medication safety?

Q2 What does a valid medication order require?

Q3 What three checks are required when administering medications?

Q4 Should Madeline have taken Giuseppe's vital signs prior to administering his medications? Why or why not?

Later that morning, the RN told Madeline that the bed was needed and asked her to quickly shower Mr Esposito, do his vital signs and get him ready for discharge.

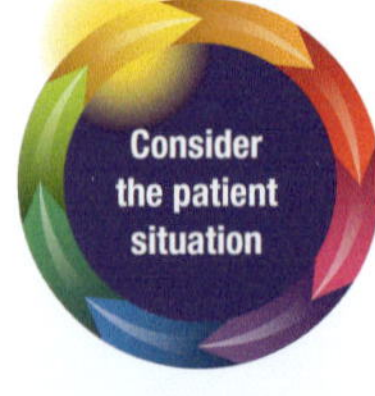

1. CONSIDER THE PATIENT SITUATION

In the first stage of the clinical reasoning cycle, the nurse begins to gain an initial impression. He or she anticipates and takes notice of the patient's concerns and begins to think about the situation.

A simple question such as 'How are you feeling?' often elicits meaningful patient information. The problem is that in healthcare, as in everyday life, we don't always listen carefully to the person's response to this question.

Madeline entered Giuseppe's room and explained that Bella would be in to pick him up soon but that she was going to take him to have a shower first. She also asked how he was feeling. He replied, 'I'm much better now that I don't have the "runs". I still feel sick in the stomach though, and I'm right off my food. I'll feel better when I get home, I should think. This gastro thing has really knocked me.'

Madeline sat Giuseppe on the side of the bed as she collected his things for the shower. As he sat there, he said, 'Geez, I'm a bit dizzy, girly.' Madeline wasn't sure what to do but decided to leave Giuseppe sitting for a few minutes because she was concerned that if she took him to the shower he might fall.

2. COLLECT CUES/INFORMATION

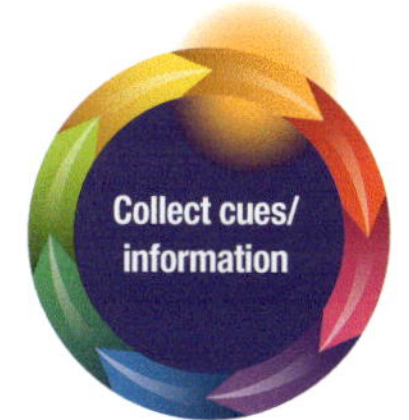

(a) Review current information

During the second stage of the clinical reasoning cycle, the nurse begins to collect relevant information about the patient. He or she starts by reviewing the information that is currently available via the patient's clinical documentation, medical and nursing notes, handover report and other available information.

As Madeline began to think about why Giuseppe was feeling dizzy, she reviewed his charts. The fluid balance chart was incomplete, as it had not been maintained since the IV tissued the previous day. Madeline noticed that, on the previous day, Giuseppe was in a positive balance (2400 mL in—mostly IV fluids and small amounts of oral fluids; total output 700 mL—he had been voiding small amounts infrequently).

It appears on face value that Giuseppe is in a positive balance. Do you think this is an accurate reflection of his fluid status? Why?

Since his admission, Giuseppe's blood pressure had been between 120/70 mmHg and 110/60 mmHg. His temperature had been 38ºC on admission but 36.4–37ºC over the last 24 hours. Giuseppe's respiratory rate had been 16–20 per minute. Madeline read Giuseppe's progress notes but there was no mention of him feeling dizzy before.

(b) Gather new information

The next stage of the clinical reasoning cycle is to collect relevant cues and information. This requires the nurse to determine which cues are relevant for a particular person at a particular point in time.

Madeline considered Giuseppe's dizziness and decided to take his blood pressure sitting and standing before getting him up for the shower. She used the manual sphygmomanometer attached to the wall beside his bed.

Q1 Why did Madeline take a sitting and a standing BP?

Q2 Why do you think Madeline chose to use the manual sphygmomanometer instead of the electronic one?

Q3 Giuseppe's blood pressure was 110/65 mmHg sitting and 92/ 58 mmHg standing. What might this reading indicate?

Madeline also checked Giuseppe's pulse rate; it was 96, weak and thready.

Q4 From the following list, identify three other cues that you believe Madeline should have collected?

- a Appetite
- b Condition of oral mucosa
- c Oral intake
- d Pain
- e Cognitive state
- f Level of thirst

Something to think about . . .

When the correct cues are not collected, all of the actions that follow may be incorrect. Making decisions based on incomplete information is a leading cause of clinical errors. Early subtle cues, when missed, can lead to adverse patient outcomes (Liaw et al., 2018).

Q5 Are there any questions you would have asked Giuseppe if you had been in this situation?

(c) Recall knowledge

While cue collection involves reviewing current and gathering new information, it also requires recall of related knowledge. This includes a broad and deep knowledge of physiology, pathophysiology, pharmacology, epidemiology, therapeutics, culture, context of care, ethics and law, and so on; as well as an understanding of evidence-based practice. For students, this can be challenging because it requires not only a strong foundation of knowledge but also the ability to synthesise and apply their knowledge to clinical situations that are often complex and fluid.

Madeline tried to recall what she had learnt about gastroenteritis, quality use of medicines, and the medications Giuseppe was taking.

Quick Quiz!

To ensure that you have a good understanding of these important topics, test yourself with the following questions.

Q1 List the four key members of the medication safety team.

Q2 'Therapeutic index' refers to:
- a The way drugs are categorised into groups (e.g. analgesics)
- b The margin between effectiveness and toxicity of drugs
- c The register that is kept of drugs that are and are not therapeutic for particular patient groups
- d The relative potency of a medication

Q3 Vomiting and diarrhoea may cause a significant loss of which electrolyte from the gastrointestinal tract?
- a Calcium
- b Magnesium
- c Potassium
- d Sodium

Q4 The organ responsible for the excretion of most drugs and their metabolites is the:
- a Liver
- b Gut
- c Kidney
- d Lungs

Q5 Dehydration results in:
- a An increased glomerular filtration rate
- b A decreased glomerular filtration rate
- c No change to the glomerular filtration rate

Q6 What is the action of the diuretic frusemide?
- a It blocks the absorption of sodium, chloride and water from the fluid in the Bowman's capsule, causing an increase in urine output (diuresis).
- b It blocks the absorption of sodium, chloride and water from the filtered fluid in the kidney tubules, causing an increase in urine output (diuresis).
- c It enhances the absorption of sodium, chloride and water from the filtered fluid in the kidney tubules, causing a decrease in urine output (oliguria).
- d It blocks the absorption of potassium, magnesium and water from the filtered fluid in the kidney tubules, causing an increase in urine output (diuresis).

Q7 Frusemide may cause serum potassium levels to:
- a Increase
- b Decrease
- c Stay the same

Q8 Enalapril should be used with caution in patients with:
- a Hypervolaemia (fluid overload)
- b Hypertension
- c Hypovolaemia and/or dehydration
- d Asthma

Q9 Atorvastatin belongs to which class of drugs?
- a Antihypertensive drugs
- b Lipid regulating drugs
- c Antiarrhythmic drugs
- d Vasodilators

Q10 Adverse effects of atorvastatin include:
- a Hypertension and hypercholesterolaemia
- b Acute liver failure
- c Nausea and diarrhoea
- d Bleeding

Prior to administering Giuseppe's medications, Madeline had reviewed the *Australian Medicines Handbook* (Rossi, 2021). She recalled reading that enalapril can cause significant hypotension in patients that are dehydrated and can also have adverse side effects, such as palpitations, tachycardia, dizziness, malaise, vertigo, confusion, pruritus, nausea and vomiting. Madeline also recalls reading that frusemide should be ceased in patients experiencing hypovolaemia and/or dehydration. She recalls frusemide can have adverse reactions, including fluid and electrolyte disturbances, headache, visual disturbances, dizziness, vertigo, restlessness, nausea, vomiting and diarrhoea.

Q11 Which signs and symptoms of a potential adverse reaction to enalapril or frusemide did Giuseppe have?

3. PROCESS INFORMATION

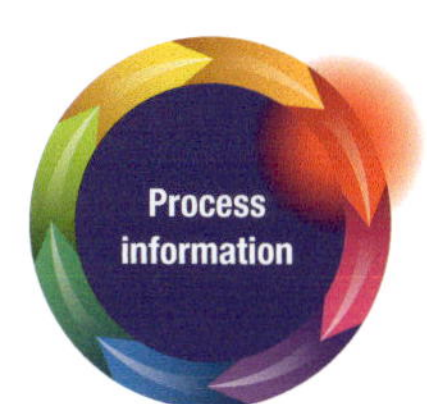

(a) Interpret

The next step of the clinical reasoning cycle is to interpret the data (cues) collected through careful analysis and to identify aberrations from normal. Always ask the question: 'Are these cues normal for this person, at this time and in this place?'

Q Which of the following would be considered to be within normal parameters for Giuseppe?

- a Temperature: 36.4–37°C
- b Pulse: 96 beats/min
- c Respiratory rate: 16–20 breaths/min
- d Blood pressure: 110/65 mmHg sitting and 92/58 mmHg standing

(b) Discriminate

At this stage, the nurse narrows down the information to what is most important.

Q From the following list, select five cues that you believe are *most relevant* to Giuseppe *at this time*.

- a Blood pressure
- b Respiratory rate
- c Temperature
- d Dizziness
- e Pulse rate
- f Level of consciousness
- g Urine output

(c) Relate

The next step for Madeline was to cluster together the cues that she had collected and try to make sense of them by looking for relationships or patterns. Some people call this stage 'connecting the dots' or 'putting two and two together'.

Q Label the following statements either *true* or *false*.

- a Giuseppe may have been hypotensive due to insensible fluid loss (vomiting and diarrhoea).
- b Giuseppe's dizziness and nausea could have been a side effect of one of his medications.
- c Giuseppe's weak and thready pulse may have been caused by his hypotension and negative fluid balance.
- d Giuseppe's tachycardia and hypotension may have been from anxiety and stress.
- e Giuseppe's negative fluid balance may have been caused by vomiting, diarrhoea and inadequate oral intake.

(d) Infer

In this stage of the clinical reasoning cycle, the nurse thinks about all the cues that have been collected and makes inferences based on the analysis and interpretation of those cues.

From what Madeline knew about Giuseppe's history, signs and symptoms, as well as the information she had recalled, she considered potential inferences.

Q Giuseppe could have been experiencing which of the following? (Select the two that you think are most correct.)

- a Signs and symptoms of dehydration
- b An exacerbation of his gastroenteritis
- c An allergic reaction to one of his medications
- d An adverse drug reaction

(e) Predict

Next the nurse must anticipate potential outcomes depending on a particular course of action (or inaction). Madeline was worried and not sure what course of action to take. Because of her inexperience and uncertainty, she wanted to just 'wait and see'. However, she began to think about what might happen if she did nothing.

Q If Madeline did nothing, what might happen to Giuseppe? (Select the two correct answers.)

a He could go into septic shock.
b His condition would probably improve over the next few days.
c He could experience serious complications once discharged.
d He could develop life-threatening hypotension.

(f) Match

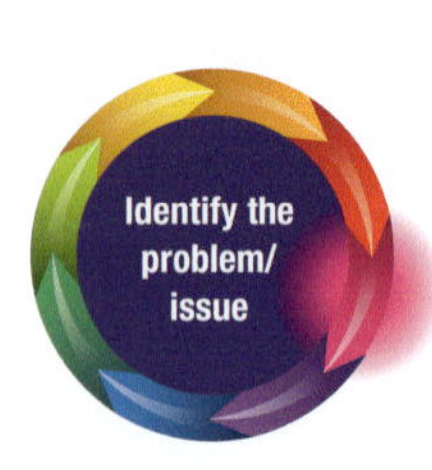

In this stage, the nurse matches the current situation to past situations, or current patient to past patients, using mental prompts such as: 'I remember when this happened before and... '; 'This is similar to... '; and 'Last time I saw this... '. However, keep in mind 'matching' is usually an expert thought process.

Over time, Madeline will develop a repertoire of experiences with which she can compare presenting clinical situations, but this will take repeated opportunities to engage in clinical reasoning (in real or simulated contexts).

Diagnosing is a pivotal step in clinical reasoning as care planning and nursing interventions follow directly from this phase. Safe and effective healthcare depends on accurate communication and documentation of nursing diagnoses.

4. IDENTIFY THE PROBLEM/ISSUE

Diagnosing is the fourth stage of the clinical reasoning cycle. It is when the nurse synthesises all of the information he or she has collected in order to identify critical patient problem(s). There are two types of nursing diagnoses: actual and risk. An actual diagnosis consists of the patient problem, the related aetiology (causal relationship between a problem and its related or risk factors) and supporting evidence (e.g. cues). A risk nursing diagnosis is a clinical judgment about a potential problem where the presence of risk factors indicates that a problem has the potential to develop unless nurses intervene appropriately (Levett-Jones, 2021).

Q What would be one actual and one risk nursing diagnosis for Giuseppe?

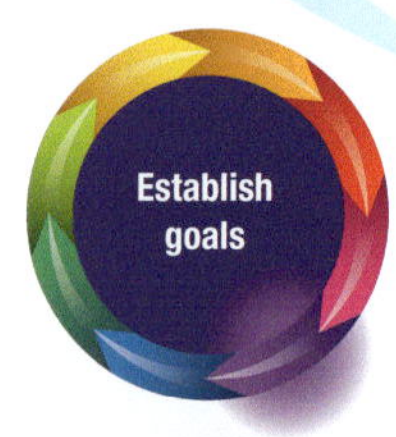

5. ESTABLISH GOALS

Madeline was concerned about Giuseppe's blood pressure and dizziness in particular and she knew she needed to refer to a more experienced nurse before she could work out what to do for Giuseppe.

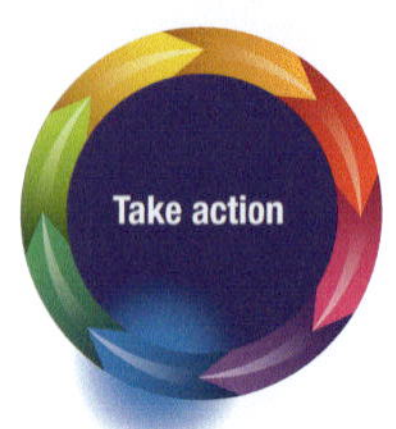

6. TAKE ACTION

The next stage of the clinical reasoning cycle requires knowledge, clinical skills, effective communication skills and clinical reasoning ability. The nurse has to decide which actions take priority, who should be notified and when to notify them (Liaw et al., 2018).

Something to think about...

Too often, nurses observe and document but fail to follow up on clinical abnormalities. For example, in an integrative literature review by Mok, Wang and Liaw (2015) it was reported that 84 per cent of hospital cardiopulmonary arrests could have been avoided if clinical signs of deterioration had not been overlooked. These types of situations can eventuate when nurses do not have adequate clinical reasoning skills.

Madeline used ISBAR (Identify, Situation, Background, Assessment, Request/Recommendation) when speaking to the RN about Giuseppe's condition.

Something to think about...

At times the most appropriate nursing action is to relay your concerns about a deteriorating patient to senior staff. To do this, you need to be confident and skilled in communicating with members of the interprofessional healthcare team so that you can signal your need for immediate help when required. Use of acronyms such as ISBAR is effective in streamlining the way healthcare professionals communicate and in increasing patient safety (Levett-Jones et al., 2010).

National Safety and Quality Health Service (NSQHS) Standards

Communicating for safety standard

The importance of effective communication to patient safety is emphasised in the NSQHS Standards (ACSQHC, 2021), where it is specified that health professionals must facilitate structured and effective communication between health service organisations, within health service organisations, between clinicians, and between clinicians and consumers.

Q In the following table, match the appropriate communication strategy with the components of the ISBAR acronym.

Communication strategy

- State your request.
- Summarise the patient's current condition or situation. Explain your assessment of the problem including your risk diagnoses for Giuseppe.
- Provide nurse's name, position, location. Provide patient's name, age, gender.
- Outline the patient's medical diagnosis, relevant history, investigations, what has been done so far.
- Briefly explain the reason for your concern.

ISBAR	Communication strategy
Identify	
Situation	
Background	
Assessment	
Request/recommendation	

7. EVALUATE

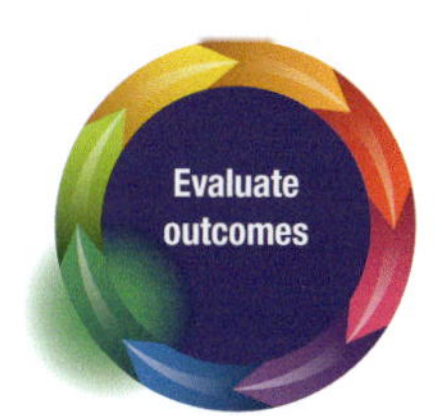

In this stage of the clinical reasoning cycle, the effectiveness of one's actions is assessed.

Because of Madeline's clear, succinct and relevant communication, the RN felt compelled to review Giuseppe. She took his vital signs again and noted a greater than 20 mmHg drop in systolic pressure when standing and a marked increase in pulse rate from lying to standing. The RN returned to the nurses' station and accessed Giuseppe's blood results on the intranet identifying that he was hypokalaemic and hypernatraemic, and his urea/creatinine ratio was 1:5, suggesting hypovolaemia.

The RN conducted an ECG but did not identify any abnormalities. The RN consulted the clinical pharmacist who was on the ward and phoned the medical officer.

What is hypokalaemia and hypernatraemia? What may have caused this electrolyte imbalance? How does measuring urea and creatinine determine a patient's fluid volume status?

Patient Safety Competency Framework (PSCF)

Domain 9—Medication safety

The PSCF emphasises the requirement for nursing students to work within their scope of practice with regards to medication administration. By raising concerns about Mr Giuseppe Esposito in a timely manner, and with clarity and confidence, Madeline has worked within her scope of practice and communicated effectively at a standard expected of a nursing student.

Source: *The Patient Safety Competency Framework for Nursing Students*, https://patientsafetyfornursingstudents.org

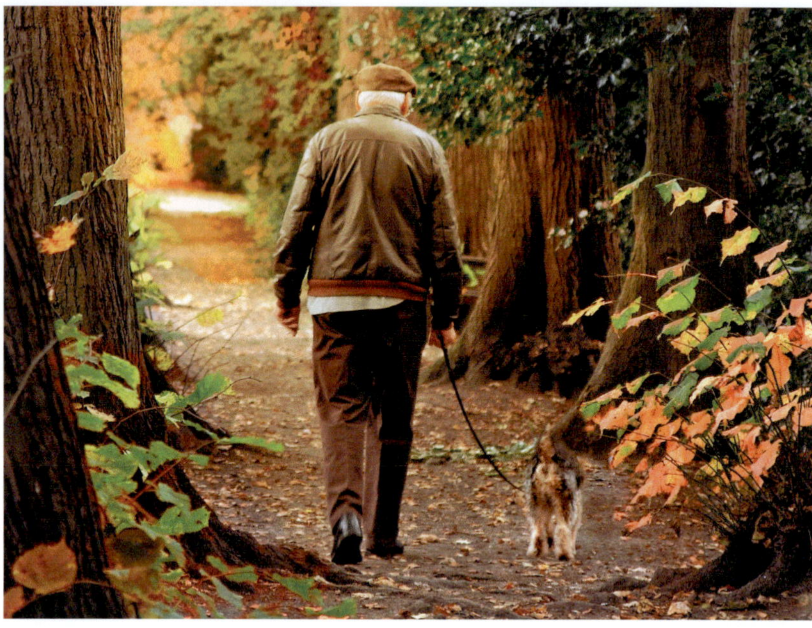

Giuseppe returns to his farm following discharge © Anneka/ Shutterstock

Communication errors are identified as the root cause of 70 per cent of sentinel events in healthcare settings (The Joint Commission, 2015). Access this website to explore why interprofessional communication is essential to safe medication practices: https://patientsafetyfornursingstudents.org/resources/medication-safety

Following a medical review, Giuseppe's frusemide was ceased and his enalapril dose was reduced to 10 mg nocte. He was also given 1 litre of Hartmann's solution with 20 mmol KCL (potassium chloride) intravenously. The RN was directed to repeat the ECG four hours after the Hartmann's infusion was complete and a repeat electrolyte/urea/creatinine (EUC) test was ordered for the following morning. (Rossi, 2021).

When telling the afternoon staff what had happened to Giuseppe, the RN said to the nurses, 'I am so glad Madeline was on the ball. I dread to think what might have happened if we'd sent him home like that.'

Giuseppe's condition improved over the next three days and he was discharged under the care of his local GP. He agreed to stay with Bella for a few days before going back to his farm.

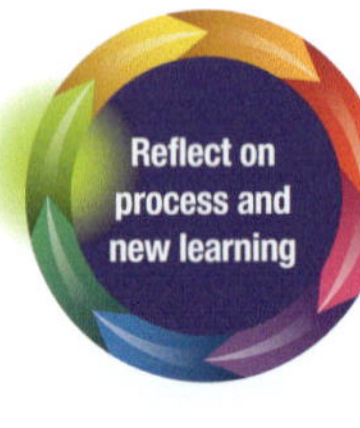

8. REFLECT

The final stage of the clinical reasoning cycle is 'reflection'. Reflection in this context refers to the process of 'looking back' and reviewing what you have learnt from the scenario. It also means 'looking forward' and deciding what you will do if presented with a similar situation in clinical practice.

Consider the following questions.

Q1 What are three of the most important things that you have learnt from this scenario?

Q2 What actions will you take in your clinical practice as a result of your learning from this scenario?

Q3 How will you demonstrate person-centred care when administering medications?

Q4 What have you learnt from this scenario about communication, clinical leadership and teamwork that you can apply to your clinical practice?

FURTHER READING

Bolster, D. & Manias, E. (2010). Person-centred interactions between nurses and patients during medication activities in an acute hospital setting: Qualitative observation and interview study. *International Journal of Nursing Studies, 47*(2), 154–65.

NPS Medicinewise Learning—Medication Safety Module. Retrieved from: https://learn.nps.org.au/mod/page/view.php?id=4277

Patient Safety for Nursing Students website: https://patientsafetyfornursingstudents.org/resources/medication-safety

Reid-Searl, K., Moxham, L., Walker, S. & Happell, B. (2010). Nursing students administering medication: Appreciating and seeking appropriate supervision. *Journal of Advanced Nursing, 66*(3), 532–41.

REFERENCES

Australian Commission on Safety and Quality in Health Care (ACSQHC). (2017). *Australia Joins International Push to Halve Medication Errors*. Retrieved from: https://www.safetyandquality.gov.au/media_releases/australia-joins-international-push-to-halve-medication-errors#:~:text=this%20suggests%20at%20least%20230%2c000,of%20at%20least%20%241.2%20billion

Australian Commission on Safety and Quality in Health Care (ACSQHC). (2019). *Person-Centered Care*. Retrieved from: https://www.safetyandquality.gov.au/our-work/partnering-consumers/person-centred-care

Australian Commission on Safety and Quality in Health Care (ACSQHC). (2021). *National Safety and Quality Health Service Standards* (2nd edn). Sydney, Australia.

Johnson, M. & Young, H. (2011). The application of Aronson's taxonomy to medication errors in nursing. *Journal of Nursing Care Quality, 26*(2), 128–35.

Levett-Jones, T. (2021). Diagnosing. In A. Berman, S. Snyder, T. Levett-Jones et al. (Eds), *Kozier and Erb's Fundamentals of Nursing* (3rd edn). Sydney: Pearson.

Levett-Jones, T., Dwyer, T., Reid-Searl, K., Heaton, L., Flenady, T., Applegarth, J., Guinea, S. & Andersen, P. (2017). *The Patient Safety Competency Framework (PSCF) for Nursing Students*. Sydney, NSW. Retrieved from: http://psframework.wpengine.com/wp-content/uploads/2018/01/PSCF_Brochure_UTS-version_FA2-Screen.pdf

Levett-Jones, T., Gilligan, C. Outram, S. & Horton, G. (2020). Key attributes of 'patient safe' communication. In T. Levett-Jones (Ed.), *Critical Conversations for Patient Safety: An Essential Guide for Health Professionals*. Sydney: Pearson.

Levett-Jones, T., Hoffman, K., Dempsey, Y., Jeong, S., Noble, D., Norton, C. A., Roche, J. & Hickey, N. (2010). The 'five rights' of clinical reasoning: An educational model to enhance nursing students' ability to identify and manage clinically 'at risk' patients. *Nurse Education Today, 30*(6), 515–20.

Liaw, S., Cooper, S. & Levett-Jones, T. (2018). Development and psychometric testing of a Clinical Reasoning Evaluation Simulation Tool (CREST) for assessing ability to recognize and respond to clinical deterioration. *Nurse Education Today. 62*, 74–79. doi.org/10.1016/j.nedt.2017.12.009

Manias, E. (2020). Communicating to promote medication safety. In T. Levett-Jones (Ed.), *Critical Conversations for Patient Safety: An Essential Guide for Health Professionals*. Sydney: Pearson.

Manias, E., Rixon, S., Williams, A., Liew, D. & Braaf, S. (2015). Barriers and enablers affecting patient engagement in managing medications within specialty hospital settings. *Health Expectations, 18*(6), 2787–98.

Mok, W., Wang, W. & Liaw, S. (2015). Vital sign monitoring to detect patient deterioration: An integrative literature review. *Journal of Nursing Interventions, 21*(S2), 91–98.

Nursing and Midwifery Board of Australia (NMBA). (2016). *Registered Nurse Standards for Practice*. Retrieved from: www.nursingmidwiferyboard.gov.au/Codes-Guidelines-Statements/Professional-standards.aspx

Nursing and Midwifery Board of Australia (NMBA). (2019) *Supervision Guidelines for Nursing and Midwifery*. Retrieved from: www.nursingmidwif eryboard.gov.au/Registration-and-Endorsement/Supervised-practice.aspx

Reason, J. (2000). Human error: Models and management. *British Medical Journal, 320*, 768–70.

Reid-Searl, K., Moxham, L., Walker, S. & Happell, B. (2010). Nursing students administering medication: Appreciating and seeking appropriate supervision. *Journal of Advanced Nursing, 66*(3), *532–41*.

Rossi, S. (Ed.). (2021). *Australian Medicines Handbook* (8th edn). Adelaide: Australian Medicines Handbook Pty Ltd.

Rossiter, R., Scott, R. & Walton, C. G. (2020). Key attributes of therapeutic communication. In T. Levett-Jones (Ed.), *Critical Conversations for Patient Safety: An Essential Guide for Health Professionals*. Sydney: Pearson.

The Joint Commission. (2015). *Sentinel Event*. Retrieved from: https://patientsafetyfornursingstudents.org/resources/medication-safety

Westbrook, J., Li, L., Lehnbom, C., Baysari, M., Braithwaite, .J, Burke, R., Conn, C. & Day, R. O. (2015). What are incident reports telling us? A comparative study at two Australian hospitals of medication errors identified at audit, detected by staff and reported to an incident system. *International Journal for Quality in Health Care, 27*(1), 1–9.

World Health Organization. (2016). *Medication Errors: Technical Series on Safer Primary Care*. Retrieved from: https://apps.who.int/iris/bitstream/handle/10665/252274/9789241511643-eng.pdf;jsessionid=fdb1be2683396d2da592f947714ebf5e?sequence=1

Chapter 3

Caring for a person with fluid and electrolyte imbalance

TRACY LEVETT-JONES and PETER SINCLAIR

LEARNING OUTCOMES

Completion of the activities in this chapter will enable you to:

- explain why an understanding of fluid and electrolyte balance is essential to safe and effective nursing practice (**recall** and **application**)
- identify the clinical manifestations of hypovolaemia, dehydration, hypervolaemia and electrolyte imbalance that guide the collection and interpretation of appropriate cues (**gather, review, interpret, discriminate, relate** and **infer**)
- identify risk factors for fluid and electrolyte imbalance (**match** and **predict**)
- examine clinical information to identify the main nursing diagnoses for a patient with a fluid and electrolyte imbalance (**synthesise**)
- describe the priorities of care for a patient with a fluid and electrolyte imbalance (**goal setting** and **taking action**)
- identify clinical criteria for determining the effectiveness of nursing actions taken to manage fluid and electrolyte imbalance (**evaluate**)
- apply what you have learnt about fluid and electrolyte imbalance to new situations (**reflection** and **translation**).

INTRODUCTION

The two linked scenarios introduced in this chapter focus on the care of an older person who experiences fluid and electrolyte imbalance. You will be introduced to Mr Arthur Barrett and follow his healthcare journey from admission, through the post-operative period, to discharge. Alterations in fluid status are common in post-operative patients; they manifest rapidly and can have potentially fatal consequences, particularly in an older person with multiple co-morbidities. Maintaining the delicate fluid and electrolyte equilibrium of post-operative patients is essential to safe and effective nursing care. Excellent clinical reasoning skills will help you to recognise and manage people at risk of fluid and electrolyte imbalance early, with the aim of preventing deterioration and adverse patient outcomes.

KEY CONCEPTS

dehydration
hypovolaemia
hypervolaemia
electrolyte imbalance
kidney disease

SUGGESTED READINGS

P. LeMone, G. Bauldoff, P. Gubrud-Howe, M.-A. Carno, T. Levett-Jones, … D. Stanley (Eds). (2020). *LeMone and Burke's Medical–Surgical Nursing: Critical Thinking in Person-Centred Care* (4th edn). Melbourne: Pearson Australia.
Chapter 3: Nursing care of people having surgery
Chapter 9: Nursing care of people with altered fluid, electrolyte and acid–base balance
Chapter 27: Nursing care of people with kidney disorders

SCENARIO 3.1 The fluid shift begins…

SETTING THE SCENE

Mr Arthur Barrett is a 74-year-old man diagnosed with cancer of the colon. He had sought medical treatment after noticing rectal bleeding, and occasional constipation and diarrhoea. Noting that Mr Barrett was anaemic and that he had a family history of bowel cancer, his GP performed a digital rectal examination. Although unable to identify a palpable rectal mass, the GP referred Mr Barrett to a gastroenterologist and a colonoscopy was subsequently performed. The colonoscopy revealed left-sided colon cancer and a bowel resection was scheduled.

Access *Cancer in Australia 2019* to find out more about the incidence, mortality, death rate and survival rate for colorectal cancer: https://www.aihw.gov.au/reports

The epidemiology of colorectal cancer

Epidemiology is the study of the distribution and determinants of disease, injury and other health-related outcomes in populations. In Australia, colorectal cancer is one of the most prevalent cancers with men having a one-in-twelve and women having a one-in-seventeen risk of being diagnosed before the age of 85 (Australian Institute of Health and Welfare, 2019).

The aetiology and pathogenesis of colorectal cancer

Colorectal cancer is a malignant tumour that starts in the bowel wall. Usually, the tumour is confined locally for a relatively long period before spreading through the bowel wall and metastasising to lymph nodes and other parts of the body. The aetiology of colorectal cancer is complex and involves hereditary and environmental factors. Modifiable dietary and lifestyle factors have been estimated to account for 70 per cent of the risk for colorectal cancer in Western populations.

Person-centred care

Mr Barrett was born in Geraldton, a country town in Western Australia. He was the oldest child of a large family, with four sisters and two brothers. Arthur left school at age 15 and worked on the land for a number of years before marrying Megan. They had two children, a son and a daughter. Arthur and Megan had a strong marriage and a happy life together. Meg died three years ago from breast cancer and last year Arthur's son was killed in a farming accident. Once an active and jovial man, Arthur has been very lonely and sad since their deaths. This period of his life has been hard and he is struggling to come to terms with his recent diagnosis of bowel cancer.

If you do not know a person's past, then you cannot understand their present (Kerr & Wilkinson, 2005).

Pre-operative care

Mr Barrett was admitted the day before his surgery as he was considered to be 'high risk'. Review his admission observations, co-morbidities and medical orders.

Admission observations

Temperature	36.7°C
Pulse rate	90
Respiratory rate	18
Oxygen saturation level	97%
Blood pressure	150/90 mmHg
BGL	8 mmol/L

Co-morbidities

- COPD (chronic obstructive pulmonary disease) which Mr Barrett has had for 15 years. He uses a salbutamol inhaler and smokes occasionally.
- Osteoarthritis: Mr Barrett takes the over-the-counter (OTC), non-steroidal anti-inflammatory drugs (NSAIDs) ibuprofen and paracetamol PRN.
- Type 2 diabetes (diet-controlled).

Medical orders

Mr Barrett's doctor ordered the following:

- Two PicoPreps to be given the night before surgery
- Clear fluid diet until midnight and then nil orally
- Enoxaparin sodium 40 mg SCI
- Metronidazole 500 mg IV and cephalothin 2 g IV

What are sodium phosphate bowel preparations such as PicoPreps and why are they used with extreme caution in older people?

Q1 Why might Mr Barrett be considered 'high risk'?

Q2 What other information would you need if you were caring for Mr Barrett pre-operatively?

Q3 What risk assessments should be undertaken pre-operatively?

1. CONSIDER THE PATIENT SITUATION

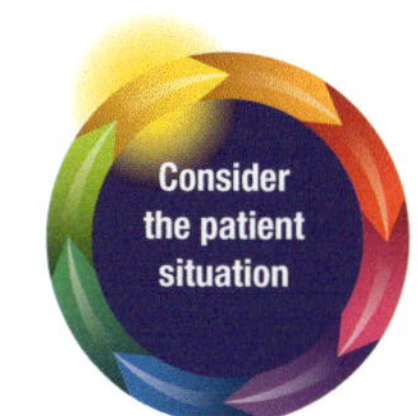

Day 1 post-operatively

You are allocated to the care of Mr Barrett on the morning shift and receive the following handover:

We have Mr Arthur Barrett in room 22. He's 74 years old. He had a partial colectomy and formation of a colostomy secondary to bowel cancer. He's under Dr Ng. His surgery was uneventful and he was stable throughout. He has a morphine PCA and an IVT of normal saline running at 84 mL/hr. His last reported pain score was 5/10. He didn't have a good night as his BP dropped and he needed two 300 mL fluid challenges. He's still dry though. He has an IDC on hourly measures and they have been averaging about 25–30 mL/hr since midnight. He has a bellovac in situ which has drained 300 mL since yesterday. His wound has a dry dressing and it's intact. He has a drainage bag over the stoma—no drainage. His oxygen therapy is still at 6 L/min via a Hudson mask. His sats are OK. The obs are due again at 0800. He is on 4th hourly BGLs and they have been OK. His daughter should be in later today.

Quick Quiz!

This handover report uses a number of abbreviations and terminologies. Although this is useful for providing a lot of information concisely, it can cause problems if the terms are not clearly understood. Test your understanding of abbreviations and terminologies by selecting the correct response for each of the identified terms.

Q1 Partial colectomy:
- a Removal of the colon
- b Removal of a section of the large bowel
- c Removal of a section of the small bowel

Q2 PCA:
- a Patient care assistant
- b Pre-cancer anaesthetic
- c Patient-controlled analgesia

Q3 IVT:
- a Intra-operative therapy
- b Intravenous therapy
- c Intravascular therapy

Q4 Fluid challenge:
- a Administration of a large amount of IV fluids over a short period of time under close monitoring to evaluate the patient's response
- b Rapid ingestion of water under close monitoring to evaluate the patient's response

Q5 Bellovac:
- a Urinary drainage system
- b Vacuum dressing
- c Vacuum drain

Q6 IDC:
- a Independent drainage catheter
- b Indwelling catheter
- c Intermittent drainage catheter

Q7 Stoma:
- a An opening into the body from the outside created by a surgeon
- b An opening out of the body from a fistula

Q8 BGL:
- a Blood glucose level
- b Basic saturation level
- c Blood gas levels

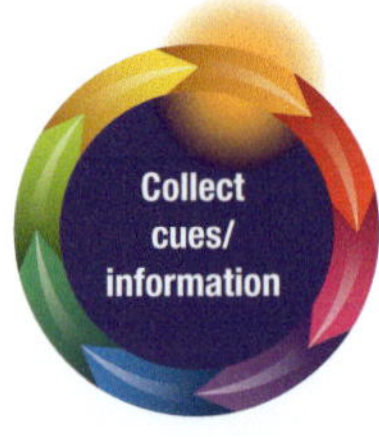

2. COLLECT CUES/INFORMATION

(a) Review current information

Now that you have considered Mr Barrett's situation, the next stage of the clinical reasoning cycle is to collect relevant cues and information. Start by reviewing Mr Barrett's current post-operative observations:

Temperature	37°C
Pulse rate	112 (weak and thready)
Respiratory rate	22
Blood pressure	90/50 mmHg
Oxygen saturation level	96%
Hourly urine output (average)	26 mL/hr
Specific gravity of urine	1.022
BGL	4 mmol/L

(b) Gather new information

Something to think about . . .

Remember: *When the correct cues are not collected, all of the actions that follow may be incorrect. Making decisions based on incomplete information is a leading cause of clinical errors. Early subtle cues, when missed, can lead to adverse patient outcomes (Levett-Jones et al., 2010).*

Q What other clinical information do you need? From the following list, identify four cues that you believe are *most* relevant to your assessment of Mr Barrett at this time.

a Appetite (nil)
b Condition of oral mucosa (dry and tongue furrowed)
c Level of thirst (reports that he is very thirsty)
d Pain level (3 out of 10)
e Cognitive state (restless and anxious)
f Colour (pale)
g Skin condition (poor skin turgor)

To revise your knowledge of the urinary system, access *Meet the Kidneys!* at the Khan Academy: https://www.khanacademy.org/science/health-and-medicine/human-anatomy-and-physiology/introduction-to-the-kidneys/v/meet-the-kidneys

(c) Recall knowledge

While cue collection involves reviewing current information and gathering new information about Mr Barrett, it also requires recall of knowledge about related physiology and pathophysiology.

Quick Quiz!

Test your knowledge of physiology and pathophysiology related to fluid balance.

Q1 When a person's glomerular filtration rate drops:
a The anterior pituitary gland responds by secreting antidiuretic hormone.
b The adrenal glands respond by secreting renin.
c The adrenal glands respond by reducing the secretion of aldosterone.
d The juxtaglomerular cells in the kidney respond by secreting renin.

Q2 Antidiuretic hormone is secreted:
a By the anterior pituitary gland in response to increased serum albumin
b By the posterior pituitary gland in response to increased serum osmolality
c By the posterior pituitary gland in response to decreased serum sodium levels
d By the collecting ducts of the kidneys in response to dehydration

Q3 Oliguria:
- a May be defined as an absence of urine production
- b Is common after major surgery and, as such, is nothing for the nurse to be concerned about
- c Is generally defined as more than 30 mL/hr of urine excretion and is uncommon in the immediate post-operative period
- d Is generally defined as less than 30 mL/hr of urine excretion and, left untreated, may lead to acute kidney injury

Q4 When assessing a patient's fluid status, which of the following groups include the *most* important nursing observations?
- a Weight, urine output, bowel sounds
- b Chvostek's sign, fluid intake, blood pressure
- c Serum potassium, bowel sounds, urine output
- d Urine output, blood pressure, weight

Q5 Insensible fluid loss occurs through all of the following routes *except*:
- a Skin
- b Lungs
- c Kidneys
- d Gastrointestinal tract

Q6 Extracellular fluid loss refers to fluid loss from the interstitial fluid compartment and/or:
- a Intravascular compartment
- b Intracellular compartment
- c Retention of fluid in the plasma
- d Loss of magnesium and albumin from the kidneys

Q7 In assessing a patient with dehydration, you would expect the urine output to be:
- a Increased with elevated specific gravity
- b Increased with decreased specific gravity
- c Decreased with elevated specific gravity
- d Decreased with decreased specific gravity

Q8 A third-space fluid shift may occur as a result of all of the following *except*:
- a Hypoalbuminaemia
- b An allergic reaction
- c Hypertension
- d Hypovolaemia

3. PROCESS INFORMATION

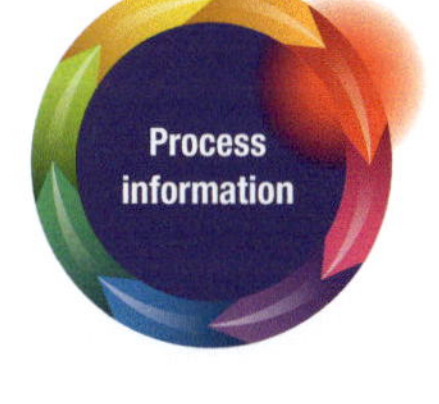

(a) Interpret

The next step of the clinical reasoning cycle is to interpret the data (cues) that you have collected by careful analysis and by applying your knowledge of fluid balance. By comparing normal versus abnormal, you will come to a more complete understanding of Mr Barrett's signs and symptoms. Begin by comparing Mr Barrett's pre- and post-op observations in the following table.

	Pre-op	Post-op
Temperature	36.7°C	37°C
Pulse rate	90	112 (weak and thready)
Respiratory rate	18	22
Blood pressure	150/90 mmHg	90/50 mmHg
Oxygen saturation level	97%	96%
Hourly urine output (average)	N/A	26 mL/hr
Specific gravity of urine	1.016	1.022
BGL	7 mmol/L	4 mmol/L

National Safety and Quality Health Service (NSQH) Standards

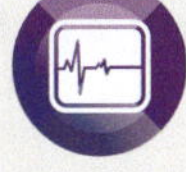

Recognising and responding to acute deterioration standard

The NSQHS Standards specify that each health service organisation must have processes for clinicians to graphically document and track changes in observations to detect acute deterioration over time (ACSQHC, 2021).

Q1 Which two of the following are considered to be within normal parameters for Mr Barrett?

- a Temperature: 37°C
- b Pulse rate: 112 beats/min
- c Respiratory rate: 22 breaths/min
- d Blood pressure: 90/50 mmHg
- e Specific gravity of 1.022

In handover, a number of statements were made that need further clarification. Analyse each of the following statements and physiological parameters. Compare normal versus abnormal, and identify what you would consider 'normal' for Mr Barrett at this time.

Q2 'His sats (SaO_2) are OK.' A 'normal' oxygen saturation level for Mr Barrett would be:

- a 80–85%
- b 85–90%
- c 90–95%
- d 95–100%

Q3 'He has an IDC on hourly measures and these are still a bit low.' For Mr Barrett, a 'normal' urine output would be at least:

- a 41 mL/hr
- b 82 mL/hr
- c 60 mL/hr
- d 10 mL/hr

Hint: See Table 3.2 in the epilogue to this chapter.

Q4 'His BGLs are okay.' A 'normal' BGL for Mr Barrett would be:

- a 4–8 mmol/L
- b 2–4 mmol/L
- c 1–3 mmol/L
- d 8–10 mmol/L

(b) Discriminate

From the cues and information you now have, you need to narrow down the information to what is most important.

Q From the following list, select four cues that you believe are *most relevant* to Mr Barrett's fluid status *at this time*.

- a Blood pressure
- b Respiratory rate
- c Temperature
- d Pulse
- e Condition of wound
- f Oxygen saturation level
- g Condition of oral mucosa
- h Level of consciousness
- i Urine output

(c) Relate

It is important to cluster cues together and identify relationships between them (based on the information you have collected so far).

Q Which of the following statements are 'true' and which are 'false'?

- a Mr Barrett is probably hypoxic as a result of the extended anaesthetic period and his COPD.
- b Mr Barrett could be hypotensive and tachycardic from the pre-operative bowel prep.
- c Mr Barrett could be tachycardic and hypotensive from a third-space fluid shift.
- d Mr Barrett is febrile and tachycardic because of a post-operative wound infection.

Something to think about . . .

A third-space fluid shift occurs when too much fluid moves from the intravascular space (blood vessels) into the interstitial space (the area between the cells), the bowel or the peritoneal cavity. Fluid sequestered in these spaces is physiologically useless and the loss of fluids from the intravascular compartment can lead to hypotension and reduced cardiac output (Holcomb, 2009). Learn more about third-spacing here: https://www.straightanursingstudent.com/third-spacing

(d) Infer

It is time to think about all the cues that you have collected about Mr Barrett's condition, and to make inferences based on your analysis and interpretation of those cues.

Q From what you know about Mr Barrett's history, surgery, signs and symptoms (as well as your knowledge about fluid balance), identify two of the following inferences that are correct.

- a Mr Barrett is normotensive and bradycardic.
- b Mr Barrett is oliguric and tachycardic.
- c Mr Barrett is hypertensive and afebrile.
- d Mr Barrett is polyuric and hypotensive.
- e Mr Barrett is hypotensive and afebrile.

(e) Predict

At this stage, you begin to consider the consequences of your actions or inaction by predicting potential outcomes for your patient.

Q If you do not take the appropriate actions at this time, what could happen to Mr Barrett if his fluid imbalance is not corrected? (Select the three correct answers.)

- a Mr Barrett could go into shock.
- b Mr Barrett's condition will gradually improve over the next few days.
- c Mr Barrett could develop acute kidney injury.
- d Mr Barrett could develop pulmonary oedema.
- e Mr Barrett could die.

4. IDENTIFY THE PROBLEM/ISSUE

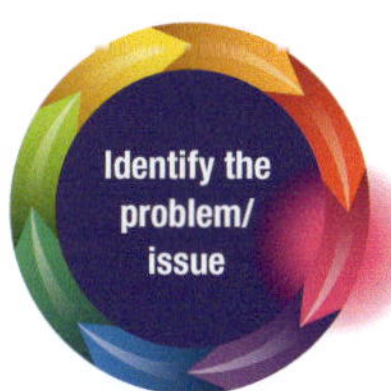

Now bring together (synthesise) all of the facts you've collected and inferences you've made to make a nursing diagnosis of Mr Barrett's main problems or issues.

Q1 From the following, identify the correct nursing diagnoses for Mr Barrett.

- a Hypervolaemia related to fluid intake and surgical blood loss, evidenced by tachycardia, hypertension and cognitive changes
- b Dehydration related to GIT fluid losses (PicoPrep) and limited oral fluid intake, evidenced by decreased skin turgor, dry mucous membranes and thirst
- c Hypervolaemia related to excess fluid output and inadequate fluid intake
- d Acute kidney injury related to third-space fluid shift, evidenced by oliguria and decreased specific gravity of urine
- e Hypovolaemia related to inadequate fluid intake and surgical blood loss, evidenced by tachycardia, hypotension, oliguria, elevated specific gravity of urine and cognitive changes

Do you know the difference between hypovolaemia and dehydration?

Hint: Think about the causes and consequences of third-space fluid shifts.

Q2 Identify four factors that may have led to Mr Barrett's deterioration.

5. ESTABLISH GOALS

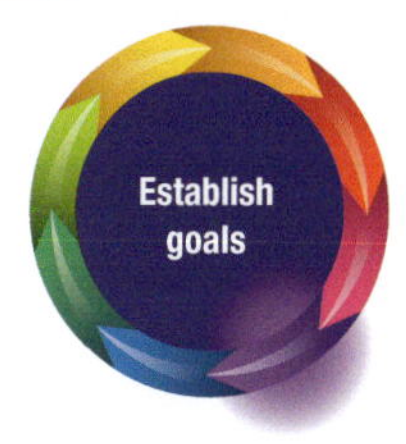

The therapeutic goal for the management of hypovolaemia and dehydration is to return the intravascular fluid compartment to normal in order to prevent the potentially life-threatening complication of hypovolaemic shock.

Q Before implementing any actions to improve Mr Barrett's condition, it is important to clearly specify what you want to happen and when. From the following list, choose the most important and realistic short-term goals for Mr Barrett's management at this time.

a For Mr Barrett to be normotensive with urine output at least 30–40 mL/hr within the next 24 hours
b For Mr Barrett to be normotensive with urine output greater than 80–100 mL/hr within the next 2 hours
c For Mr Barrett to be normotensive with urine output at least 40–45 mL/hr within the next 2–4 hours
d For Mr Barrett to be normotensive with urine output greater than 80–100 mL/hr within the next 24 hours

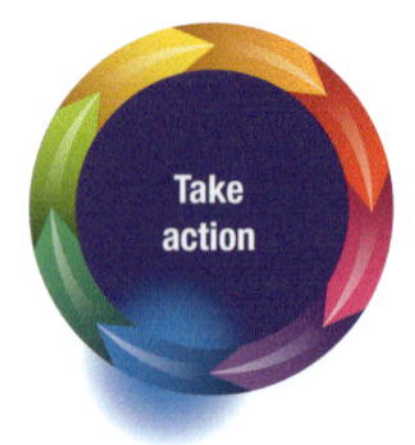

6. TAKE ACTION

Nursing 'action' is the behaviour following on from a judgment or decision. This stage of the cycle requires knowledge, clinical skills, communication skills and clinical reasoning ability. The nurse has to decide which actions take priority, who should be notified and who is best placed to undertake the nursing action(s). At all times, the nurse's practice must be informed by a sound evidence base and relevant policies and guidelines (Vierula et al., 2020).

Note: All of these actions are important, but you need to select those that are the most important to the management of Mr Barrett's deteriorating condition at this time!

Q1 The treatment of hypovolaemia and dehydration consists of restoring fluid volume, correcting any electrolyte imbalances and monitoring for improvement or deterioration in the person's condition. From the following list, choose the five *most immediate actions* you should take at this stage.

a Notify Mr Barrett's doctor of his condition.
b Monitor Mr Barrett's level of consciousness.
c Monitor Mr Barrett's pain score.
d Monitor the condition of Mr Barrett's drain, stoma and wound.
e Check that the IV cannula is not kinked or blocked.
f Administer a fluid challenge and increase Mr Barrett's IV fluid rate *as ordered.*
g Monitor Mr Barrett's vital signs and oxygen saturation level.
h Strictly monitor Mr Barrett's hourly urine output.

Q2 In the following tables, match the rationales for care to the corresponding nursing action.

Airway and breathing

Rationale

- To measure level of oxygenation
- To ensure adequate oxygen delivery

Nursing action	Rationale
Maintain oxygen therapy via nasal prongs or Hudson mask	
Check oxygen saturation level regularly	

Circulation

Rationale

- To identify changes in Mr Barrett's condition
- This is the best indication of changes in fluid status
- To enable administration of IV fluids as ordered

- To monitor changes in fluid status
- Sodium, potassium, urea and creatinine are indicators of fluid status and renal function

Nursing action	Rationale
Maintain patent IV access	
Review biochemistry and haematology levels	
Check specific gravity of urine	
Weigh Mr Barrett daily	
Monitor pulse rate and blood pressure regularly	

Disability

Rationale

- Anxiety and restlessness may indicate worsening fluid status
- To maintain psychosocial wellbeing

Nursing action	Rationale
Check cognitive status regularly	
Reassure patient	

7. EVALUATE

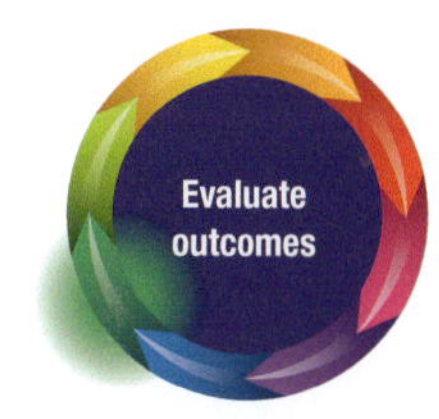

It is now 1100 hours, two hours since Mr Barrett was given a 300 mL fluid challenge and had his IV rate increased to 125 mL/hr. Each of Mr Barrett's signs and symptoms provide you with cues to make a determination of whether or not your nursing actions have been effective and whether his condition is improving.

Nursing and Midwifery Board of Australia (NMBA) *Registered Nurse Standards for Practice* The NMBA's *Registered Nurse Standards for Practice* (2016) state that registered nurses must accurately conduct comprehensive and systematic assessments, analyse information and communicate outcomes as the basis for safe nursing practice.

Q1 Rate each of the following signs and symptoms as *unchanged, improving* or *deteriorating*:

- a Cognitive status: Mr Barrett restless and anxious
- b Level of thirst: Mr Barrett reports some thirst
- c Pulse rate: 90 beats/min
- d Urine output: 36 mL/hr
- e Oral mucosa: mouth is dry and tongue furrowed
- f Oral intake: tolerating sips of water
- g Blood pressure: 110/70 mmHg
- h Colour: pale
- i Skin condition: skin turgor poor

Q2 You now need to synthesise these parameters to decide whether Mr Barrett's fluid status has improved overall. With regards to Mr Barrett's current signs and symptoms, which of the following statements are *most correct*?

a Mr Barrett's fluid status has improved significantly.

b Mr Barrett's fluid status has improved significantly but still requires careful monitoring.

c Mr Barrett's fluid status has improved slightly but still requires careful monitoring. You will need to contact the doctor again if further improvement is not seen in the next four hours.

d Mr Barrett's fluid status has not improved but you will monitor his condition carefully for the next four hours.

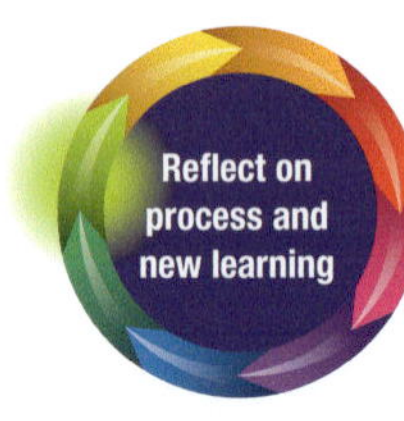

8. REFLECT

The final stage of the clinical reasoning cycle is 'reflection'. Reflect on your learning from this scenario and consider the following questions.

Q1 Could Mr Barrett's deterioration have been prevented? If so, how?

Q2 What are three of the most important things that you have learnt from this scenario?

Q3 What actions will you take in clinical practice as a result of your learning from this scenario?

SCENARIO 3.2 The pendulum swings in the other direction

CHANGING THE SCENE

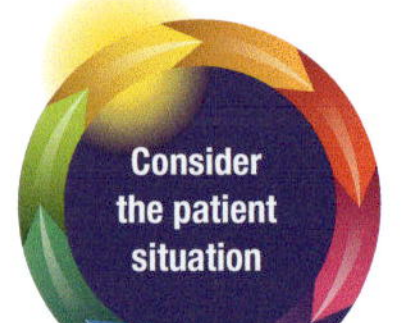

1. CONSIDER THE PATIENT SITUATION

Day 2 post-operatively

It is now 1430 hours and Mr Barrett is day 2 post-op. You are the registered nurse responsible for his care.

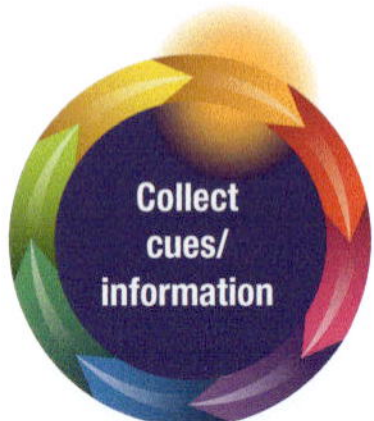

2. COLLECT CUES/INFORMATION

(a) Review current information

You review Mr Barrett's charts and identify the following:

Temperature	37°C
Pulse rate	121 beats/min (full, bounding and irregular)
Respiratory rate	32 breaths/min
Blood pressure	184/95 mmHg
Oxygen saturation level	90%
Hourly urine output (average)	15–30 mL/hr
BGL	6.9 mmol/L
IV rate	125 mL/hr

(b) Gather new information

When you enter Mr Barrett's room at 1500 hours to take his observations, you note that he has a dry irritating cough, and he is talking to himself, plucking at the bed sheets and attempting to get out of bed. When you ask, 'Are you alright, Mr Barrett?', he doesn't look at you but holds his head and mumbles, 'My head hurts.' Then he vomits a small amount of clear fluid.

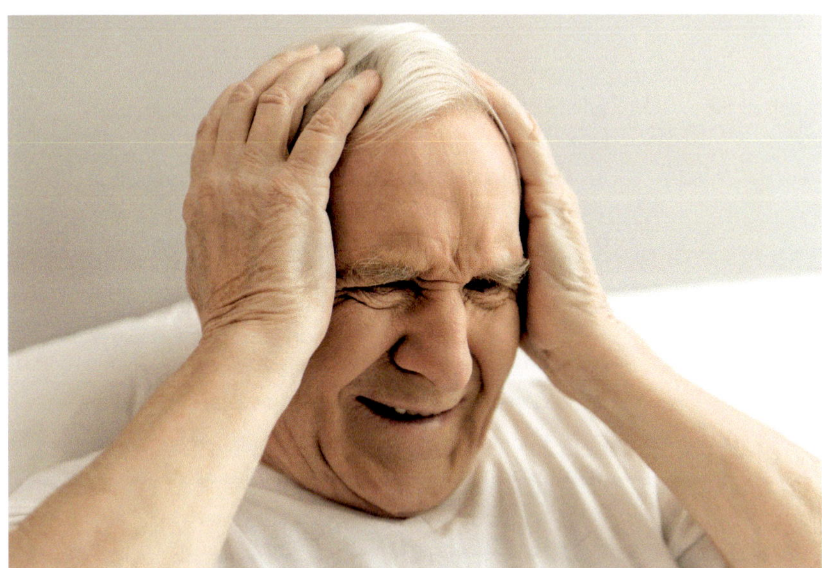

Mr Barrett complaining that his 'head hurts' © Vadim Guzhva/123RF

The nurse caring for the patient in the next bed shakes her head and says to you, 'Just what we need today, another one with dementia.'

Q1 This nurse's comment is an example of (select two correct answers):

a Ascertainment bias
b Diagnostic momentum
c Pattern matching
d Intuition

Q2 From the following list, select the four clinical assessments that are *most relevant* at this stage.

a Temperature: 37.2°C
b Level of consciousness: responsive but slightly confused
c Oxygen saturation level: 90%
d Condition of wound: dressing dry and intact, no ooze, no redness around the area
e Respiratory rate: 32 breaths/min
f Urine specific gravity: 1.001

(c) Recall knowledge

Something to think about . . .

Third-spacing has two phases—loss and reabsorption. In the loss phase, increased capillary permeability leads to the movement of proteins and fluids from the intravascular space to the interstitial space. This phase lasts 24 to 72 hours after the event that precipitated the increased capillary permeability (e.g. surgery, trauma, burns, sepsis or ascites). During the reabsorption phase, tissues begin to heal, fluid shifts back into the intravascular space and hypovolaemia resolves. Patients should be monitored carefully at this stage as hypervolaemia can occur as many litres of interstitial fluid move back to the intravascular space (Holcomb, 2009, p. 10).

Quick Quiz!

Q1 When the inflammatory stage of wound healing resolves (24–72 hours post-operatively), what is likely to happen to your patient?

a Plasma from the interstitial compartment typically returns to the circulating blood volume.
b Plasma from the intravascular compartment typically returns to the intracellular compartment.
c Plasma from the intracellular compartment typically returns to the intravascular compartment.

Quick Quiz! continued

Q2 Type 2 diabetes can influence fluid balance. Which of the following statements are *true* and which are *false*?

- a Diabetes can cause impaired renal function.
- b Hypoglycaemia results in increased serum osmolarity, resulting in nocturnal diuresis.
- c Hyperglycaemia results in increased serum osmolarity, resulting in excessive diuresis.
- d Diabetes can cause impaired liver function.

Q3 Confusion in the older post-operative person can result from which of the following? (Select the five correct responses.)

- a Constipation
- b Pain
- c Leukopaenia
- d Fluid and electrolyte imbalance
- e Infection
- f Hypoxia
- g Haemoptysis

Q4 Fluid shifts can contribute to tachypnoea because:

- a Hypovolaemia causes anxiety.
- b Dehydration causes carbon dioxide retention.
- c Insensible fluid losses cause hypoxia.
- d Fluid shifts into the alveolar spaces causing pulmonary oedema and impacting on oxygenation levels.

Q5 Which of the following is *true* of altered sodium (Na^+) levels?

- a Decreased sodium concentration can be a consequence of over-hydration.
- b Decreased sodium levels are a consequence of dehydration and excessive dietary intake.
- c Decreased sodium concentration can be a consequence of dehydration and excessive exercise.
- d Increased sodium levels are a consequence of excessive vomiting and diarrhoea.

Q6 Older people are at risk of fluid imbalance because they have an increased likelihood of all of the following *except*:

- a Impaired renal function
- b Chronic dehydration
- c Morbid obesity
- d Malnutrition

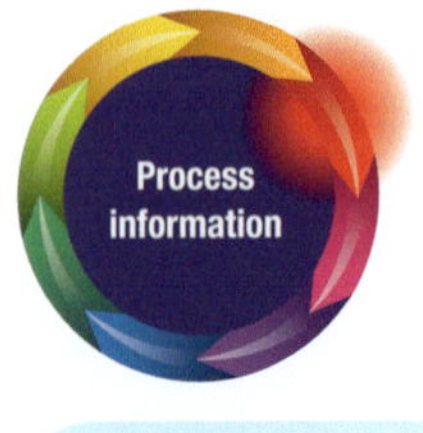

3. PROCESS INFORMATION

(a) Interpret

Can you define the terms 'hyponatraemia' and 'hypokalaemia'?

Q1 Based on Mr Barrett's current signs and symptoms, do you think he is in a positive or a negative fluid balance?

Interpret the information in the following pathology chart and answer these questions.

Q2 Today (day 2), is Mr Barrett hypernatraemic or hyponatraemic?

Q3 Today (day 2), is Mr Barrett hyperkalaemic or hypokalaemic?

Q4 What do Mr Barrett's urea and creatinine levels indicate?

Pathology results—Arthur Barrett

	Pre-op	Day 1	Day 2	Normal values
Sodium	140 mmol/L	138 mmol/L	128 mmol/L	136–144 mmol/L
Potassium	3.9 mmol/L	3.6 mmol/L	3.3 mmol/L	3.6–5.0 mmol/L
Urea	3.0 mmol/L	4.1 mmol/L	2.9 mmol/L	3.6–8.4 mmol/L (55+ years)
Creatinine	130 μmol/L	130 μmol/L	400 μmol/L	110 μmol/L (males)

Q5 Which of these signs and symptoms might indicate that Mr Barrett is hyponatraemic? (Select the three correct answers.)

- a Confusion
- b Abdominal cramps

- c Headache
- d Nausea and vomiting
- e Muscle weakness

Mr Barrett's hyponatraemia and hypokalaemia have probably resulted from the increased fluid volume rather than an actual loss of electrolytes.

Q6 Hypokalaemia can cause which of the following signs and symptoms? (Select four correct answers.)

- a Nausea
- b Irregular pulse
- c Arrhythmias
- d Diarrhoea
- e Cardiac arrest
- f Irritability
- g Cramps
- h Hypotension

(b) Discriminate, (c) Relate and (d) Infer

Something to think about...

Nurses have a unique advantage in the identification of deteriorating patients. Rather than 'treat' and 'retreat', nurses are a constant presence when caring for patients. They detect trends, compare normal vs abnormal, and recognise gaps in the information at hand. Their ability to recognise clinically 'at risk' patients is crucial. By recognising early warning signs you will be able to identify patients at risk of serious adverse events.

Q With reference to the following table, and based on what you now know about Mr Barrett's condition, identify four early warning signs that he is demonstrating and that would signal the need for an immediate clinical review.

Early warning signs
a. Respiratory rate: breaths/min 10 or less or 25 or more
b. SpO_2: < 95%
c. Pulse rate: beats/min 50 or less or 120 or more
d. Systolic blood pressure: <100 mmHg or >180 mmHg
e. Chest pain
f. Newly reported pain or uncontrolled pain
g. Blood glucose level: < 4 or > 20 mmol/L
h. Urine output: <100 mL over 4 hours or less that 0.5 mL/kg/hour via a IDC
i. Newly reported confusion

Source: Based on T. Jacques, G. Harrison, M. McLaws & G. Kilborne (2006). Signs of critical conditions and emergency responses (SOCCER): A model for predicting adverse events in the inpatient setting. *Resuscitation, 69*(2), 175-83.

National Safety and Quality Health Service (NSQH) Standards

Recognising and responding to acute deterioration standard

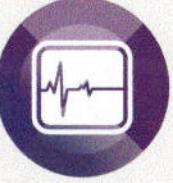

The NSQHS Standards highlight the importance of early recognition of patient deterioration. However, serious adverse events, such as unexpected death or cardiac or respiratory arrests, are often preceded by observable physiological abnormalities which aren't always recognised or managed appropriately (ACSQHC, 2021).

(e) Predict

Positive patient outcomes depend on close surveillance and timely identification of deterioration, followed by prompt and effective nursing actions.

Q If you do not take the appropriate actions at this time, what could happen to Mr Barrett if his fluid imbalance is not corrected? (Select the three that apply.)

a Mr Barrett could die.
b Mr Barrett could go into shock.
c Mr Barrett could become hypoxic.
d Mr Barrett's condition will gradually improve over the next few days.
e Mr Barrett could develop pulmonary oedema.

Patient Safety Competency Framework (PSCF)

Domain 7–Preventing, minimising and responding to adverse events

The PSCF specifies that nurses must have the skills required to respond appropriately to adverse events. This includes the ability to recognise and manage patient deterioration, to participate in analysis of events in order to identify system failures and appropriate solutions, and to provide honest and timely communication about the facts of the adverse event.

Source: *The Patient Safety Competency Framework for Nursing Students*, https://patientsafetyfornursingstudents.org

(f) Match

Q Have you ever seen someone with the same signs and symptoms as Mr Barrett? If so, what was done to manage the situation?

4. IDENTIFY THE PROBLEM/ISSUE

Q Based on all of the information you have about Mr Barrett, complete these nursing diagnoses:

a Hypervolaemia related to excess IV fluids, evidenced by cognitive changes and _______________.
b Hypervolaemia related to the reabsorption phase of the third-space fluid shift and return of fluids from the interstitial space to the intravascular component, evidenced by hypertension and _______________.
c Early-stage pulmonary oedema related to excess IV fluids and resolution of third-space fluid shift, evidenced by hypoxia, dry irritating cough and _______________.
d Electrolyte imbalance related to hypervolaemia, evidenced by irregular pulse _______________ and _______________.

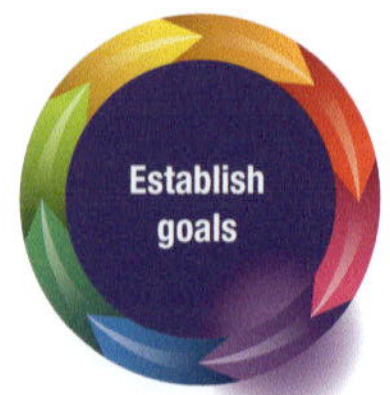

5. ESTABLISH GOALS

Before implementing any actions to improve Mr Barrett's condition, it is important to clearly specify what you want to happen and when.

Q From the following list, choose the four most immediate goals for Mr Barrett's management.

a For Mr Barrett to be self-caring and ambulant
b Vital signs to be within normal parameters
c Oral food and fluid intake established
d Oxygen saturation level >94%
e Cognitive status improving
f Stoma functioning
g Urine output satisfactory
h Lung sounds normal
i Electrolytes returning to normal levels

6. TAKE ACTION

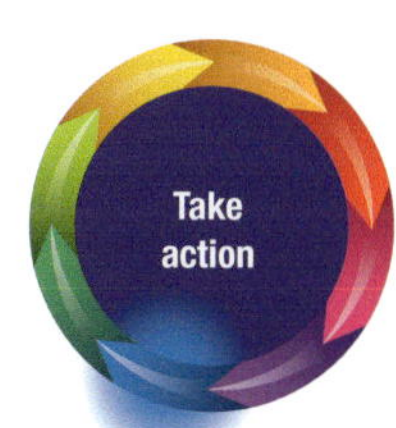

Q1 From the following list, choose the five most *immediate* actions you would take at this stage. *Note*: Many of these actions are correct but you need to focus on immediate priorities.

a Contact attending doctor using ISBAR to request a medical review
b Administer an antiemetic
c Administer oxygen 6–8 L/min
d Document vital signs QID
e Sit Mr Barrett in a semi-Fowler's position
f Check Mr Barrett's weight each day
g Decrease IV rate TKVO pending medical orders
h Monitor cognitive status
i Monitor for improvement in serum electrolytes
j Regular position change to prevent pressure areas
k Take an ECG

Hint: Think ABC!

Timing is critical in clinical reasoning. Critical incidents occur not only when early signs and symptoms fail to be recognised or acted upon but also when nursing/medical interventions are commenced too late.

Q2 From the following list, choose the three nursing actions that you anticipate taking following a clinical review of Mr Barrett.

a Increase the IV rate following doctor's orders.
b Administer a diuretic (probably IV frusemide) following doctor's orders.
c Give anginine tablets following doctor's orders.
d Reduce the IV rate as ordered by medical officer.
e Take blood for biochemistry and haematological profile.
f Prepare to give a fluid challenge.

A useful acronym, particularly when you have significant concerns about a particular course of action, is CUS:

- I am Concerned about my patient's condition.
- I am Uncomfortable with my plan of action.
- I am worried this will impact on my patient's safety.

7. EVALUATE

Q From the following list, identify four signs and symptoms that will indicate to you that Mr Barrett's condition has improved following clinical review and initiation of appropriate nursing actions.

a Decreased BP
b Increased BP
c Decreased urine output (as a result of the diuretic)
d Increased urine output (as a result of the diuretic)
e Increased oxygen sats
f Decreased oxygen sats
g Decreased pulse and respiratory rate
h Increased pulse and respiratory rate

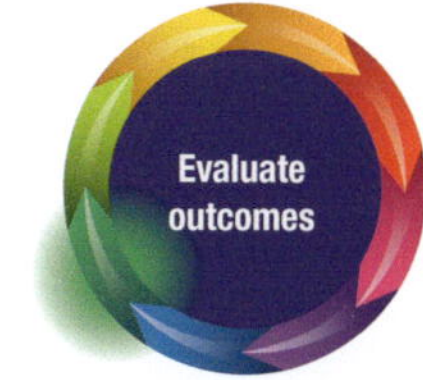

Nursing and Midwifery Board of Australia (NMBA) *Registered Nurse Standards for Practice* The NMBA's *Registered Nurse Standards for Practice* (2016) state that registered nurses must evaluate and monitor progress towards expected goals, revise the care plan based on the evaluation, and discuss further priorities with the relevant person(s).

8. REFLECT

Reflective practice is a crucial professional activity and one that is intrinsic to learning. Reflection is a deliberate, orderly and structured intellectual activity. It allows you to process and critically review your learning experience with a view to refinement, improvement or change.

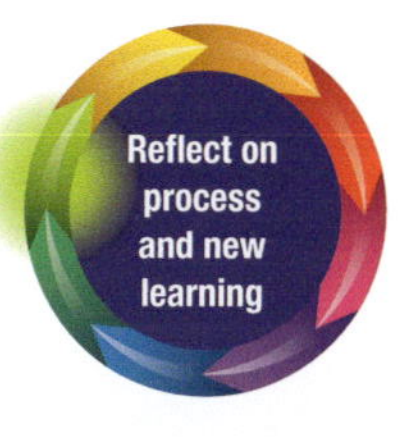

Contemplate what you have learnt from this scenario and how this learning will inform your practice. Use the following questions to frame your reflection.

Q1 How could Mr Barrett's deterioration have been prevented?

Q2 What have you learnt from the scenario that you can apply to your future practice?

Q3 Why are older post-operative patients at risk of fluid and electrolyte imbalance?

EPILOGUE

The two scenarios presented in this chapter illustrate situations that are all too common in clinical practice. Mr Barrett's deterioration resulted from several factors, including a failure to recognise the seriousness of his condition and to establish his baseline kidney function pre-admission. Identification of pre-existing kidney disease is critical as it enables the treating team to reduce the risk of further kidney damage and prevent related post-operative complications.

Consider what might have happened had Mr Barrett been reviewed by a practice nurse in a general practice setting five years prior to his diagnosis of colorectal cancer. Might he have been identified to be at risk of chronic kidney disease (CKD) based on the risk factors outlined in Table 3.1?

Table 3.1 *Risk factors for CKD*

Risk factors for CKD?	
CKD risk factors	• Diabetes • High blood pressure • Age over 60 years • Smoking • Obesity • Family history of kidney disease • Aboriginal or Torres Strait Islander origin • Established cardiovascular disease • History of acute kidney injury

Mr Barrett had five risk factors for CKD: diet-controlled diabetes, history of hypertension, smoking, aged over 60 and BMI 31.4. Once a person at risk of CKD has been identified, further screening should be conducted using the Kidney Health Check. This simple three-step process includes (1) a blood test to measure eGFR; (2) a urine albumin:creatine ratio (ACR) to check for the presence of albuminuria; and (3) blood pressure measurement (Kidney Health Australia, 2021).

Glomerular filtration rate (GFR) is determined through a formula that takes into consideration the person's serum creatinine level, age and gender. In Australia, whenever a biochemistry screen is ordered, the estimated glomerular filtration rate (eGFR) is tested to screen for and detect early kidney damage. The eGFR is also used to categorise the stages of chronic kidney disease (see Figure 3.1).

A person is diagnosed as having CKD if their eGFR is <60 mL/min/1.73 m^2 for a period of three months or longer, with or without evidence of kidney damage; or if they have evidence of kidney damage (with or without decreased GFR) for longer than three months (i.e. microalbuminuria, proteinuria, haematuria, or pathological or anatomical abnormalities). Timely identification of CKD can prevent complications, slow disease progression and reduce cardiovascular risk, as well as reducing mortality and morbidity.

Let's imagine Mr Barrett had a kidney health check five years ago and his blood pressure was 130/82 mmHg and ACR 7.8 mg/mmol (indicating microalbuminuria). A creatinine level of 110 µmol/L at the age of 69 would have given Mr Barrett an eGFR of 58 mL/min/1.73 m^2. With a repeat eGFR confirming this level three months later, Mr Barrett would have been diagnosed with stage 3a CKD and he would have been closely monitored for further decline in kidney function, particularly acute increases in serum

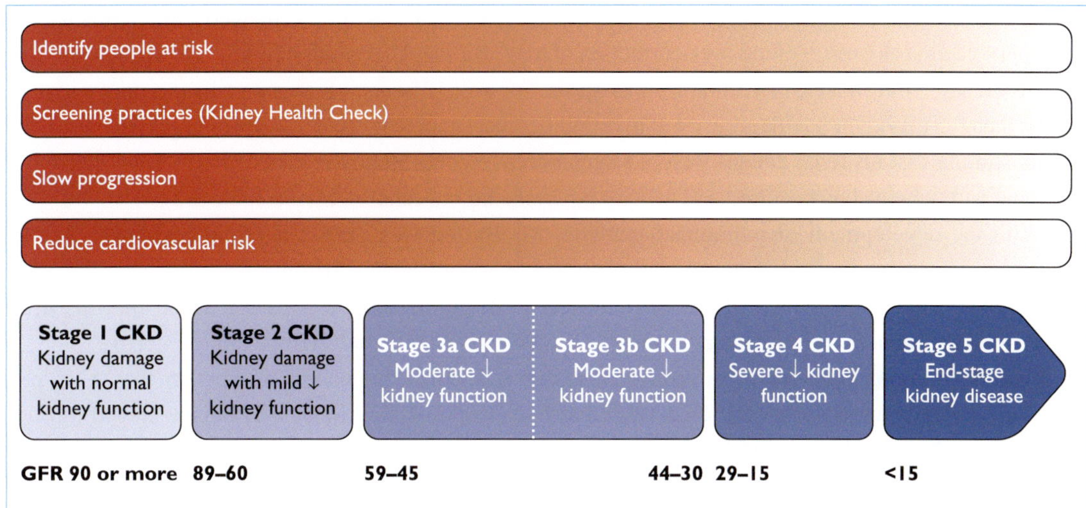

Figure 3.1
The chronic kidney disease trajectory
Source: Used with permission of The University of Newcastle.

creatinine and/or decreases in urine output. Importantly, knowledge of Mr Barrett's pre-existing kidney disease would have enabled the treating team to reduce the risk of acute kidney injury (AKI) when he was admitted to hospital for surgery.

AKI can be precipitated by numerous factors, including nephrotoxic medications, sepsis and hypovolaemia. The presence of CKD during any acute insult to the kidneys results in further decreased renal function; this is called 'acute on chronic kidney disease', sometimes referred to as 'acute on chronic'. It is important to remember that eGFR is not valid in AKI as its measurement is reliant on a steady-state creatinine (Bennett, Sinclair & Schoch, 2019). Consequently, classification systems that consider levels of severity based on serum creatinine increases and urine output are used (see Table 3.2).

In Scenario 3.1, Mr Barrett's urine output dropped to between 25 and 30 mL/hr for at least eight hours. Using the criteria shown in Table 3.2 and according to the **R**isk, **I**njury, **F**ailure, **L**oss, **E**nd-Stage Kidney Disease (RIFLE) (Bellomo et al., 2004) and Acute Kidney Injury Network (AKIN) (Mehta et al., 2007) staging criteria, this classifies him as *at risk of* AKI secondary to renal hypoperfusion. Continued hypoperfusion and associated renal tissue hypoxia resulted in damage to his renal parenchyma and the development of acute tubular necrosis.

Table 3.2 *Comparison of AKI staging by RIFLE and AKIN systems*

RIFLE stage[a]	RIFLE serum creatinine increase[b]	RIFLE and AKIN urine output criteria[c]	AKIN serum creatinine increase[d]	AKIN stages
Risk	≥150 to 200%	<0.5 mL/kg/hr for >6 hrs	≥0.3 mg/dL or ≥150 to 200%	1
Injury	>200 to 300%	<0.5 mL/kg/hr >12 hrs	>200 to 300%	2
Failure	>300%	<0.3 mL/kg/hr for ≥24 hrs or anuria ≥12 hrs	>300%[d] or acute RRT	3

a The remaining RIFLE stages are Loss (persistent AKI = complete loss of kidney function >4 weeks) and ESKD (>3 months).

b Serum creatinine increase from baseline

c Urine output criteria are identical in the corresponding RIFLE and AKIN stages.

d Increase in Cr> 4 mg/dL and acute rise ≥0.5 mg/dL

Source: P. M. Palevsky & P. T. Murray (May 2009). Acute kidney injury and critical care nephrology. *Nephrology self-assessment program: NephSAP*, Table 1, p. 174. Copyright 2009 by American Society of Nephrology. Reproduced with permission of American Society of Nephrology via Copyright Clearance Center.

In Scenario 3.2, when Mr Barrett was day 2 post-operatively, his condition changed from hypovolaemia to hypervolaemia as a result of the over-correction of his fluid status, resolution of his third-space fluid shift and his kidneys being unable to maintain homeostasis. For over 12 hours, Mr Barrett's urine output remained at less than 0.5 mL/kg/hr but the severity of his condition was not recognised. His specific gravity was 1.001 demonstrating that his renal tubules were no longer able to concentrate the glomerular filtrate, damage to his renal parenchyma had occurred and he was experiencing pre-renal AKI (see Table 3.2).

With the development of pulmonary oedema, Mr Barrett was placed on fluid restriction and IV frusemide was administered. Consequently, his urine output began to improve. However, delays in identification and management of Mr Barrett's acute on chronic kidney disease meant that his urine output was less than 30 mL per hour for an extended period of time before it began to improve.

One of the major post-operative priorities for any individual, regardless of whether they have pre-existing kidney disease, is to ensure the continued perfusion of the kidneys. This is achieved through avoiding insults to the kidney, vigilant monitoring, and the careful management of fluid status throughout a person's hospital stay and particularly in the first 72 hours post-operatively.

By day 3 post-operatively, Mr Barrett's urine output had improved and he was discharged from hospital seven days later. However, his baseline creatinine had increased from 130 µmol/L pre-op to 210 µmol/L on discharge. He was referred to a nephrologist for follow-up and three months later blood tests confirmed the deterioration in his kidney function, with his eGFR declining to 27 mL/min/1.73 m^2. This indicated that Mr Barrett had progressed to stage 4 CKD and renal replacement therapy options (i.e. dialysis) had to be considered.

Currently, one in ten Australians are unaware they have the early signs of kidney disease. Take the kidney risk test to see if you are at risk:

https://kidney.org.au/kidneyrisktest

Mr Barrett's clinical deterioration was preventable. Had the healthcare professionals caring for him identified his underlying CKD earlier, recognised that he was predisposed to AKI and managed his post-operative complications in a timely manner, acute on chronic kidney disease would not have resulted. Mr Barrett's story should be used as a precedent to highlight how clinical reasoning errors and failure to escalate in a timely manner can lead to serious and preventable adverse patient outcomes.

FURTHER READING

Kidney Health Australia (2020). Chronic Kidney Disease (CKD) Management in Primary Care (4th edn). Kidney Health Australia, Melbourne. https://kidney.org.au/health-professionals/ckd-management-handbook

Martin, G. S., Kaufman, D. A., Marik, P. E., Shapiro, N. I., Levett, D. Z., Whittle, J.,... & Miller, T. E. (2020). Perioperative Quality Initiative (POQI) consensus statement on fundamental concepts in perioperative fluid management: Fluid responsiveness and venous capacitance. *Perioperative Medicine*, *9*, 1–12. doi.org/10.1186/s13741-020-00142-8

REFERENCES

Australian Commission on Safety and Quality in Health Care (ACSQHC). (2021). *National Safety and Quality Health Service Standards* (2nd edn). Sydney, Australia.

Bellomo, R., Ronco, C., Kellum, J. A., Mehta, R. L. & Palevsky, P. (2004). Acute renal failure — definition, outcome measures, animal models, fluid therapy and information technology needs: The Second International Consensus Conference of the Acute Dialysis Quality Initiative (ADQI) Group. *Critical Care*, *8*(4), 1–9.

Bennett, P., Sinclair, P. & Schoch, M. (2019).Chapter 27: Caring for people with kidney disorders. In P. LeMone, K. Burke, G. Bauldoff, P. Gubrud-Howe, T. Levett-Jones, T. Dwyer,... D. Raymond (Eds)., *Medical–Surgical Nursing: Critical Thinking in Client Care* (4th edn). Sydney: Pearson.

Holcomb, S. S. (2009). Third-spacing: When body fluids shift. *Nursing 2009*, *4*(2), 9–12.

Jacques, T., Harrison, G., McLaws, M. & Kilborne, G. (2006). Signs of critical conditions and emergency responses (SOCCER): A model for predicting adverse events in the inpatient setting. *Resuscitation*, *69*(2), 175–83.

Kerr, D. & Wilkinson, H. (2005). *In the Know: Implementing Good Practice—Information and Tools for Anyone Supporting People with a Learning Disability and Dementia*. Brighton: Pavilion Publishing.

Kidney Health Australia. (2021). Know Your Kidneys. Retrieved from: https://kidney.org.au/your-kidneys/know-your-kidneys/know-the-risk-factors/kidney-health-check

Levett-Jones, T., Dwyer, T., Reid-Searl, K., Heaton, L., Flenady, T., Applegarth, J., Guinea, S. & Andersen, P. (2017). *The Patient Safety Competency Framework (PSCF) for Nursing Students*. Sydney, NSW. Retrieved from: http://psframework.wpengine.com/wp-content/uploads/2018/01/PSCF_Brochure_UTS-version_FA2-Screen.pdf

Levett-Jones, T., Hoffman, K., Dempsey, Y., Jeong, S., Noble, D., Norton, C.,... Hickey, N. (2010). The 'five rights' of clinical reasoning: An educational model to enhance nursing students' ability to identify and manage clinically 'at risk' patients. *Nurse Education Today, 30*(6), 515–20.

Mehta, R. L., Kellum, J. A., Shah, S. V., Molitoris, B. A., Ronco, C., Warnock, D. G. & Levin, A. (2007). Acute Kidney Injury Network: report of an initiative to improve outcomes in acute kidney injury. *Critical Care*, *11*(2), 1–8.

Nursing and Midwifery Board of Australia (NMBA). (2016). *Registered Nurse Standards for Practice*. Retrieved from: www.nursingmidwiferyboard.gov.au/Codes-Guidelines-Statements/Professional-standards.aspx

Vierula, J., Hupli, M., Talman, K. & Haavisto, E. (2020). Identifying reasoning skills for the selection of undergraduate nursing students: A focus group study. *Contemporary Nurse*, 56(2): 120–31.

Chapter 4

Caring for a person experiencing pain

TRACY LEVETT-JONES and BERNADETTE BUGEJA

LEARNING OUTCOMES

Completion of the activities in this chapter will enable you to:

- explain why an understanding of pain is essential to competent clinical practice (**recall** and **application**)
- identify the clinical manifestations of acute and persistent pain that are used to guide the collection and interpretation of cues (**gather, review, interpret, discriminate, relate** and **infer**)
- examine myths related to pain management (**recall**)
- explain the benefits of pre-emptive and multimodal analgesia (**recall**)
- identify complications from poorly managed pain (**match** and **predict**)
- review clinical information to identify the main nursing diagnoses for someone experiencing acute or persistent pain (**synthesise**)
- describe the priorities of care for a patient with acute or persistent pain (**goal setting** and **taking action**)
- identify clinical criteria for determining the effectiveness of nursing actions taken to prevent and manage pain (**evaluate**)
- adopt a holistic approach to pain management (**taking action**)
- apply what you have learnt about pain management to clinical practice (**reflection** and **translation**).

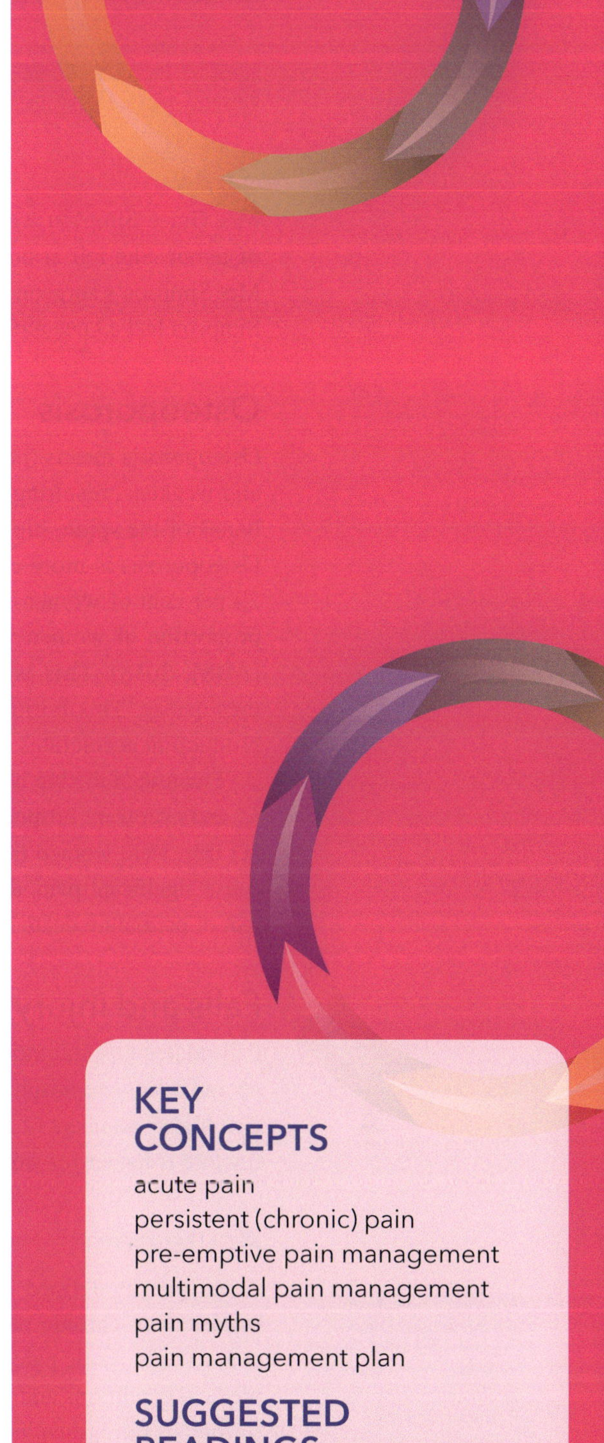

INTRODUCTION

In this chapter, you will be introduced to Mrs Grace Simpson, a 74-year-old woman admitted to hospital with a hip fracture following a fall at home. It is the therapeutic management of Mrs Simpson's pain, both in the acute care setting and following discharge, that is the focus of the two scenarios.

For many years, pain was accepted as inevitable and indifference to its seriousness was common. Contemporary approaches to pain now recognise that effective pain management is a fundamental human right and integral to ethical, professional and cost-effective clinical practice (Schug et al., 2020). Pain management requires sophisticated clinical reasoning ability, a sound knowledge base, highly developed clinical skills and a commitment to person-centred care.

Pain is a complex, individual, multifactorial experience influenced by a person's culture, previous pain experiences, beliefs, mood and coping ability. Although pain may be an indicator of injury and tissue damage, it may also be experienced in the absence of an identifiable cause. Response to pain and the degree of disability it causes varies between people. Similarly, individuals respond differently to the management strategies used to alleviate pain. Complications resulting from poorly managed pain are significant, widespread and at times life-threatening. Research has identified a link between acute pain, especially when not managed appropriately, and persistent pain that lasts for months or years (Commonwealth of Australia [Department of Health], 2019). Sound clinical reasoning skills will help you to recognise and appropriately manage your patients' pain, thus preventing short- and long-term complications from poorly managed pain.

KEY CONCEPTS

acute pain
persistent (chronic) pain
pre-emptive pain management
multimodal pain management
pain myths
pain management plan

SUGGESTED READINGS

P. LeMone, G. Bauldoff, P. Gubrud-Howe, M.-A. Carno, T. Levett-Jones, . . . D. Stanley (Eds). (2020). *LeMone and Burke's Medical-Surgical Nursing: Critical Thinking in Person-Centred Care* (4th edn). Melbourne: Pearson Australia.

Chapter 8: Nursing care of people in pain

Chapter 38: Nursing care of people with musculoskeletal trauma

SCENARIO 4.1 Caring for a person experiencing acute pain

SETTING THE SCENE

Mrs Grace Simpson was admitted to hospital following a fall in which she fractured her right neck of femur. She fell at home and was not discovered until her son returned from work six hours later. Mrs Simpson's surgeon told her family that the fracture was related to her history of osteoporosis. Mrs Simpson had a knee replacement 12 months ago and has a history of angina.

Osteoporosis

Osteoporosis means 'porous bones'; it is a musculoskeletal disorder in which the bone density thins and weakens, resulting in an increased risk of fracture. The most common sites of fracture are the bones of the spine, hip and wrist. In 2017–18, an estimated 924,000 Australians had osteoporosis. Osteoporosis is more common in females and people aged 75 years and over. In the same period, 29 per cent of women aged 75 and over had osteoporosis compared with 10 per cent of men. The proportion of women with osteoporosis also increases with age (Australian Bureau of Statistics [ABS], 2018). This is because there is a sharp decline in the female hormone oestrogen after menopause. This hormone plays a vital role in maintaining bone mass density and the decreased production accelerates calcium loss in bones.

Fracture of the hip is one of the most serious outcomes of osteoporosis. In 2016, 20,027 people aged 65 and over were hospitalised due to a hip fracture, of whom 72 per cent were aged 80 and over and 71 per cent were women (Australian Institute of Health and Welfare [AIHW], 2019a). Such fractures can cause significant pain, disability and reduced quality of life; they are also associated with an increased risk of premature death (Bliuc et al., 2013).

Falls and injury in Australia

Fall-related hospitalisation is common in older people. In 2016–17, an estimated 125,021 people aged 65 and over were hospitalised for a fall-related injury, and of these, 65 per cent were women. There are also higher numbers of hip fractures in women and the average length of hospital stay following a hip fracture is longer for women (AIHW, 2019b).

Acute pain

Acute pain is defined as pain that has a recent onset and limited duration. This is in contrast to persistent or chronic pain, which persists beyond the time of healing of the original injury (Schug et al., 2020). Acute pain is a response to trauma and includes pain related to medical procedures, acute medical conditions and physiological causes such as childbirth. If poorly managed, it can lead to more serious health issues, including chronic pain. (Commonwealth of Australia [Department of Health], 2019). Acute pain occurs across the life span and the majority of patients within the acute hospital setting will experience pain.

Pain generated from damage of the tissues, skin, ligaments and visceral organs is referred to as 'nociceptive' pain. This type of pain generally responds well to simple analgesics and opioids. Pain generated from damage to the nervous system itself is referred to as 'neuropathic' pain. This type of pain is much more difficult to treat and often requires adjuvant medications.

> Adjuvant medications are those used in pain management where their original purpose was for another condition. Examples include antidepressants and anticonvulsants which can be used for the treatment of neuropathic pain.

Person-centred care

Mrs Simpson grew up in the Blue Mountains in New South Wales and was a primary school headmistress for many years. She is a widow and lives with her eldest son, Alan. Mrs Simpson is the matriarch of her family, and is loved and respected by her children and grandchildren. Although fiercely independent and stoic in many ways, Mrs Simpson is acutely aware that her body is 'letting her down' even though mentally she remains 'sharp as a tack'.

Nursing and Midwifery Board of Australia (NMBA) *Registered Nurse Standards for Practice* Effective communication is central to person-centred care and effective therapeutic relationships. The NMBA's *Registered Nurse Standards for Practice* Standards (2016) state that registered nurses must communicate effectively, and be respectful of each person's dignity, culture, values, beliefs and rights.

1. CONSIDER THE PATIENT SITUATION

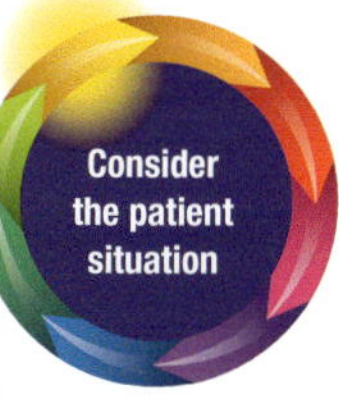

It is now 0800 hours and Mrs Simpson is day 1 post-operatively. You are given the following handover report:

0700 hours: Mrs Simpson, day 1, has a morphine PCA (Patient Controlled Analgesia) pump. She was given a single-shot nerve block in theatre but this wore off in recovery. She was quite unsettled and complained of pain on and off during the night. She vomited twice and ondansetron was given at 0300. She seems a bit more settled now and has drifted off to sleep. Obs stable, but BP a bit elevated. Urine output OK. Wound dressing dry and intact. IV 8-hourly.

Handover practices are often highly variable and unreliable. Breakdown in the transfer of information or in communication at handover has been identified as a preventable cause of patient harm (Moroney, 2020).

2. COLLECT CUES/INFORMATION

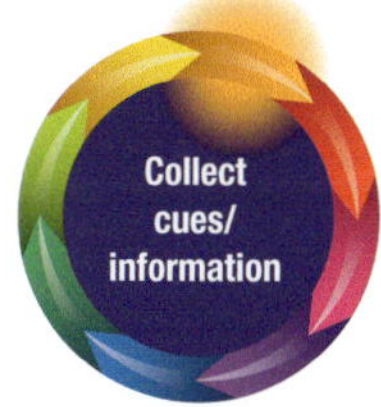

(a) Review current information

You review Mrs Simpson's charts and note that her blood pressure is 145/90 mmHg, pulse rate 98 and urine output 35–40 mL/hr. On the PCA chart, a lockout period of 10 minutes and a dose of 1 mg/mL are documented. You identify that Mrs Simpson made multiple and repeated PCA attempts during the night (not all of them successful). She was using about 4 mg of morphine per hour until 0400 hours and from then on used less than 1 mg/hr. When assessed during the night, Mrs Simpson reported pain scores of between 5 and 8 using the verbal numerical rating scale.

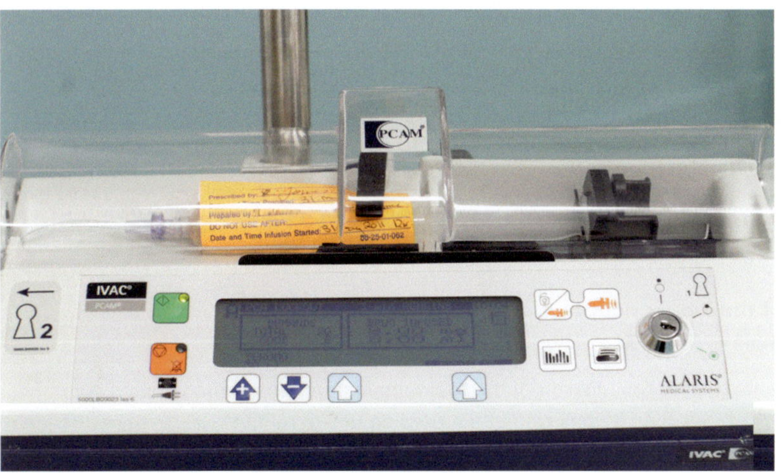

PCA showing 20 attempts but only 8 mg infused

Q The information you have to date leads you to think that overnight Mrs Simpson:

a Has pushed her PCA button too many times
b Has not pushed her PCA button enough
c Has needed a dose of morphine more frequently than the lockout period would allow
d Has needed a smaller dose of morphine than was prescribed

(b) Gather new information

You decide to assess Mrs Simpson's pain.

Q1 What are the two most accurate methods of assessing a person's pain?

a Asking the patient to describe and locate their pain
b Careful observation of physiological signs
c Asking the patient to rate their pain using a visual or numerical rating scale
d Reviewing the patient's chart

PCAs have been shown to be more effective in treating pain than intermittent IM or IV injections, providing increased patient control over pain relief and lower levels of pre-operative anxiety (Patak et al., 2013).

Something to think about...

Margo McCaffery's seminal definition of pain states that pain is whatever the patient says it is, existing whenever the patient says it does (McCaffery, Rolling Ferrell & Paseo, 2000). This definition implies that the patient is in the best position to describe and inform the nurse about his or her pain. Nurses must therefore elicit the patient's assessment of their pain, accept and believe that assessment, and take appropriate actions to manage the pain.

It is essential to reflect on and question one's assumptions and preconceptions about people who are experiencing pain, as failure to do so may negatively impact on your clinical reasoning ability and consequently your patient's clinical outcomes.

Q2 Why is pain often referred to as the fifth vital sign?

- a To ensure that nurses remember to assess their patient's pain when they undertake routine observations
- b To emphasise the importance of regular assessment and ongoing management of pain
- c So that pain assessment is always accurate and complete
- d To allow pain scores to be communicated from one nurse to another

You observe that Mrs Simpson is pale and drawn in appearance. When you ask her about her pain, she reveals that she is reluctant to use the PCA as one of the night duty nurses told her that she should be feeling better by now, that she could become addicted to the morphine or even stop breathing, and that the morphine was causing her nausea.

Something to think about...

Nurses' beliefs cause them to process clinical situations and act in particular ways. Their overarching philosophies serve as perspectives that condition the ways in which they judge and ultimately deal with patients experiencing pain. In a study by McCaffery, Rolling Ferrell and Paseo (2000), nurses' opinions of their patients and their personal beliefs about pain significantly influenced the quality of their pain assessment and management.

(c) Recall knowledge

Quick Quiz!

To ensure that you have a good understanding of the key concepts related to pain, test yourself with the following questions.

Q1 Morphine is:

- a A non-steroidal anti-inflammatory (NSAID)
- b An antiemetic
- c An opioid
- d An antipyretic

Q2 Pain can result in stimulation of the stress response. For each of the following, indicate whether pain would *increase* or *decrease* the likelihood of the physiological response.

- a Heart rate
- b Serum cortisol level
- c Blood pressure
- d Gastric motility
- e Risk of deep vein thrombosis

Q3 Which of the following instructions should nurses give their patients regarding use of a PCA?

- a Use the PCA every hour on the hour.
- b Use the PCA only when the pain is severe.
- c Avoid overuse of the PCA because of the risk of addiction.
- d Use the PCA regularly to prevent and manage pain.

Q4 Which of the following are examples of opioids?

- a Codeine
- b Paracetamol
- c Ketoprofen
- d Oxycodone
- e Tramadol
- f Morphine
- g Digesic
- h Ibuprofen

3. PROCESS INFORMATION

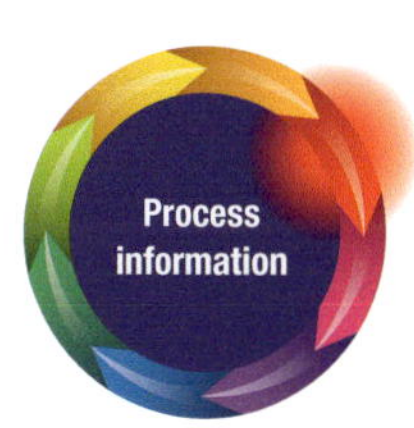

(a) Interpret

The next step of the clinical reasoning cycle is to interpret the data (cues) that you have collected by careful analysis, all the while applying your knowledge about pain.

Q Select *true*, *false* or *infrequently* for the following dose-related side effects of morphine.

- a Difficulty being roused
- b Nausea and vomiting
- c Substance misuse or addiction
- d Opioid tolerance
- e Pruritus
- f Respiratory depression
- g Pupillary dilation

Something to think about . . .

It is not unusual for nurses to be overly concerned about the risks of respiratory depression and opioid addiction when caring for people who have a PCA. In reality, these side effects are uncommon. Patients in severe pain can tolerate very high doses of opioids without becoming excessively sedated or experiencing respiratory depression. Although you would routinely and regularly check Mrs Simpson's respiratory rate and oxygen saturation level, you can be confident that if she is awake and conversing she is not likely to be experiencing respiratory depression.

Similarly, while tolerance may occur with long-term use of opioids, addiction is rare in the normal course of events for post-operative patients. Research shows that addiction occurs in less than one per cent of hospitalised patients treated with opioids (Patak et al., 2013). It is important to be clear about making the distinction between tolerance and addiction. Tolerance occurs when the body no longer responds as well to the opioid's pain-relieving properties at the current dose. For example, some cancer patients with severe pain may need increasing amounts of morphine to maintain an adequate level of pain relief. Addiction, on the other hand, is an overwhelming compulsion to continue use of the medication, even when pain relief is no longer needed.

(b) Discriminate and (c) Relate

Q There are many myths about pain and pain management. From the following, identify those that are *true* and those that are *false*.

- a 'Clock watching', 'knowing too much' and asking for more medication often indicate narcotic addiction.
- b Severe pain always presents with physiological signs.
- c Pre-emptive analgesia is more effective than PRN analgesia.
- d Pain is an inevitable consequence of injury and cannot be completely relieved.
- e People with dementia are unable to rate their pain levels.
- f Older men are stoic about pain.

> Nurses should pre-empt their patient's pain and provide analgesia before rather than after pain develops, for example, prior to deep breathing and coughing exercises or painful dressing changes.

(d) Infer

Q A continuing pain score of 5–8 is:

- a Indicative of a low pain threshold and of significant concern
- b Not unusual for a person who has had major surgery
- c Indicative of severe pain that is poorly managed
- d Typical for a person who is day 1 post-operatively and nothing to be concerned about

(e) Match

Nurses have a professional, ethical and legal responsibility to manage pain effectively. Have you ever been in a clinical situation where you felt concerned about how a patient's pain was managed? If so, what actions did you take or could you have taken?

> The International Council of Nurses code of ethics for nurses (2012) states that, 'Nurses have four fundamental responsibilities: to promote health, to prevent illness, to restore health and to alleviate suffering.' People experiencing pain often feel vulnerable, powerless and fearful. Nurses must therefore prevent rather than just treat pain, and ensure that their patients are informed, educated and supported.

(f) Predict

Q Complications of poorly managed acute pain may include which of the following? (Select the six correct answers.)

- a Hypercoagulopathy
- b Delayed wound healing
- c Pneumonia
- d Bleeding tendencies
- e Impaired immune response
- f Paralytic ileus
- g Improved wound healing
- h Increased gastric motility
- i Persistent pain

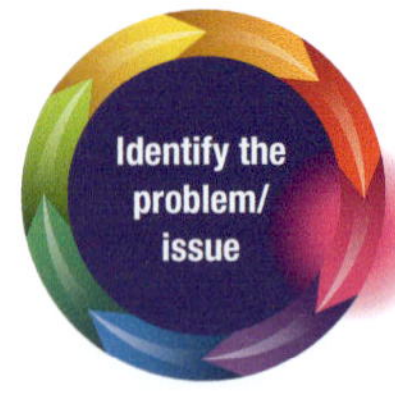

4. IDENTIFY THE PROBLEM/ISSUE

Why is pre-operative patient education about pain management strategies essential?

Q Mrs Simpson is currently experiencing a number of problems. From the following list, select two *incorrect* nursing diagnoses.

- a Exacerbation of acute pain related to provision of misinformation about PCA use, evidenced by pain scores of 5–8, pallor, intermittent sleeping overnight, nausea, tachycardia and hypertension
- b Acute post-operative pain related to a low pain threshold, evidenced by pain scores of 5–8
- c Post-operative pain related to inappropriate PCA use, evidenced by reluctance to use PCA and incorrect understanding of potential PCA side effects
- d Acute pain related to tissue injury secondary to surgery, evidenced by restlessness, pallor, tachycardia, hypertension and pain score of 5–8
- e Risk of addiction related to excessive PCA use
- f Risk of delayed wound healing, associated with poor acute pain management

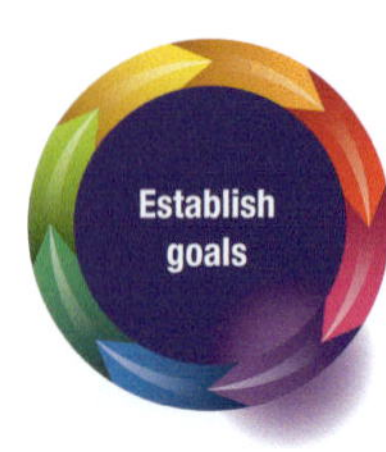

5. ESTABLISH GOALS

Q1 With regard to Mrs Simpson's pain, your goals should include which of the following? (Select all that apply.)

- a That she reports her pain severity as 0 on a 0 to 10 scale
- b That she reports her pain severity as less than 4 on a 0 to10 scale
- c That her level of pain allows her to take deep breaths and participate in activities of daily living (ADLs) without any discomfort
- d That her level of pain allows her to participate in activities of daily living (ADLs) without too much discomfort

Q2 You are concerned that, by encouraging Mrs Simpson to use her PCA more often, her nausea and vomiting will recur. Which of the following will achieve the goal of managing Mrs Simpson's pain while reducing her nausea and vomiting? (Select the three correct answers.)

Simple analgesics include paracetamol and NSAIDS. On occasion, adjuvant medications are also prescribed.

- a Prophylactic administration of antiemetics
- b Slow titration of opioids
- c Discontinuation of morphine PCA
- d PRN administration of antiemetics
- e Administration of simple analgesics to reduce the need for opioids and because they have a synergistic effect

6. TAKE ACTION

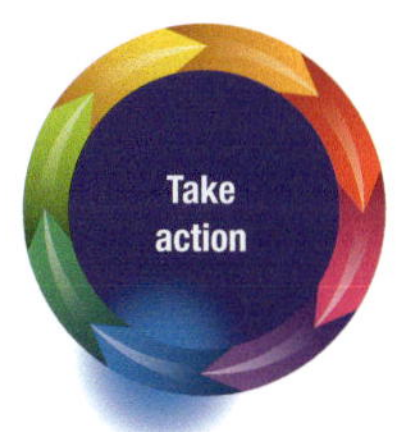

Currently Mrs Simpson's pain is not at a satisfactory level. You decide to undertake a more comprehensive physical assessment and a detailed pain assessment because you want to be sure that her pain is related to the site of surgery only. You are aware that Mrs Simpson's pain could be caused by a number of other problems (e.g. full bladder, internal bleeding).

Q1 Using the PQRST method of pain assessment, categorise each of the questions below with a P, a Q, an R, an S or a T.

P = Provokes
Q = Quality
R = Radiates
S = Severity
T = Time

a Did the pain start elsewhere and is now localised to one spot?
b How severe is the pain on a scale of 0 to 10?
c Is it sharp, dull, aching, stabbing, burning, crushing?
d What time did the pain start? How long has it lasted? What is causing the pain?
e Does anything make it worse?
f Where is the pain?
g Can you describe your pain?
h Does the pain radiate or is it just in one place?
i How does your pain affect your movement, sleep, concentration, relationships, mood?

Q2 List the following nursing actions according to the order in which you would execute them.

a Provide education about the use of the PCA.
b Make Mrs Simpson more comfortable in the bed.
c Obtain an order for simple medications such as IV paracetamol.
d Adjust PCA lockout to five minutes (following medical orders).
e Check whether Mrs Simpson has been ordered any other medications for pain.
f Contact pain team (if available) or medical officer.

As a result of your assessment, you determine that Mrs Simpson's pain is most likely related to her surgery. Because there are no contraindications, you reassure Mrs Simpson that it is quite safe for her to use her PCA regularly. The pain team orders IV paracetamol and changes the PCA lockout to five minutes.

> A pain team provides a multi-disciplinary approach to pain management. It consists of health professionals who are specifically trained in the assessment and management of pain. The team is also responsible for staff training, quality control and auditing.

Q3 You are aware that multimodal analgesia has which of the following effects? (Select the three correct responses.)

a Increases the need for opioids by 20–30%
b Reduces the risk of over-sedation and respiratory depression from excessive opioids
c Increases pain relief, while minimising the potential for side effects due to reduced reliance on a single medication
d Increases the risk of complications such as constipation, pruritus and post-operative nausea and vomiting
e Reduces the need for opioids by 20–30%

Something to think about . . .

The concept of multimodal analgesia involves the use of different classes of analgesics and different sites of analgesic administration to provide better pain relief with reduced analgesic-related side effects. This method of pain management interrupts the pain transmission pathway at numerous points, from the peripheral to the central nervous system. Multimodal analgesia often employs combinations of COX-2 specific inhibitors, local anaesthetics, opioids, non-steroidal anti-inflammatory medications and paracetamol. Both NSAIDs and paracetamol reduce the total daily requirements of opioids, although paracetamol may be better tolerated in the older post-operative patient (Schug et al., 2020).

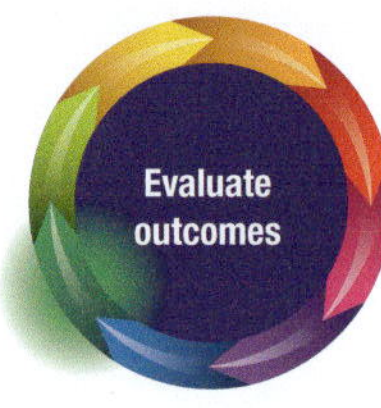

7. EVALUATE

Q Once you have given the prescribed IV paracetamol and changed the PCA lockout to five minutes, it is essential to reassess Mrs Simpson's pain to determine the effect of the analgesics. Which of the following are *true* statements?

a Mrs Simpson's report of pain and response to interventions are the best indicators of treatment effectiveness.
b Mrs Simpson's behaviour and physiological status are the best indicators of analgesia effectiveness.
c Mrs Simpson should be advised to wait until her pain reaches a score of 4 before using the PCA.
d Mrs Simpson's pain should be reassessed 30 to 60 minutes later.
e Pain assessment using the 0 to 10 scale is the preferred way of determining the effectiveness of analgesics.
f Mrs Simpson's pain should be reassessed four hours later.

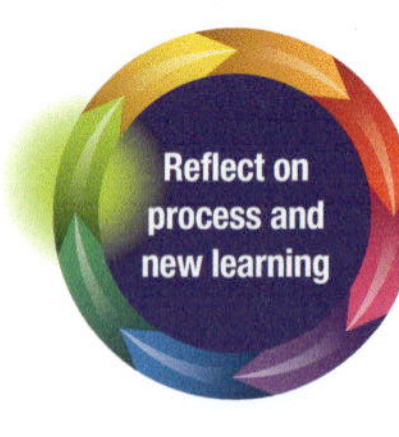

8. REFLECT

In the last stage of the clinical reasoning cycle, it is important to consider what you have learnt and how your learning will inform your future practice. Reflect on your learning from this scenario and consider the following questions.

Q1 What are three of the most important things that you have learnt about acute pain management from this scenario?
Q2 In what way is patient education important to effective pain management?
Q3 Why is pain management legally and ethically imperative?
Q4 What actions will you take in your clinical practice as a result of your learning from this scenario?

SCENARIO 4.2 Caring for a person experiencing persistent pain

CHANGING THE SCENE

Scenario 4.1 was situated in an acute orthopaedic ward and the focus was on the management of acute pain. Once Mrs Simpson's pain had been effectively addressed, her post-operative recovery progressed without further complications. Seven days following her surgery, Mrs Simpson was transferred to a rehabilitation unit. During the two weeks of rehabilitation and with daily physiotherapy and hydrotherapy, she gradually became more ambulant and independent.

Before her discharge, Mrs Simpson's home was assessed by an occupational therapist to ensure that it was safe for her to return home. Rails and a shower chair were installed in the bathroom and a rail was installed to help her negotiate the stairs to her back door.

It is now four months since Mrs Simpson returned home. Her family has noticed that she 'just isn't herself'; she is often 'teary' and tells them that she is frightened she might fall again, especially when Alan (her son) is at work. Mrs Simpson confides in her son that, although her hip is getting better, it is the constant pain in her lower back that is making her miserable. Alan phones the general practitioner (GP), as he is becoming increasingly concerned about his mother's pain and the impact it is having on her quality of life. The GP informs him that his mother has severe osteoarthritis, a degenerative condition that is common in older people. However, the GP comments that Mrs Simpson is 'not as stoic as some older people'. He feels that the analgesics he prescribed should be adequate and he suggests to Alan that because his mother is not keeping busy she is spending too much time thinking about her pain. Alan accepts this advice but wants someone to see his mother at home. The GP agrees to organise a community nurse to visit.

The GP's attitude is an example of fundamental attribution error; that is, the tendency to be judgmental and to blame patients for their illnesses rather than examine the situational factors that may be responsible (Croskerry, 2003).

Osteoarthritis

Osteoarthritis is one of the most common forms of arthritis. It is a degenerative condition that is caused mainly by accumulated wear of the cartilage. Cartilage cushions the ends of bones where they meet to form a joint. As the cartilage degenerates, the normal function of the joint is disrupted, causing pain. The disease affects mainly the hands, spine and weight-bearing joints such as the hips, knees and ankles. In Australia, osteoarthritis affects more than 2.2 million Australians and is a major cause of disability, psychological distress and poor quality of life. The prevalence of osteoarthritis increases sharply from the age of 45 and women (10%) are more commonly affected than men (6.1%) (AIHW, 2020a). In 2015–16, osteoarthritis accounted for over $3.5 billion of Australia's health expenditure (AIHW, 2019c).

Persistent (chronic) pain

Persistent pain affected 3.24 million Australians in 2018, of whom 53.8 per cent were women and 1.03 million were 65 years and over. The cost of persistent pain in Australia in 2018 was $73.2 billion. (Deloitte Access Economics, 2019). However, provision of evidence-based care could lead to substantial savings and better health outcomes.

Patient Safety Competency Framework (PSCF)

Domain 6–Evidence-based practice

Evidence-based practice is the conscientious and explicit use of contemporary research, current evidence, clinical expertise and patient values to make decisions about patient care. Evidence-based practice requires the ability to search for, critically appraise, utilise and translate research into practice.

Source: *The Patient Safety Competency Framework for Nursing Students*, https://patientsafetyfornursingstudents.org

Pain in older people, is often under-reported, under-recognised by healthcare professionals and undertreated. Pain in older people may present as mood and behavioural changes, reduced socialisation, impaired mobility, reduced function, and loss of independence.

1. CONSIDER THE PATIENT SITUATION

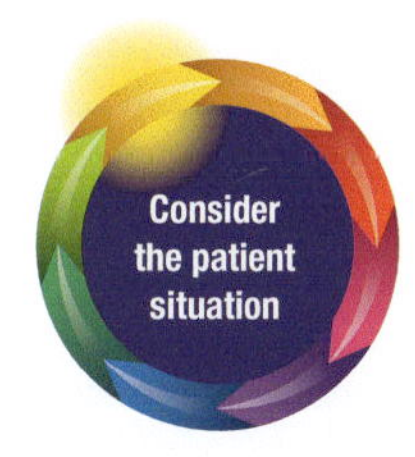

You are the community nurse asked to visit Mrs Simpson to discuss her pain and possible management options. When you arrive, Mrs Simpson offers to make you a cup of tea. You accept, seeing this as an opportunity to begin to assess her functional capacity.

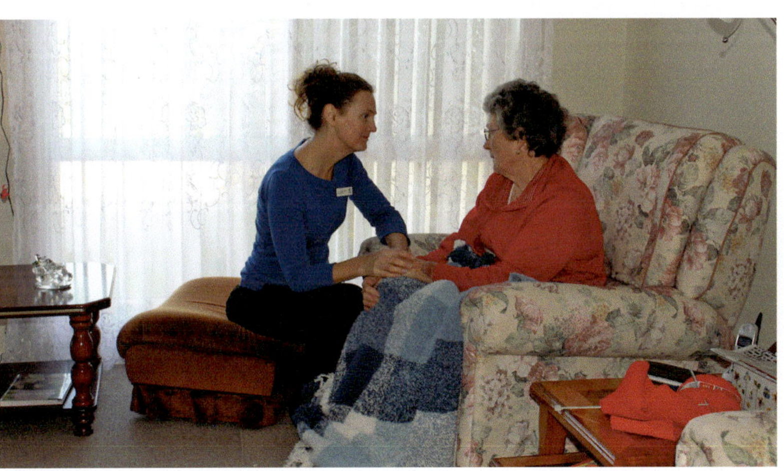

Community nurse visiting Mrs Simpson

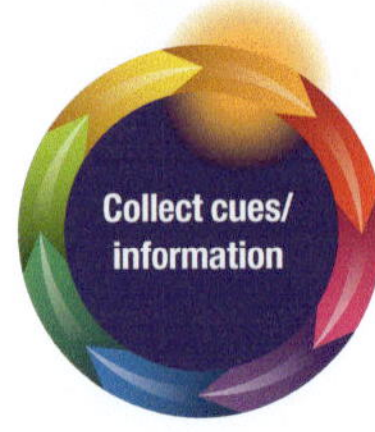

2. COLLECT CUES/INFORMATION

(a) Review current information

As you drink your tea, Mrs Simpson begins to share her story with you.

National Safety and Quality Health Service (NSQHS) Standards

Comprehensive care standard

The NSQHS Standards emphasise that safe care must be delivered based on a comprehensive care plan and in partnership with patients, carers and families (ACSQHC, 2021).

Mrs Simpson's mother died at the age of 75 following a fall and a fractured femur; this plays on Mrs Simpson's mind a lot as she is nearly the same age. When Mrs Simpson was first discharged from hospital, she attended hydrotherapy sessions three or four times a week but it was very expensive, and getting in and out of the community transport vehicle was difficult and painful. Her grandchildren used to call in quite often on their way home from work, but lately she has told them not to bother as she is 'fine' and really 'too tired' for visitors in the afternoon. Mrs Simpson sits on her own most of the day with a hot-water bottle on her back. She doesn't sleep well and her pain has made her feel as if life is just too difficult. She wonders how much more she can take. Mrs Simpson's GP prescribed panadeine forte—one to be taken at night—and he advised her to take paracetamol during the day if she 'really needs it'.

You observe that Mrs Simpson is pale and drawn in appearance and that she briefly grimaces when she moves in her chair. Her responses to your questions are given quietly and with little facial expression.

(b) Gather new information

You decide to assess Mrs Simpson's pain.

Q1 What are the four most accurate methods of assessing Mrs Simpson's pain in this situation?

- a Asking Mrs Simpson to describe and locate her pain
- b Observing Mrs Simpson's behaviours and facial expressions
- c Asking Mrs Simpson to tell you what provokes her pain and makes it feel better
- d Asking Mrs Simpson to score her pain using the verbal numerical rating scale
- e Using a validated assessment tool such as the Brief Pain Inventory
- f Taking Mrs Simpson's vital signs
- g Reviewing reports from the physiotherapist and occupational therapist about Mrs Simpson's functional capacity

In a person with persistent pain, intensity rating scales alone are not as useful as scales which measure both intensity and the amount of interference to everyday activities that the pain causes.

Q2 Persistent pain often results in which five of the following?

- a Grimacing on movement
- b Fatigue
- c Laughing
- d Sleep deprivation
- e Listlessness
- f Restlessness
- g Depression
- h Irritability
- i Pain score of 7–8 out of 10

(c) Recall knowledge

Quick Quiz!

To ensure that you have a good understanding of the key concepts related to persistent pain, test yourself with the following questions.

Q1 Persistent pain is pain that lasts longer than:

- a 12 months
- b 2 years
- c 1 month
- d 3 months

Q2 The following statements are either *true* or *false*.

- a Persistent pain always has an identifiable cause.
- b Persistent pain often occurs in the absence of identifiable tissue injury.
- c Persistent pain is more prevalent in men than women.
- d Persistent pain rarely occurs in young people.
- e The majority of people with persistent pain remain in full-time employment.

Q3 Of the people who experience persistent pain:

- a 33% cannot identify an event that caused their pain
- b Most will be able to recall the event that led to their pain
- c 10% cannot identify an event that caused their pain
- d All will be able to recall the event that led to their pain

Q4 Identify the seven main causes of persistent pain from the list below.

- a Lower back pain
- b Neurological conditions
- c Headache and migraines
- d Arthritis
- e Mental illness
- f Cancer
- g Gastrointestinal conditions
- h Post-surgical pain
- i Work-related accidents

Q5 With regards to physical activity, which of the following statements are correct?

- a It is harmful for people with pain.
- b It should be avoided if someone has persistent pain.
- c It must be undertaken only if weight loss is required.
- d It should be encouraged but be undertaken within a person's physical limits.

Q6 Complete the following table identifying how persistent pain differs from acute pain.

	Acute pain	Persistent pain
Diagnosis	Usually clear	
Duration	Temporary (a few days or weeks)	
Pain descriptors	Sharp, stabbing	

More Australians have persistent pain than many other common long-term conditions, with one in five people aged 45 and over living with persistent pain (AIHW, 2020b).

3. PROCESS INFORMATION

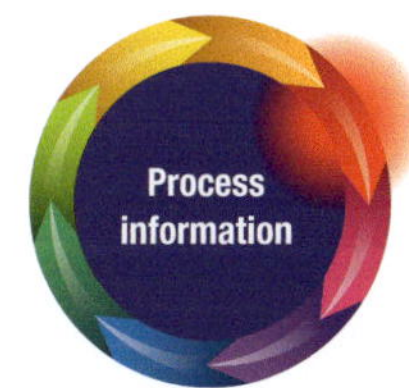

(a) Interpret

The next step of the clinical reasoning cycle is to interpret the data (cues) that you have collected by careful analysis, while at the same time applying your knowledge about persistent pain.

Review Mrs Simpson's Brief Pain Inventory.

The Brief Pain Inventory (BPI), initially developed to assess pain in people with cancer, is now widely used for people with all types of persistent pain, including osteoarthritis (Williams, Smith & Fehnel, 2006). It is a self-administered test which looks at the severity of a person's pain (averaging the worst and least pain with the current pain) and the extent to which the pain interferes with a person's life (examining how pain influences walking, mood, sleep, the ability to concentrate and the person's relationship with others).

Mrs Simpson's modified Brief Pain Inventory

STUDY ID #:__________ HOSPITAL #: __________

DO NOT WRITE ABOVE THIS LINE

The Modified Brief Pain Inventory

Date:____/____/____ Time:_______

Name: _______*Simpson*_______ (Last) _______*Grace*_______ (First) _______________ (Middle Initial)

1. Throughout our lives, most of us have had minor aches and pains from time to time. Have you had pain, other than these everyday kinds of pain, today?

   1. (Yes) 2. No

2. Please rate your pain by circling the one number that best describes your pain *at its worst* in the past 24 hours:

   0 1 2 3 4 5 6 7 (8) 9 10

   1 = No pain; 10 = Worst pain possible

3. Please rate your pain by circling the one number that best describes your pain *at its least* in the past 24 hours:

   0 1 2 3 (4) 5 6 7 8 9 10

   1 = No pain; 10 = Worst pain possible

4. Please rate your pain by circling the one number that best describes your pain *on average*:

   0 1 2 3 4 5 (6) 7 8 9 10

   1 = No pain; 10 = Worst pain possible

5. Please rate your pain by circling the one number that best describes your pain *right now*:

   0 1 2 3 4 5 (6) 7 8 9 10

   1 = No pain; 10 = Worst pain possible

6. What treatments or medications are you receiving for your pain?

   Panadeine forte and panadol

7. In the past 24 hours, how much relief have pain treatments or medications provided?

   0% (10) 20 30 40 50 60 70 80 90 100%

   0% = No relief; 100% = Complete relief

8. On the diagram, shade the area where you feel pain. Put an X on the area that hurts the most.

Page 1 of 2

STUDY ID #:__________ HOSPITAL #:__________

DO NOT WRITE ABOVE THIS LINE

Date:____/____/____ Time:______

Name: _______*Simpson*_______ _______*Grace*_______ ______________

Last First Middle Initial

9. Circle the one number that describes how, during the past 24 hours, pain has interfered with your:

A. *General activity*

0	1	2	3	4	5	6	(7)	8	9	10
Does not interfere										Completely interferes

B. *Mood*

0	1	2	3	4	(5)	6	7	8	9	10
Does not interfere										Completely interferes

C. *Walking ability*

0	1	2	3	4	5	6	7	(8)	9	10
Does not interfere										Completely interferes

D. *Relations with other people*

0	1	2	3	(4)	5	6	7	8	9	10
Does not interfere										Completely interferes

E. *Sleep*

0	1	2	3	4	(5)	6	7	8	9	10
Does not interfere										Completely interferes

F. *Enjoyment of life*

0	1	2	3	4	5	6	(7)	8	9	10
Does not interfere										Completely interferes

Measures:

Pain severity (BPI): 6/10 (add first four numbers and divide by 4)
Pain interference (BPI): 6/10 (add last six numbers together and divide by six)

Page 2 of 2

It is important to remember that pain assessment tools do not always capture fluctuations in pain, like those that can occur in osteoarthritis. A comprehensive pain history should be taken as well.

Q1 With reference to Mrs Simpson's Brief Pain Inventory, which are *true* and which are *false?*

a Mrs Simpson's pain severity score is 3.
b Mrs Simpson's pain interference score is 6.
c Mrs Simpson's analgesics have little impact on her level of pain.
d Mrs Simpson's pain ranges from 2 to 9.

Q2 On the body map on the Brief Pain Inventory, Mrs Simpson indicated the location of her pain. How would you report this pain?

a As localised
b As radiating
c As referred

(b) Discriminate and (c) Relate

It is generally accepted that people in persistent pain will have higher mood interference scores than the general population; however, older people do not always report their mood accurately.

Q With reference to Mrs Simpson's Brief Pain Inventory results, generally Mrs Simpson's pain interferes most with which of the following?

a Walking
b Housework
c Relationships
d Enjoyment of life
e Sleep
f Mood
g General activity

(d) Infer

Q With reference to Mrs Simpson's Brief Pain Inventory results, what is your interpretation of the impact of Mrs Simpson's pain on her quality of life (QOL)?

a Pain is having a slight impact on Mrs Simpson's QOL.
b Pain is having a moderate impact on Mrs Simpson's QOL.
c Pain is having a severe impact on Mrs Simpson's QOL.

(e) Match

Have you ever experienced persistent pain or do you know someone who has? Reflect on the physical and psychosocial impact of that pain and how it influenced the person's (or your) quality of life.

(f) Predict

What are the potential consequences for Mrs Simpson if her pain were to be dismissed, ignored or inadequately managed.

Something to think about . . .

Ongoing pain can be difficult to live with and older people suffer significant complications associated with under-managed pain. Sadly, healthcare professionals too often accept pain in the older person as an inevitable consequence of ageing, and fail to take into account the impact of pain on the person's physical and emotional wellbeing.

People in lower socioeconomic groups, living in regional areas, from non-English-speaking backgrounds and older people have a higher incidence of persistent pain.

Q From the list below, identify five issues associated with poorly managed persistent pain.

a Social isolation
b Depression
c Pneumonia
d Weight loss
e Dementia
f Loss of muscle strength
g Increased sensitivity to light
h Suicidal thoughts
i Improved physical fitness

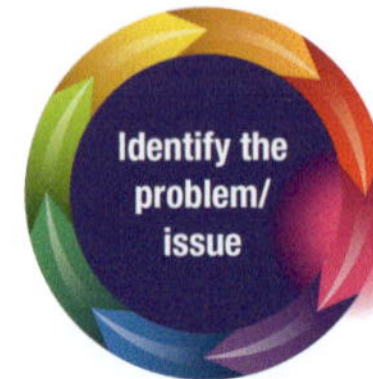

4. IDENTIFY THE PROBLEM/ISSUE

Q From the information you have gathered and interpreted about Mrs Simpson's pain, complete the nursing diagnoses below.

a Persistent pain related to osteoarthritis of _______________, as evidenced by Mrs Simpson's pain severity report of _______________.
b Disruption of social and family relationships related to persistent pain, evidenced by Mrs Simpson's pain interference score of _______________.
c Decreased quality of life related to persistent pain, evidenced by low mood and _______________.

5. ESTABLISH GOALS

Establish goals

Even though there may not be a 'cure' for persistent pain, there are many ways to help manage the pain and improve Mrs Simpson's quality of life. The primary goal of persistent pain management is to reduce any disability caused by the pain; to achieve or maintain fitness, movement and function; and for Mrs Simpson to be able to continue with normal everyday activities.

In regards to Mrs Simpson's pain, the management goals should be SMART:

Specific
Measureable
Achievable
Realistic
Timely

It is important to ask Mrs Simpson to begin by identifying three goals: one short-term (achievable within two weeks), one medium-term (achievable within two months) and one long-term (achievable within six months). The goals need to be specific and realistic, and most importantly they must be goals that Mrs Simpson wants to achieve. It is best to link goals, so that those that are completed in the short term can contribute to the realisation of the longer-term goals. The goals may not initially have a pain focus; for example, Mrs Simpson enjoys learning about her genealogy, but she has not been able to document her family tree as she finds sitting and concentrating difficult because of her pain. Therefore, the plan of care should provide strategies that will help Mrs Simpson achieve this goal.

People who identify goals that have meaning to them are more likely to work towards those goals and achieve them.

Nursing and Midwifery Board of Australia (NMBA) *Registered Nurse Standards for Practice* Collaborative goal setting is central to safe person-centred care and effective therapeutic relationships. The NMBA's *Registered Nurse Standards for Practice* (2016) state that nurses must work in partnership with patients to determine priorities for action and/or referral.

People with persistent pain require a structured approach and a pain management plan that takes into account the areas mentioned above. Mrs Simpson's plan is best developed by her with your assistance; that way, it will be more personally meaningful. The plan should identify the actions to be taken by Mrs Simpson to achieve her goals and the actions required of healthcare professionals to support her to do so.

Q The following plan provides examples of possible goals for Mrs Simpson. Complete the table by adding one more short-, medium- and long-term goal for Mrs Simpson. (*Note*: The 'actions' columns will be completed later in the scenario.)

Goal	Review date
Short term 1. Sitting for up to five minutes without flaring pain 2. Hanging out the washing without flaring pain 3.	2 weeks
Medium term 1. Sitting for up to 20 minutes without flaring pain 2. Joining local seniors Tai Chi club and attending once a week 3.	2 months
Long term 1. Sitting for up to 40 minutes without flaring pain 2. Attending the local library's genealogy classes 3.	6 months

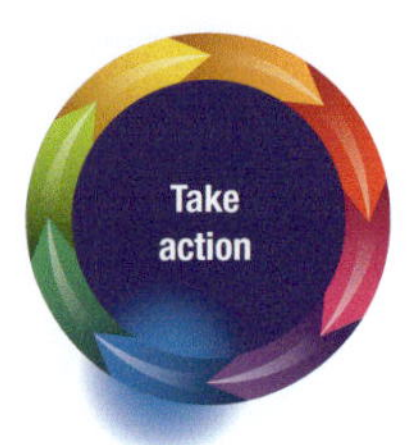

Watch this TED talk on 'The mystery of chronic pain' (TED Conferences, 2011): www.ted.com/talks/elliot_krane_the_mystery_of_chronic_pain.

6. TAKE ACTION

Approaches to persistent (chronic) pain management

Our knowledge of the mechanism of pain—how it affects the body and how to prevent and manage it—has developed greatly in the past 30 years. We now understand that pain, no matter what type, is produced in the brain. Acute pain lasting for less than three months is generally considered to be associated with acute tissue damage or injury. After three months, tissue injury has usually healed and pain that persists beyond this point is less about tissue or structural damage and more about sensitivity in the nervous system. Persistent or chronic pain is, therefore, more complex to treat and requires a different management approach from that of acute pain.

Persistent pain is best addressed by taking a broad approach and reviewing all the things that can affect the nervous system and may be contributing to a person's pain. Passive approaches to treatment are less effective than active approaches for people in persistent pain.

Medical management

The understanding of the processes behind the development of persistent pain has evolved over the past 30 years and there is now a greater emphasis on the use and benefits of pre-emptive pain management.

Medication is useful in the management of acute pain but may have a limited role in the ongoing management of persistent pain. Medications that allow the person to become active and maintain function are initially useful but should be tapered and ceased. Other medical interventions, such as surgery, may not be useful in the treatment of persistent pain, and surgeons will take into consideration the underlying biological issues as well as broader approaches to persistent pain.

Thoughts and emotions

Ongoing pain can cause stress, anxiety and depression. It is important to remember that these emotions will, in turn, affect the person's pain and can in some circumstances make the pain worse. Both pain and these thoughts and emotions are produced in the brain, so looking at ways to reduce stress and manage anxiety and depression can wind down the nervous system and reduce pain.

Diet and lifestyle

Lifestyle can have a positive or negative effect on the nervous system. Diet and lifestyle may contribute to nervous system wind-up and contribute to pain. Smoking, alcohol, fatty foods and low levels of activity create physical ill-health and affect the nervous system.

The person's story

There is often a deeper meaning to a person's ongoing pain and it is worthwhile allowing them to explore this if they wish. By looking at all the things that were happening in their lives when the pain started, such as relationships, life circumstances and emotional wellbeing, a person may be able to identify a deeper meaning to their pain, and this awareness may be included in their treatment approach. It is important to remember that a person should be *invited* to examine their personal story and not be forced to do so.

Activity

For many people in pain, physical activity is reduced or decreased and function can be lost. Activity is physically, mentally and emotionally therapeutic. It is important for people with persistent pain to undertake activity at a sensible pace and within their comfort levels, without fear and without their brain using pain to stop them. Over time, people whose persistent pain is effectively managed will gradually improve function and fitness and be able to achieve much more with their bodies.

Interprofessional collaboration

The management of persistent pain is a complex process and often includes a layered approach, involving a number of healthcare professionals. Most pain centres have pain specialists, psychologists, nurses and physiotherapists, while some also include dieticians, occupational therapists, social workers, and complementary and alternative therapy practitioners. All of these healthcare professionals work together to assess the person's needs and help them develop a realistic management plan. It is also important to consider both pharmacological and non-pharmacological approaches.

Pharmacological management of persistent pain

Mrs Simpson is currently taking panadeine forte 1 nocte and paracetamol PRN during the day. After consultation with Mrs Simpson's GP and the pain service, this is changed to paracetamol six-hourly and oxycodone in small doses for breakthrough pain. The aim of these medications is to enable Mrs Simpson to undertake activities of daily living and to improve her ability to undertake physical activity.

The pain service advises that the oxycodone should be trialled for a week to determine its effectiveness and potential side effects, such as constipation. They recommend that this medication should not be used as a long-term management strategy. Mrs Simpson is asked to maintain a pain diary (see an example in the 'Evaluate' section of this scenario). This will enable the community nurse, the pain service and Mrs Simpson's GP to track her progress and the effectiveness of the medications prescribed.

The pain service also suggests Mrs Simpson consider taking chondroitin and glucosamine, as a Cochrane review identified that, when taken together, these complimentary therapies may reduce pain in people with osteoarthritis (Singh et al., 2015). However, it takes time to take effect and must be taken daily over a two-week period at least.

It is also recommended that Mrs Simpson take omega 3, as it has anti-inflammatory properties and may improve mood and general wellbeing (Goldberg & Katz, 2007). Again this must be taken daily and for a period of at least two weeks before any benefits become obvious. The best source of omega 3 is a diet high in large oily fish, such as salmon, but dietary supplements may also be used.

Non-pharmacological management of persistent pain

During her admission in the rehabilitation unit, Mrs Simpson was reviewed by a physiotherapist who identified that she had poor posture and poor abdominal tone; her sitting tolerance was less than 3 minutes and her walking tolerance was less than 10 metres.

You refer Mrs Simpson to the physiotherapist from the pain service and he teaches Mrs Simpson stretching and strengthening exercises for her lower limbs, abdomen and back. Mrs Simpson is given a daily program and her progress will be reviewed each week. The physiotherapist suggests that Mrs Simpson consider Tai Chi classes, as they improve strength and flexibility and also allow older people to remain socially connected. Tai Chi has been shown to have a positive effect on a person's muscle strength and may improve balance, which has been a major concern for Mrs Simpson (Logghe et al., 2010). Improving her balance will also decrease Mrs Simpson's fear of falling.

Mrs Simpson is also referred to the psychologist who works with the pain service so that she has the opportunity to explore some of the issues surrounding her pain. It is important to reinforce that her pain is not 'in her head' but 'real' and causing her distress. This distress in turn can exacerbate her pain. Providing Mrs Simpson with an opportunity to learn techniques to manage stress, anxiety and low mood may be beneficial for her pain management.

Q Consider the pain management plan again and add potential actions (that of Mrs Simpson and of the healthcare professionals) in the 'actions' columns.

Pain Management Plan for Mrs Grace Simpson			
Goal	**Review date**	**Mrs Simpson's actions**	**Healthcare professionals' actions**
Short term 1. Sitting for up to five minutes without flaring pain 2. Hanging out the washing without flaring pain	2 weeks		
Medium term 1. Sitting for up to 20 minutes without flaring pain 2. Joining local seniors Tai Chi club and attending once a week	2 months		
Long term 1. Sitting for up to 40 minutes without flaring pain 2. Attending the local library's genealogy classes	6 months		

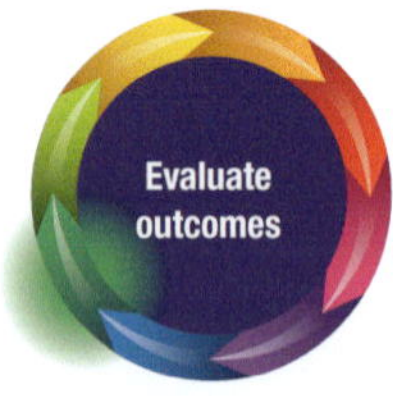

7. EVALUATE

Evaluation of the effectiveness of the pain management plan may take up to six weeks. The plan will need regular review and may need revision. Remember that, just as the plan was developed in collaboration with Mrs Simpson, its effectiveness will also be determined by her.

Maintaining a pain diary will allow Mrs Simpson to take control of her management plan and allow health professionals to review the impact of the strategies that are implemented.

Evaluation of the effectiveness of the medication regime includes assessing the benefits and side effects, including the impact on general wellbeing. The role of the community nurse is to review the pain diary and to begin to taper and cease opioids when Mrs Simpson's pain score reaches less than 4 out of 10. The Brief Pain Inventory should be used to evaluate changes in pain severity and pain interference. Seeking input from other members of the pain service will also be important in the evaluation of the pain management plan.

It is now four weeks since your initial visit to Mrs Simpson. Review Mrs Simpson's pain diary and evaluate the effectiveness of her current pain management plan and related strategies.

Grace Simpson

Five-day medication and pain diary—Grace Simpson

Please fill in this diary over five consecutive days. Include a pain score, aids used, prescribed and over-the-counter medicines, and other substances taken (e.g. alcohol and caffeinated drinks). Note any side effects.

Rate your pain on a score of 0 to 10

0 1 2 3 4 5 6 7 8 9 10

No pain — Worst pain imaginable

Date	Time	Pain score before	Substance/ aid	Notes/observations
13/9	10 am	6	oxycodone	I began to feel better by 1 pm
13/9	3 pm	5	paracetamol	Pain score 3 by 4.30 pm
13/9	9 pm	6	oxycodone	Couldn't sleep. Still awake at 11.30 pm
14/9	7 am	6	oxycodone	Very stiff and sore
14/9	10 am	5	stretches	Less stiff but still sore
	1 pm	3		
	5 pm	6	paracetamol	Keep forgetting to take
	8 pm	7	oxycodone	Overdid it today; very sore
15/9	7 am	5	paracetamol	
	10 am	5	stretches	Less stiff but still in a little pain
	12 pm	4	paracetamol	Pain score 3 by 2 pm
	6 pm	6	paracetamol and oxycodone	Sat in chair all afternoon and now more pain
	8 pm	3		Feeling better
	9 pm	2	paracetamol and oxycodone	

Q1 Mrs Simpson's pain diary indicates that:

- a Mrs Simpson is not taking her medications as instructed.
- b Mrs Simpson has increased her physical activity.
- c Mrs Simpson completed her stretches on 13/9 and 14/9.
- d Mrs Simpson has reached all her short-term goals.

Q2 Mrs Simpson's pain diary indicates that:

- a Paracetamol is ineffective.
- b Caffeine exacerbates Mrs Simpson's pain.
- c Oxycodone has a negative impact on Mrs Simpson's pain score.
- d Stretching reduces Mrs Simpson's pain score.

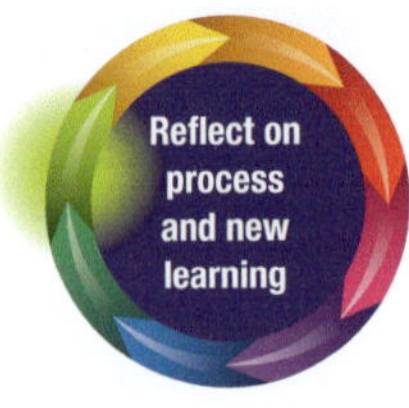

8. REFLECT

In the last stage of the clinical reasoning cycle, it is important to consider what you have learnt and how your learning will inform your future practice. Reflect on your learning from this scenario and consider the following questions.

Patient Safety Competency Framework (PSCF)

Domain 2–Therapeutic communication

Therapeutic communication is an essential skill for nurses. It includes the ability to use verbal and non-verbal communication skills to convey respect and empathy, and to encourage the individual to express their feelings and needs while at the same time maintaining professional boundaries.

Source: *The Patient Safety Competency Framework for Nursing Students*, https://patientsafetyfornursingstudents.org

Q1 What are three of the most important things that you have learnt about persistent pain management from this scenario?

Q2 In what way is therapeutic communication and person-centred care important for effective assessment of persistent pain?

Q3 In what way is interprofessional communication and teamwork important for effective management of persistent pain?

Q4 What actions will you take in your clinical practice as a result of your learning from this scenario?

EPILOGUE

The comprehensive and interprofessional approach taken to address Mrs Simpson's persistent pain resulted in a gradual but consistent improvement. Within two months, she had resumed her genealogy classes and was once again enjoying spending time with her grandchildren. Although Mrs Simpson still had some pain on and off during the day, her sleep pattern improved considerably. Sadly, a year later when Alan took his mother her morning cup of tea, he was shocked to discover that she had died in her sleep. The autopsy revealed a massive stroke. When going through her papers, Alan discovered this poem written by his mother in the last weeks of her life. He read it aloud at her funeral:

A new day wakening; the glow of sunrise
Sparking on cobwebs strung with dewdrops
Faint, wafting perfumes as multi-hued flowers unfurl
Songbirds display their talents
For those who would listen
Trees with branches entwined
Swaying to the caress of a gentle breeze
The hours march on gathering along their way
The laughter of children
Friendly words, helping hands, passing smiles
Minutes filled with useful, caring endeavours
Memories of loved ones, happy times, proud moments
A diversity of music, books, art
Wonderment at the beauty of nature
So that at day's end we may
Pull up the coverlet of sleep
And rest finally and peacefully in God's arms.

FURTHER READING

Australian Pain Management Association: www.painmanagement.org.au/resources.html
Painaustralia website: www.painaustralia.org.au
The Australian Pain Society: www.apsoc.org.au

REFERENCES

Australian Bureau of Statistics (ABS). (2018). *National Health Survey: First Results, 2017–2018*. Retrieved from: www.abs.gov.au/statistics/health/health-conditions-and-risks/national-health-survey-first-results/latest-release#data-download

Australian Commission on Safety and Quality in Health Care (ACSQHC). (2021). *National Safety and Quality Health Service Standards* (2nd edn). Sydney, Australia.

Australian Institute of Health and Welfare (AIHW). (2019a). *Trends in Hospitalised Injury Due to Falls in Older People 2007–08 to 2016–2017*. Retrieved from: https://www.aihw.gov.au/getmedia/427d3a0d-88c2-45c5-bc23-5e3986375bba/aihw_injcat_206.pdf.aspx?inline=true

Australian Institute of Health and Welfare (AIHW). (2019b). *Hospitalised Fall-Related Injury in Older People. Head and Hip Hracture Injuries: Supplementary Tables*. Retrieved from: https://www.aihw.gov.au/getmedia/427d3a0d-88c2-45c5-bc23-5e3986375bba/aihw_injcat_206.pdf.aspx?inline=true

Australian Institute of Health and Welfare (AIHW). (2019c). *Disease Expenditure in Australia 2018–19*. Cat. no. HWE 76. Canberra: AIHW. Retrieved from: https://www.aihw.gov.au/reports/health-welfare-expenditure/disease-expenditure-australia/contents/summary

Australian Institute of Health and Welfare (AIHW). (2020a). *Osteoarthritis*. Retrieved from: https://www.aihw.gov.au/reports/chronic-musculoskeletal-conditions/osteoarthritis/contents/what-is-osteoarthritis

Australian Institute of Health and Welfare (AIHW). (2020b). *Chronic Pain in Australia*. Retrieved from: https://www.aihw.gov.au/reports/chronic-disease/chronic-pain-in-australia/contents/summary

Bliuc, D., Nguyen, N., Nguyen, T., Eisman, J. & Center, J. (2013). Compound risk of high mortality following osteoporotic fracture and refracture in elderly women and men. *Journal of Bone and Mineral Research*, *28*(11), 2317–24.

Commonwealth of Australia (Department of Health). (2019). *National Strategic Action Plan for Pain Management 2019*. Retrieved from: https://www.painaustralia.org.au/static/uploads/files/national-action-plan-11-06-2019-wftmzrzushlj.pdf

Croskerry, P. (2003). The importance of cognitive errors in diagnosis and strategies to minimize them. *Academic Medicine*, *78*(8), 1–6.

Deloitte Access Economic. (2019). *The cost of pain in Australia*. Report prepared for Painaustralia. Retrieved from: file:///C:/Users/53006592/Downloads/deloitte-au-economics-cost-pain-australia-040419.pdf

Goldberg, R. J. & Katz, J. (2007). A meta-analysis of the analgesic effects of omega 3 polyunsaturated fatty acid supplementation for inflammatory joint pain. *Pain, 129*(1–2), 210–23.

International Council of Nurses (ICN). (2012). *The ICN Code of Ethics for Nurses*. Retrieved from: https://www.icn.ch/sites/default/files/inline-files/2012_ICN_Codeofethicsfornurses_%20eng.pdf

Levett-Jones, T., Dwyer, T., Reid-Searl, K., Heaton, L., Flenady, T., Applegarth, J., Guinea, S. & Andersen, P. (2017). *The Patient Safety Competency Framework (PSCF) for Nursing Students*. Sydney, NSW. Retrieved from: http://psframework.wpengine.com/wp-content/uploads/2018/01/PSCF_Brochure_UTS-version_FA2-Screen.pdf

Logghe, I., Verhagen, A., Rademaker, A., Bierma-Zeinstra, S., van Rossum, E., Faber, M. & Koes, B. (2010). The effects of Tai Chi on fall prevention, fear of falling and balance in older people: A meta-analysis. *Preventative Medicine, 51*(3–4), 222–27.

McCaffery, M., Rolling Ferrell, B. & Paseo, C. (2000). Nurses' personal opinions about patients' pain and their effect on recorded assessments and titration of opioid doses. *Pain Management Nursing*, *1*(3), 79–87.

Moroney, T. (2020). Clinical handover. In T. Levett-Jones (Ed.), *Critical Conversations for Patient Safety: An Essential Guide for Health Professionals* (2nd edn). Sydney: Pearson.

Nursing and Midwifery Board of Australia (NMBA). (2016). *Registered Nurse Standards for Practice*. Retrieved from: www.nursingmidwiferyboard.gov.au/Codes-Guidelines-Statements/Professional-standards.aspx

Patak, L., Tait, A., Mirafzali, L., Morris, M., Dasgupta, S. & Brummett, C. (2013). Patient perspectives of patient-controlled analgesia (PCA) and methods for improving pain control and patient satisfaction. *American Society of Regional Anesthesia and Pain Medicine*, *38*(4), 326–33. doi: 10.1097/AAP.0b013e318295fd50

Schug, S., Palmer, G. M., Scott, D., Alcock, M., Halliwell, R., Mott, J. F. (APM:SE Working Group of the Australian and New Zealand College of Anaesthetists and Faculty of Pain Medicine). (2020). *Acute Pain Management: Scientific Evidence* (5th edn). Melbourne: ANZCA & FPM. Retrieved from: /acute-pain-management/apmse5.pdf

Singh, J., Noorbaloochi, S., MacDonald, R. & Maxwell, L. (2015). Chondroitin for osteoarthritis. Retrieved from: https://www.cochranelibrary.com/cdsr/doi/10.1002/14651858.CD005614.pub2/full

TED Conferences (2011). *Elliot Krane: The mystery of pain* [Video file]. Retrieved from: www.ted.com/talks/elliot_krane_the_mystery_of_chronic_pain

Williams, V., Smith, M. & Fehnel, S. (2006). The validity and utility of the BPI interference measures for evaluating the impact of osteoarthritic pain. *Journal of Pain Symptom Management*, 31, 48–57.

Chapter 5

Caring for a child with type 1 diabetes

LORETTO QUINNEY, KERRY REID-SEARL and VERONICA MILLS

LEARNING OUTCOMES

Completion of the activities in this chapter will enable you to:

- explain why an understanding and applied knowledge of the basic pathophysiology of different types of diabetes mellitus is essential to competent practice (**recall** and **application**)
- outline the clinical manifestations of hypoglycaemia, hyperglycaemia and diabetic ketoacidosis (DKA) that guide the collection and interpretation of appropriate cues (**gather, review, interpret, discriminate, relate** and **infer**)
- identify risk factors for a child or adolescent with type 1 diabetes (**match** and **predict**)
- review the clinical information to identify the main nursing diagnoses for a child with type 1 diabetes who experiences hypoglycaemia and DKA (**synthesise**)
- describe the priorities of care for a child experiencing hypoglycaemia and DKA (**goal setting** and **taking action**)
- identify clinical indicators for determining the effectiveness of nursing actions taken to manage hypoglycaemia and DKA (**evaluate**)
- apply what you have learnt to new situations (**reflection** and **translation**).

INTRODUCTION

This chapter focuses on the care of a child who has type 1 diabetes mellitus. You will follow the journey of 9-year-old Haley Milangu from her initial diagnosis to discharge, and then readmission with a serious and life-threatening metabolic complication of diabetes.

Children are not 'little adults'; they have unique needs and respond in individual ways to the care provided. Thus, the care of the acutely ill child requires vigilance, commitment and well-developed clinical reasoning skills in order to identify and manage clinical deterioration.

When caring for a child, nurses must consider the societal factors that impact on the child and their family, as well as the related psychosocial factors. This is referred to as 'family-centred care'; it is an approach that acknowledges that the family is the constant in the child's life and the expert on his or her needs.

This chapter also emphasises the importance of cultural safety to the provision of quality care and addresses some of the misconceptions about Aboriginal and Torres Strait Islander peoples. Culturally safe nursing care means making decisions based on principles of social justice and includes an acceptance of human diversity (Douglas et al., 2014).

KEY CONCEPTS

diabetes
hypoglycaemia
hyperglycaemia
diabetic ketoacidosis
cultural safety
family-centred care

SUGGESTED READINGS

P. LeMone, G. Bauldoff, P. Gubrud-Howe, M.-A. Carno, T. Levett-Jones, … D. Stanley (Eds) (2020). *LeMone and Burke's Medical-surgical nursing: Critical thinking for person-centred care.* (4th edn). Melbourne: Pearson Australia. Chapter 19: Nursing care of people with diabetes mellitus

J. Mould, C. Rudd & A. Wilkinson. (2019). Communicating with children and families. In T. Levett-Jones (Ed.), *Critical Conversations for Patient Safety: An Essential Guide for Health Professionals.* (2nd edn). Melbourne: Pearson Australia.

SCENARIO 5.1 Caring for a child diagnosed with type 1 diabetes

SETTING THE SCENE

Haley Milangu is a 9-year-old girl who lives with her parents, Jenny and Bob, her two brothers, Jim and Charlie, and her grandmother, Doris. They live on a cattle property 60 kilometres from Mepunda in Central Queensland, which is a five-hour drive from the nearest regional hospital. Healthcare is provided by a nurse practitioner (NP) and remote area nurses (RANs) at the community health centre, with fortnightly visits from a general practitioner (GP).

Haley has a close network of friends at school and the highlight of her week was playing soccer in her little league team, but lately she has lost interest in physical activities and seems to be tired much of the time.

Over the last month, Jenny has noticed that Haley has become increasingly unwell, and is constantly complaining of being thirsty and hungry. She has been passing urine frequently and getting up to the toilet two or three times a night. More recently, Haley has had episodes of abdominal pain and her mother is concerned that she is losing weight.

With her level of concern increasing, Jenny takes Haley to the community health centre. After obtaining the history from Jenny, the NP performs a capillary blood glucose level (BGL) test and a urinalysis. Haley's BGL is 20 mmol/L and her urinalysis shows large amounts of glucose and a trace of ketones. The NP explains to Jenny that this could potentially indicate type 1 diabetes. She further explains that Hayley needs an immediate review and contacts the paediatrician at the regional hospital. The NP arranges for Haley to be transported by air and admitted to the hospital, accompanied by her mother.

The epidemiology of type 1 diabetes mellitus

Diabetes is the world's fastest growing chronic disease with 246 million people currently affected (Diabetes Australia, 2017). Of these, 10 to 15 per cent of people have type 1 diabetes, with the majority having type 2. In Australia, 1.8 million people are living with diabetes; this includes 1.3 million people who have been diagnosed and an estimated 500,000 cases of undiagnosed type 2 diabetes. According to the National Diabetes Services Scheme, every five minutes someone in Australia is diagnosed with diabetes—almost 300 people every day—and, despite ongoing awareness, the incidence of both type 1 and type 2 diabetes continues to rise.

Access the Diabetes Australia website to learn more about the incidence of diabetes in Australia: https://www.diabetesaustralia.com.au/about-diabetes

Although type 1 diabetes can occur at any age, it is more common in children and young people. Australia has one of the highest incidences of type 1 diabetes with 2,800 new cases diagnosed in 2018; this equates to approximately 12 cases per 100,000 population (Australian Institute of Health and Welfare [AIHW], 2019). In 2018, approximately 20,700 children and young adults up to the age of 24 had type 1 diabetes; this equates to 261 per 100,000 population (AIHW, 2019). In the past, type 2 diabetes was unusual in children, but it is becoming more common in this age group as a result of increased obesity and lack of exercise (AIHW, 2020).

The aetiology and pathogenesis of type 1 diabetes

For more information about the aetiology, pathogenesis and management of diabetes, access https://diabetesnsw.com.au/health-professionals/resources/

There have been no modifiable risk factors for type 1 diabetes identified as yet; however, it is thought that a combination of environmental and genetic factors are responsible (Diabetes Australia, 2017). At this stage, nearly 100 years following the invention of insulin, there is still no cure for, or way of preventing, type 1 diabetes.

The disease processes of type 1 and type 2 diabetes have some similarities but also important differences. Refer to the table below which compares the key factors that differentiate these diseases.

	Type 1 diabetes	Type 2 diabetes
Origin of diagnosis	Autoimmune disease related to insulin deficiency; inconclusive direct causes but related to genetic, environmental and idiopathic factors.	Metabolic disease related to insulin resistance, heredity factors, obesity (central adipose), polycystic ovarian syndrome, physical inactivity and metabolic syndrome.

	Type 1 diabetes	Type 2 diabetes
Early signs	Blood sugar level (finger prick) usually >12 mmol/L, weight loss, polydipsia, polyuria, polyphagia, glycosuria, blurred vision and tiredness.	Blood sugar level (finger prick) usually >12 mmol/L, tiredness, malaise, polyuria (especially at night), polydipsia, weight loss/gain, blurred vision and frequent slow-healing infections; sometimes asymptomatic.
Body weight	Mostly normal or thin; often a history of weight loss.	Mostly overweight or obese; often a history of weight gain.
Usual age at onset	Usually children/teens/young adults: 4–25 years (majority 4–14 years).	Usually adults >40 years. Although uncommon in children, those diagnosed with type 2 diabetes (T2D) (usually around puberty), generally have a family history of diabetes, are overweight and are physically inactive. T2D is more common in Indigenous children.
Onset	Rapid (days to weeks); often acute presentation with weight loss and ketoacidosis.	Slow (1–5 years); many people are not diagnosed for 20 years or more.
Ketones	High at diagnosis, then absent following stabilisation with insulin therapy.	Usually negative but can be positive in pregnancy if insulin is deficient or if individual is following a 'keto' diet.
Treatment	Always requires insulin to sustain life (subcutaneous injection usually via insulin pens or insulin pumps); requires dietary management, regular BGL monitoring, and exercise is highly beneficial.	Usually requires oral hypoglycaemic medications, dietary management, regular BGL monitoring, and exercise and weight loss are highly beneficial; SCI insulin may be required, usually within 7 years of onset.
Glucose channel/ receptors	The hormone insulin opens glucose receptors and helps absorb glucose into cells to be utilised by the body for energy production. (This is impeded when the endogenous beta cell production of insulin ceases.)	People with T2D are unable to open glucose receptors effectively and have reduction in cellular absorption of glucose; therefore, the use of glucose for energy production is impeded. Consequently, high levels of glucose stay in the blood stream.
Cure	None. (Pancreatic transplant and closed loop pump therapy will potentially decrease the daily management demands.)	There is no cure for type 2 diabetes, although extreme weight loss can result in 'remission'. Physical exercise, maintaining a healthy weight and dietary management are always required.

Source: Based on Diabetes Australia, 'What is diabetes'. Retrieved from: www.diabetesaustralia.com.au/about-diabetes/what-is-diabetes

Type 1 diabetes is an autoimmune disease that occurs when there is a gradual destruction of the insulin-producing beta cells in the islets of Langerhans in the pancreas. This results in a gradual and progressive decline in the production of insulin needed to assist the transport of glucose from the blood into the cells where it is utilised as energy. Blood glucose levels then rise and, because there is a lack of glucose available for cellular metabolism, the body uses fat stores as an alternative. A by-product of fat oxidation by the liver is the formation of ketone bodies, resulting in ketonaemia and ketonuria. The presence of ketones alters the acid–base balance and the person develops metabolic acidosis. Additionally, the presence of high levels of glucose shifts the osmolarity of the blood, and the kidneys increase urine output as a consequence. Thus, the person with type 1 diabetes usually presents with a combination of the following signs and symptoms: polydipsia (excessive thirst), polyuria (excessive urination), polyphagia (excessive hunger), dehydration, lethargy, tiredness, unexplained weight loss, delayed wound healing, pruritus, skin infections, blurred vision, mood swings, headaches, dizziness and leg cramps. Treatment consists of replacing the body's insulin with a regime of injected insulin (Diabetes Australia, 2017).

Admission to the emergency department

At 1200 hours, Haley arrives at the hospital's emergency department (ED) where she is assessed by nursing staff and the paediatrician. Her initial assessment includes vital signs, blood glucose and ketone levels, capillary refill, skin turgor, weight, height, level of consciousness and pain score. Dr James, the paediatrician, assesses Haley and organises for her transfer to the paediatric unit at 1500 hours. You are the paediatric nurse responsible for Haley's care. You receive the following handover from the ED nurse.

Handover report

I	Identify	*My name is Tyler Jones and I am the RN from ED. This is Haley Milangu and her mother, Jenny. Haley is 9 years old.*
S	Situation	*Haley was flown in from Mepunda at 1200 hrs and has been diagnosed with type 1 diabetes.*
B	Background	*Haley presented with a history of polyuria and polydipsia, as well as abdo pain and weight loss. She has had increasing tiredness.* *Haley's mother, Jenny, took her to the community health centre this morning; her BGL was 20 mmol/L and urinalysis showed large glucose and a trace of ketones. The NP contacted Josh James, the paediatrician, and Haley was brought to the ED.*
A	Assessment	*On arrival at the ED, Haley's BGL was 23.0 mmol/L and ketones 1.9 mmol/L. Urinalysis showed large glucose and ketones.* **Admission observations:** Temperature 37.1°C (tympanic) Pulse rate 96 Blood pressure 100/60 mmHg Respiratory rate 30 Capillary refill <2 secs Skin turgor skin fold evident for 1 sec *Haley weighs 22 kg, which is slightly below average weight range for her age; her height is 132 cm, which is slightly above average.* *Haley had a stat dose of 3 u/s NovoRapid at 1240 hrs. Bloods for serology have been taken.*
R	Request/ recommendation	*Haley has an IV cannula in her left cubital fossa. It was inserted at 1230.* **Medical orders:** 4-hourly obs Full diet, with carb counting IVT normal saline 30 mL/hr BGLs prior to meals, including morning and afternoon tea, at 2100 hrs and 0200 hrs; and a urinalysis each shift. Check ketones using finger prick test with every BGL until negative or trace levels reached. If BGL >15 mmol/L, contact MO for further orders. SCI NovoRapid (insulin aspart, a short-acting insulin) and Levemir (insulin determir, a long-acting insulin), but report all BGLs to the doctor prior to the dose being decided. *Can you arrange for the diabetes educator to see Haley and her mother today?* *Notify Dr James if you have any concerns.*

For a more detailed understanding of insulin and delivery devices, refer to www.diabetesaustralia.com.au/insulin and T. Danne, M., Phillip, B. A. Buckingham, P. Jarosz-Chobot, B. Saboo, T. Urakami, ... & E. Codner. (2018). ISPAD Clinical Practice Consensus Guidelines 2018: Insulin treatment in children and adolescents with diabetes. *Pediatric Diabetes*, 19, 115–35.

Having received the handover from the ED nurse, you introduce yourself to Haley and Jenny and begin a 'rapid assessment'. You visually inspect Haley and take her vital signs and a BGL:

Temperature	37°C (tympanic)
Pulse rate	90
Blood pressure	102/58 mmHg
Respiratory rate	25
BGL	12 mmol/L
SpO_2	98% on room air

You then begin the formal admission process which includes a physical assessment, risk assessment and history taking.

Communicating with children

Hospitals are alien places to most children and the way in which Haley is greeted and settled into the paediatric unit can have a significant impact on Haley and her family. Haley may react strongly and unpredictably to smells, sounds, people and procedures. She may have concerns about separation from her family and isolation from activities she enjoys. She may also be worried about unfamiliar people touching and examining her. Hence, therapeutic communication skills are central to establishing an effective rapport with Haley and her family, and in developing a trusting partnership.

Patient Safety Competency Framework (PSCF)

Domain 2–Therapeutic communication

Therapeutic communication is an essential skill for nurses; it includes the ability to use verbal and non-verbal communication skills to convey respect and empathy, and to encourage the individual to express their feelings and needs, while at the same time maintaining professional boundaries.

Source: *The Patient Safety Competency Framework for Nursing Students*, https://patientsafetyfornursingstudents.org

Nursing and Midwifery Board of Australia (NMBA) *Registered Nurse Standards for Practice* The NMBA's *Registered Nurse Standards for Practice* (2016) state that registered nurses must communicate effectively and be respectful of each person's dignity, culture, values, beliefs and rights.

What are some important communication strategies that the nurse could implement to allay potential anxiety when Haley first presents to the unit? Watch Natalie May (2017). *It's Not OK—Culture, Communication and Conversations in Paediatric Critical Care at #dasSMACC*, www.youtube.com/watch?v=39bZYNnpH9k for more insight into communicating with children.

Family-centred care

Until now, the primary concern has been to monitor and stabilise Haley. However, when caring for a child it is important to remember that the child and his or her family (in all the many ways 'family' can be defined) should be considered as a single unit. This is defined as 'family-centred care'.

It is imperative to understand the societal factors that impact on families and the psychosocial and physical health and wellbeing of their members. Family-centred care takes into account that the family is the anchor point in the child's life. From this vantage point, nurses adopt strategies that promote collaboration between the family and healthcare professionals and recognise that the entire family are care recipients (Walton, 2014).

Family-centred care enhances the family's confidence and capacity to care for their child's future health needs. A wide body of evidence details the benefits of this approach (Mould, Rudd & Wilkinson, 2014).

While there are immediate practicalities to contend with, there will also be ongoing challenges for all members of the Milangu family. Additionally, each member of the family will respond in an individual way to the circumstances of Haley's diagnosis.

National Safety and Quality Health Service (NSQHS) Standards

Partnering with consumers standard

The NSQHS Standards emphasise the importance of consumer-centred healthcare and the inclusion of patients and families as partners in shared decision making (ACSQHC, 2021).

Q1 Using the family background information provided below, consider the potential impact of Haley's diagnosis on the members of her family and how they can be supported to adjust and manage this situation.

***Bob** manages the cattle property the family lives on. He is an Aboriginal man with a strong spiritual connection to the land and his heritage. He and his wife have been concentrating on reducing overhead debt and the only road vehicle they own is an old four-wheel drive that requires frequent maintenance.*

***Jenny** is a qualified accountant. She runs a business from home doing the tax returns and business statements for several local property owners.*

***Haley** has been a fit and active girl until recently. She is captain of the school soccer team and plays in the regional representative side. Haley works hard to achieve above-average grades for her schoolwork. She is popular and has a strong network of friends at school.*

What is the relationship between Doris's chronic conditions and her type 2 diabetes? It is important to understand the aetiology and pathogenesis of this disease as 1 in 10 of your patients is likely to have type 2 diabetes.

***Doris** is Bob's mother and she lives with the family on the property. Doris has type 2 diabetes mellitus, poor vision and stage 2 chronic kidney disease. She had a mild stroke last year. Every alternate Friday, Jenny drives Doris and several of the senior members of the outlying communities to the Aboriginal Medical Service in Mepunda for their check-ups.*

***Jim** is Haley's older brother. He is 13 years old and works at a neighbouring station doing odd jobs after school for two afternoons a week. His dad picks him up from the station at around 6 pm. Jim has been selected for the under-16 football team.*

***Charlie** is Haley's 4-year-old younger brother. He attends play group at the local community centre four mornings a week and will begin school next year.*

Patient education

Haley's management plan includes regular monitoring of BGLs to achieve glycaemic control, and education for Haley and her parents.: The diabetes educator explains to Hayley and her family that the first stage of education will be on survival skills, and that an easy way to remember these is by using an ABCDEFGH format.

HbA1c is an index of blood glucose estimation over the previous 2- to 3-month period and is considered the most widely accepted measure for evaluation of glycaemic control (Rewers et al., 2014).

A: **A**lways take your insulin and rotate injection sites.
B: **B**lood glucose testing—know how and when to measure BGL.
C: **C**ontrol—aiming for BGL of 4.0–7.8 mmol/L and monitoring HbA1c (glycosylated haemoglobin).
D: **D**iet—meal planning, nutrition and carbohydrate counting; referral to a dietitian.
E: The importance of daily **e**xercise.
F: The importance of looking after your **f**eet.
G-H: **G**et **H**elp—recognising and managing hyper- and hypoglycaemia and sick-days.

Q1 Why is it necessary for Haley to monitor her carbohydrate intake?

Carbohydrate counting is a skill that children with type 1 diabetes should learn. Educating children about their diabetes is vital for successful management. Refer to the following links for some useful resources for children in understanding their condition:

Snacking: https://jdrf.org.au/snacking-101-an-explainer-for-people-living-with-t1d

A world without T1D: https://jdrf.org.au/get-involved

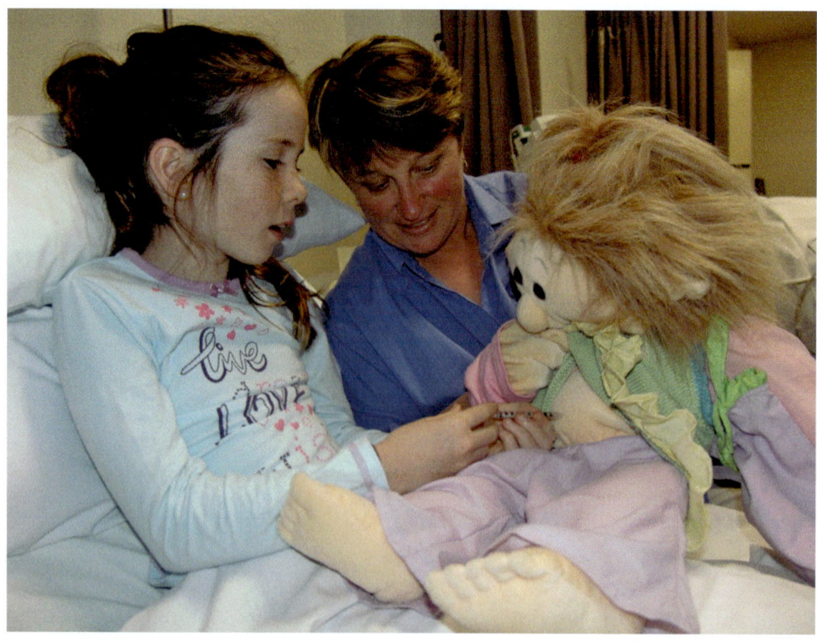

The nurse uses a puppet to actively engage Haley and teach her about insulin injections

Loretto Quinney/Kerry Reid-Searl

Refer to the clinical pathway in the following table for an overview of the education required for a child newly diagnosed with type 1 diabetes.

Stages of care	Expected condition of child	Care and education required	Clinician responsible
On admission (day 1)	**Subjective** Child will be drowsy, lethargic, anxious and usually hungry as fatigue reduces. **Objective** Treatment depends on acuity. Insulin infusion with hourly BGLs and twice daily blood tests. Expected BGL: 13–20 mmol/L Expected ketones: positive >1.5 mmol/L	Initial assessment: vital signs including capillary refill, BGL and ketones. Orientate child and family to the ward; outline what to expect and the initial plan. Provide a brief overview of diabetes and demonstrate the BGL monitor. Provide child with the Juvenile Diabetes Research (JDRF) backpack which has a BGL monitor and information book. *Note*: education will be postponed if child unwell	Ward RN Refer to diabetes educator and social worker. For more information about this backpack and booklet, access https://www.jdrf.org/t1d-resources/newly-diagnosed/children/bag-of-hope
Day following admission (day 2)	**Subjective** Child will be less tired but remain hungry, irritable and sometimes teary.	If potassium levels are >5.0 mmol/L and ketones <1.4 mmol/L), the insulin infusion will cease and subcutaneous insulin will commence.	Ward RN Paediatric consultant Paediatric registrar
	Objective Expected BGLs: 9–20 mmol/L Ketones: negative	Usual regime is a long-acting insulin at night and a rapid-acting insulin for each meal. BGL testing will continue before and after each meal. Education about how to take BGLs and self-administer insulin will start as soon as child and family feel ready.	Diabetes educator, dietitian and social worker will visit the child and family to establish a collaborative education plan.
Day before discharge (day 3)	Patient and family should be more relaxed and confident. Child will be looking forward to going home and becoming increasingly independent in managing diabetes. Expected BGLs: 3–16 mmol/L Ketones: negative	BGL monitoring continues seven times per day. The child (and family) should be able to do this independently. The child learns self-injection (with assistance from the ward RN or educator). The child is likely to experience a hypoglycemic episode during their first admission and an important part of preparing for discharge is ensuring the family can deal with potential emergencies. Day leave is encouraged for the child and family to have a trial with independently managing insulin and BGL monitoring.	Ward RN Diabetes educator will explain blood tests (e.g. HBA1c), sick-day management, hypoglycaemia education plan and register the child with the National Diabetes Services Scheme (NDSS). The diabetes educator will provide a carbohydrate-to-insulin ratio and the dietitian will provide education on carbohydrate counting. The medical team will review insulin requirements.

(continued)

Stages of care	Expected condition of child	Care and education required	Clinician responsible
Day of discharge (day 4)	The child and family are usually looking forward to discharge. Expected BGLs: 3–12 mmol/L Ketones: negative	The medical team check that the child and family are independent with the following: • Self-injection of insulin • Operation of BGL monitor and checking ketones • Recognising signs of hypoglycaemia (hypo) and management of a hypoglycaemic episode • Recognising hyperglycaemia and taking appropriate actions • Sick-day management • Suitable food choices, serving sizes and carbohydrate counting.	Diabetes educator will assist with reviewing all skills and provide contact information. Dietitian will provide final review of carbohydrate counting. Medical team will review insulin requirements, provide prescriptions for insulin and glucagon and make a daily plan for contact until outpatient appointment.

Children are sometimes told that needles just feel like a mosquito sting or that a cannula is a tiny straw going into their hand—analogies that are not helpful. How could you explain concepts such as subcutaneous injections, venepuncture or cannulation? (Mould, Rudd & Wilkinson, 2014).

It is now two days since Haley's admission and she is progressing well. Her BGLs are becoming more stable and the nurses and diabetes educator are teaching her to monitor her own BGLs and administer her own insulin. However, Haley becomes distressed during one of the teaching sessions and says, 'I don't want any more needles. Why can't I just have tablets like Nanna does for her diabetes?'

Q2 How would you explain to Haley why she needs injections when her grandmother doesn't?

Q3 How could you help Haley openly discuss her fears and frustrations?

Initially, Haley's insulin was administered by the nurses. She took particular notice of how two nurses always checked the dose of her insulin together. Haley asks you why she has two different types of insulin in the morning and evening but only one injection prior to meals.

Research by Karges et al. (2017) reveals that inconvenience, inaccuracy, pain, anxiety and social unacceptability all present barriers for children when learning to administer insulin.

Q4 What explanation will you give Haley for this?

Haley remembered the diabetes educator telling her mum about a pump that replaces the need for regular insulin injections and, distressed about all her needles, she asks you why she can't 'just have the pump now'.

Q5 How would you respond to Haley?

For more information about insulin delivery in children and adolescents, refer to: T. Danne, M., Phillip, B. A. Buckingham, P. Jarosz-Chobot, B. Saboo, T. Urakami, … & E. Codner. (2018). ISPAD Clinical Practice Consensus Guidelines 2018: Insulin treatment in children and adolescents with diabetes. *Pediatric diabetes*, 19, 115–35.

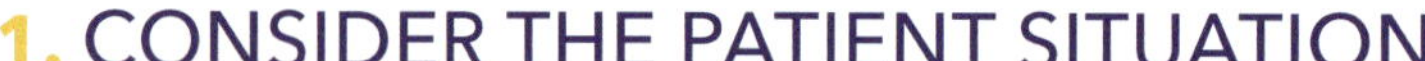

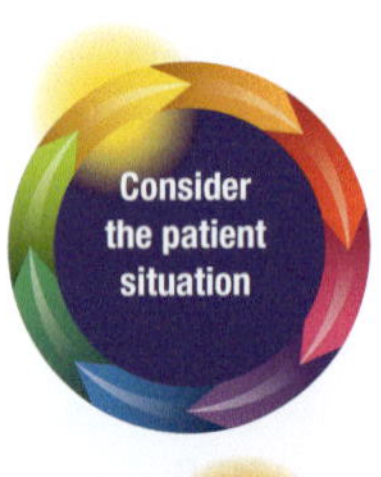

1. CONSIDER THE PATIENT SITUATION

On the afternoon of day 3, Haley is allowed to leave the paediatric unit for a few hours to attend her cousin's birthday party. Haley and her dad know that they need to be back by 1800 in time for her dinner and insulin.

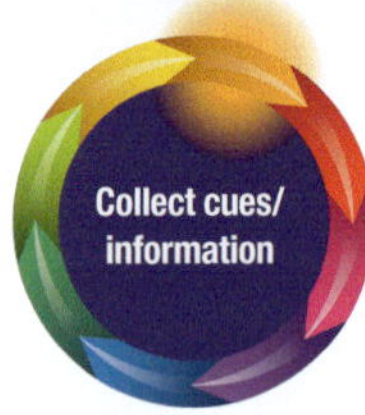

2. COLLECT CUES/INFORMATION

(a) Review current information

Haley returns to the ward at 1800 hours and her vital signs are checked:

Temperature	37.1°C (tympanic)
Pulse rate	84
Blood pressure	100/76 mmHg
Respiratory rate	20
SpO_2	100% on room air

Haley tells you all about the party and says she 'feels fine'. Bob tells you that Haley did not eat much apart from some popcorn and a drink of soda water. She is still excited about playing with her cousins and doesn't eat much of her dinner.

When it is time for Haley to check her BGL and have her insulin injection, she organises the equipment under your supervision. As she is about to undertake the measurement, another child calls out from the bathroom for help and you respond to the needs of the other child. When you return, Haley has completed the BGL and the monitor reads 16 mmol/L.

You check the insulin with another RN and, following the six rights of safe medication administration, you administer three units of NovoRapid, a rapid-acting insulin, as prescribed. Half an hour later, Bob comes and tells you that Haley is not feeling well.

How could this situation have been managed differently?

(b) Gather new information

Q1 Rapid-acting insulin is clear in appearance and begins to work:

- a Immediately
- b Within 20 minutes
- c Within 30 minutes
- d Within 1 hour.

Q2 You return to Haley's room. What cues would you collect at this time?

(c) Recall knowledge

Quick Quiz!

To ensure that you have a good understanding of the key concepts related to the care of diabetes, test yourself with the following questions.

Q1 A normal BGL is:

- a 2.5 to 3.5 mmol/L
- b 4.0 to 7.8 mmol/L
- c 5.0 to 10.0 mmol/L

Q2 Symptoms of hyperglycaemia *do not* include which of the following?

- a Higher levels of glucose concentration
- b Moodiness
- c Muscle cramps
- d Tiredness

Q3 Symptoms of hypoglycaemia *may* include which of the following?

- a Kussmaul breathing and acetone-smelling breath
- b Polyuria and glycosuria
- c Pallor, sweating and irritability
- d Oliguria and ketonuria

Q4 Contamination of the skin from glucose can give a false BGL reading when using a finger prick technique:

- a Never
- b Often
- c Sometimes

Q5 Insufficient blood obtained on a glucometer test strip may result in:

- a A false low reading
- b A false high reading
- c No difference at all

Q6 Which of the following statements are *true* and which are *false*.

- a Hypoglycaemia is a high-priority situation.
- b Hyperglycaemia can happen within minutes.
- c A hypoglycaemic child may have a seizure.
- d Hypoglycaemia can happen within minutes.
- e Hypoglycaemia evolves over hours and sometimes days.

3. PROCESS INFORMATION

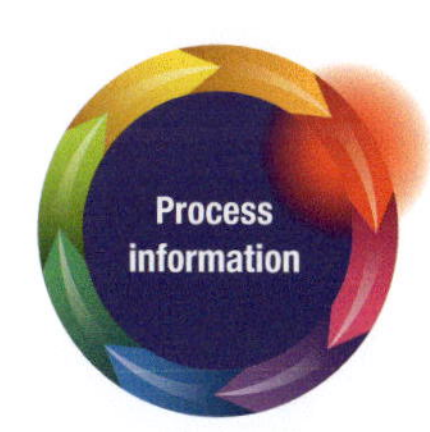

(a) Interpret

Q From the following list, identify which of Haley's cues are *normal* and which are *abnormal*. This will require careful analysis and application of your knowledge of type 1 diabetes.

- a Cold and clammy skin
- b Pallor

c Irritability
d Hunger
e Nausea
f Temperature: 36.9°C (tympanic)
g Pulse rate: 114
h Blood pressure: 96/54 mmHg
i Respiratory rate: 22
j BGL: 2.2 mmol/L
k SpO_2: 98% on room air

(b) Discriminate

Q Which of Haley's cues are of *greatest* concern at this time?

(c) Relate and (d) Infer

It is now time to cluster the cues together, identify relationships between them and make inferences based on those relationships.

Q Consider the following statements in relation to your assessment of Haley. Which of them are *true* and which are *false*?

a Haley could have a low BGL and tachycardia because she ate cakes and sweets at the party.
b Haley is probably pale and sweaty because she caught a virus from one of her cousins.
c Haley could be irritable and tachycardic because she is overtired.
d Haley could be irritable and tired because of her low BGL.
e Haley could be nauseated because she ate cakes and sweets at the party.
f Haley could have a low BGL because she was not given enough insulin when she returned from the party.
g When Haley came back from the party, her BGL measurement may have been inaccurate, leading to the administration of an inaccurate insulin dose.
h Haley could be pale and sweaty because of her low BGL.

(e) Predict

Q Select three outcomes that could occur if you do not take immediate action in relation to Haley's signs and symptoms.

a Haley's condition will gradually improve.
b Haley could become unconscious.
c Haley will develop an infection.
d Haley could have a seizure.
e Haley could become cognitively impaired.
f Haley's blood glucose could continue to rise, causing her to go into a hyperglycaemic coma.

(f) Match

Q Have you ever seen someone with the same signs and symptoms as Haley? If so, what was the problem and what was done to manage the situation?

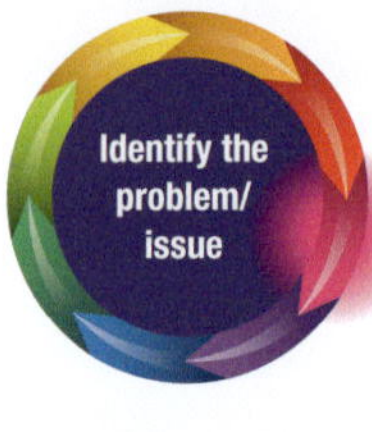

4. IDENTIFY THE PROBLEM/ISSUE

Q Re-examine the information you have about Haley and then identify the three correct nursing diagnoses for Haley:

a Hypoglycaemia related to inadequate carbohydrate intake, as evidenced by BGL of 2.2 mmol/L, pallor and irritability

b Hyperglycaemia related to inadequate carbohydrate intake, as evidenced by BGL of 2.2 mmol/L, pallor and irritability
c Hyperglycaemia related to an underlying infection, as evidenced by temperature and tachycardia
d Hypoglycaemia related to inadequate insulin administration, as evidenced by high BGL
e Hypoglycaemia related to excessive insulin administration, as evidenced by BGL of 2.2 mmol/L, pallor and irritability
f Risk of hypoglycaemic shock related to BGL of 2.2 mmol/L
g Risk of DKA related to BGL of 2.2 mmol/L
h Risk of seizure related to BGL of 2.2 mmol/L

5. ESTABLISH GOALS

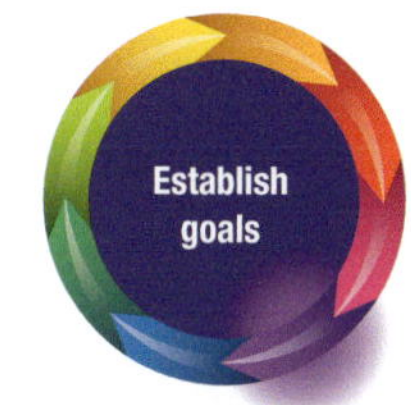

Q Before initiating any actions, it is important to be clear about your goals for Haley. Select the correct nursing goal from the following.
a For Haley's BGL to be between 4 and 7.8 mmol/L within the next 24 hours
b For Haley's BGL to be between 8 and 12 mmol/L within the next 12 hours
c For Haley's BGL to be between 2 and 4 mmol/L within the next 2 hours
d For Haley's BGL to be between 4 and 7.8 mmol/L within the next 30 minutes

6. TAKE ACTION

You realise that you need to deal with the immediate issue of Haley's hypoglycaemia; later you will need to determine the cause of this situation.

Q Select two *immediate* priorities for Haley's care from the list below.
a Leave Haley in the care of her father while you go to phone the paediatrician.
b Administer glucagon subcutaneously.
c Give a repeat dose of insulin.
d Ask one of the other nurses to find a sandwich or some biscuits for Haley.
e Give Haley some oral glucose equivalent to 15 grams of carbohydrate (e.g. glucose lollies, lemonade or orange juice) and repeat 15 minutes later if needed.
f Contact the medical officer using ISBAR and ask him or her to insert an IV so that you can administer IV glucose 5% to Haley.
g Monitor Haley's condition closely and carefully.

7. EVALUATE

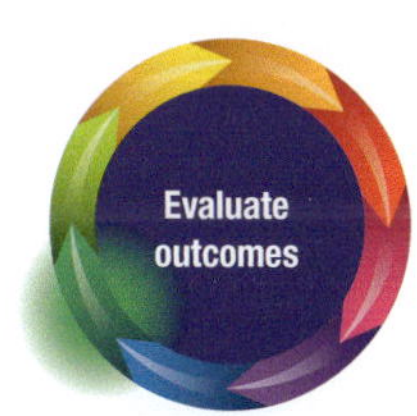

Q1 Which *two* statements provide evidence that your nursing actions have been effective in managing Haley's situation appropriately.
a Following administration of insulin, Haley's BGL is 12 mmol/L.
b Fifteen minutes after consuming the glucose drink, Haley's BGL is 4.4 mmol/L.
c Forty-five minutes after consuming the glucose drink, Haley's BGL is 3.0 mmol/L.
d Two hours after consuming the glucose drink, Haley's BGL is 3.0 mmol/L.
e Haley's observations return to normal within 1 hour.

Once Haley's condition is stable, you consider what may have precipitated her hypoglycaemic episode when she had been so stable over the last few days. Although you are aware that Haley's carbohydrate intake was not high prior to this event, the insulin dose you administered was titrated to her BGL of 16 mmol/L. You begin to wonder whether the BGL could have been inaccurate.

Q2 What factors can contribute to an inaccurate BGL result?

At handover, when you are reporting on the hypoglycaemic event that Haley experienced when she returned from the party, one of the nurses makes the comment, 'Typical. Those people don't know how to look after their kids.'

Prejudice, racism and stereotyping have a negative impact on the healthcare experiences and clinical safety of Aboriginal and Torres Strait Islander peoples (AIHW, 2011). Understanding the impact of racism can support a positive healthcare experience for Aboriginal and Torres Strait Islander peoples.

Q3 This is an example of which clinical reasoning error?

Q4 How would you respond to this comment?

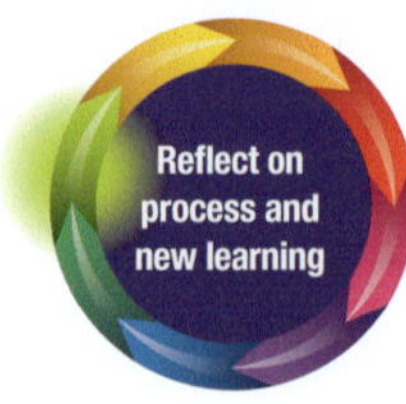

8. REFLECT

After talking to Haley and her dad later in the evening, you discover that at the party one of her cousins tripped and spilt a jug of cordial over the table. Haley had helped to clean it up. Haley does not recall washing her hands after this happened and prior to checking her BGL. Bob tells you that he is really anxious about Haley having another 'hypo'.

Q1 What have you learnt from this scenario that will help you to support and educate Haley and Bob about how to prevent and manage hypoglycaemic events in the future?

Nursing and Midwifery Board of Australia (NMBA) *Registered Nurse Standards for Practice* The NMBA's *Registered Nurse Standards for Practice* (2016) specifies that nurses can develop and shape their practice 'through reflection on experiences, knowledge, actions, feelings and beliefs'.

Q2 What actions will you take in your future practice as a result of what you have learnt from this scenario?

SCENARIO 5.2 Caring for a child with diabetic ketoacidosis (DKA)

CHANGING THE SCENE

With her family's support, Haley progresses well in managing her diabetes and she is discharged on day 4. Part of Haley's discharge plan requires Jenny to be in regular contact with the paediatrician and diabetes educator. However, despite close attention and careful monitoring, Haley's condition deteriorates six weeks later.

At 0700, Jenny tries to wake Haley for school but finds her difficult to rouse. There is a large amount of vomit in the bed. Haley's younger brother has also woken with vomiting and diarrhoea. Bob immediately drives Haley to the community health centre. The remote area nurse organises for Haley's emergency transfer to the regional hospital by air.

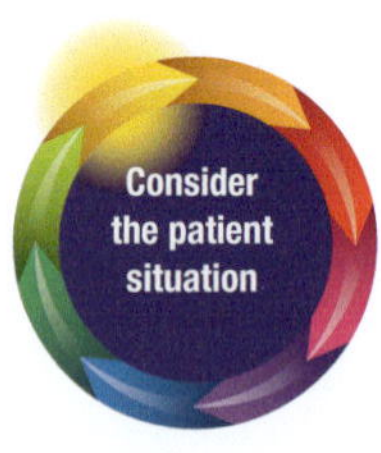

1. CONSIDER THE PATIENT SITUATION

You are the RN on the morning shift in the ED and receive the following handover report from the retrieval nurse:

This is 9-year-old Haley Milangu who was diagnosed six weeks ago with type 1 diabetes. She was very difficult to wake this morning—probably DKA. Her other siblings have symptoms of GI upset.

Initial observations

Temperature	38.4°C (tympanic)
Pulse rate	123
Blood pressure	95/72 mmHg
Respiratory rate	32 (regular and deep)
BGL	28 mmol/L
SpO_2	100%

Haley's skin is hot and flushed and she is complaining of a dry mouth. Her breath has an acetone smell. She is aware of where she is but slips into a deep sleep easily and needs to be roused. This seems to be getting worse. An IV of normal saline has been started and we gave Haley a stat dose of 6 units of NovoRapid an hour ago.

Patient Safety Competency Framework (PSCF)

Domain 7—Preventing, minimising and responding to adverse events

Competent nurses demonstrate the ability to anticipate and respond to human and systems factors that have the potential to jeopardise patient safety, and take appropriate actions to prevent reoccurrence of errors and near misses.

Source: *The Patient Safety Competency Framework for Nursing Students*, https://patientsafetyfornursingstudents.org

Diabetic ketoacidosis (DKA)

Diabetic ketoacidosis (DKA) is a potentially life-threatening complication of diabetes mellitus where a cascade of pathophysiology is generated from the absence of insulin. It is the result of inadequate insulin and usually (but not always) associated with an extremely elevated serum glucose level. DKA can occur as the first manifestation of diabetes in previously undiagnosed patients, or as an acute exacerbation of the disease initiated by stress, insufficient insulin intake, illness or infection (Wolfsdorf et al., 2018).

In undiagnosed diabetes, a lack of insulin results in the inability to transfer glucose across the cell membrane, so there is a high concentration of glucose in the blood. The elevated serum glucose results in the kidney increasing the volume of urine excreted to maintain osmolarity and a serious fluid imbalance can result (Bullock & Hales, 2018). In patients with known diagnosis, DKA can manifest secondary to an infection, stress or change in metabolism such as occurs in puberty. In these circumstances, the body releases counter-regulatory hormones such as glucagon, catecholamines, growth hormone and serum cortisol, which significantly impede the effectiveness of insulin (London et al., 2016).

Absence of glucose as a cellular energy source causes the body to 'implement a safety strategy' to maintain cellular function, so protein and fat are used as energy sources (Parrish, 2017). The utilisation of fat as an energy source results in the build-up of ketones, a metabolite produced by the liver from fatty acids. The accumulation of ketones results in metabolic acidosis, and the life-threatening condition known as DKA can develop. An acidotic state will cause a change in the respiratory pattern as the body compensates and tries to correct the shift in pH. Electrolyte levels are often affected and, in particular, hypokalaemia can occur (Craig et al., 2014). This is caused by a movement of potassium out of the intracellular space into the extracellular space to correct the acidosis. The potassium is then excreted by the kidneys, resulting in an overall body deficit of potassium. Although serum potassium levels may initially be normal or high, levels will drop as the insulin treatment causes the potassium to shift back into the cells and the patient will be at risk of life-threatening hypokalaemia (Wolfsdorf et al., 2018). Haley's condition may be further complicated by the potassium loss that occurs with gastrointestinal upsets.

For further information about DKA, review LeMone et al. (2019).

2. COLLECT CUES/INFORMATION

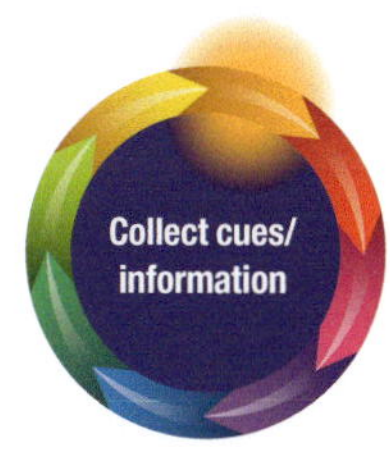

(a) Review current information

You review the information provided by the retrieval nurse to gain a deeper understanding of Haley's condition. You also leave a phone message for the paediatrician.

(b) Gather new information

You then conduct a set of admission observations:

Temperature	38.4°C (tympanic)
Pulse rate	140
Blood pressure	80/50 mmHg
Respiratory rate	32 (regular and deep)
Capillary BGL	30 mmol/L
Capillary ketones	1.2 mmol/L
SpO_2	100% on room air

Q What other information do you need to collect at this time? From the following list, select the four cues that are of *least* importance at this time.

a Appetite
b BMI
c Condition of oral mucosa
d Cognitive state
e Urine output
f Serum urea and electrolytes
g Level of thirst
h Serum glucose
i Serum ketones
j Respiratory pattern
k FBC

These questions require a solid knowledge base. If unsure of any of the answers, refer to your textbook or Chapters 11–13 of: https://www.ispad.org/page/ISPADGuidelines2018

(c) Recall knowledge

Test your knowledge of Haley's current condition and related terminology.

Quick Quiz!

Q1 GI refers to:
a Glucose intolerance
b Gastrointestinal
c Gut intestinal

Q2 U/E refers to:
a Usual enquiry
b Urea and electrolytes
c Urine and electrodes

Q3 Haley's pattern of breathing is called 'Kussmaul breathing'. It is a physiological response to:
a High levels of glucose
b Metabolic acidosis
c Deteriorating cerebral perfusion
d Altered electrolyte levels

Q4 An elevated WBC may indicate which of the following?
a A sign of ketosis
b Underlying infection
c An elevated metabolic rate
d A stress response to DKA

Q5 Which of the following pathways *do not* occur in diabetic ketoacidosis (DKA)?
a Hyperglycaemia → glycosuria polyuria → dehydration → marked electrolyte loss
b Hyperglycaemia → cellular dehydration → diminished level of consciousness
c Fat breakdown → ketone accumulation → pH shift to acidosis
d Hyperglycaemia → increased viscosity of the blood → decreased urine output

Q6 The three main causes of DKA are:
a Too much insulin, infection, lack of fluid intake
b Noncompliance, ignorance, early discharge
c Lack of exercise, unstable home environment, lack of education
d Inadequate or missed insulin dose, illness or infection, and undiagnosed or untreated diabetes

Q7 Normal arterial pH is:
a 7.25–7.33
b 7.35–7.43
c 7.45–7.53
d 7.55–7.63

3. PROCESS INFORMATION

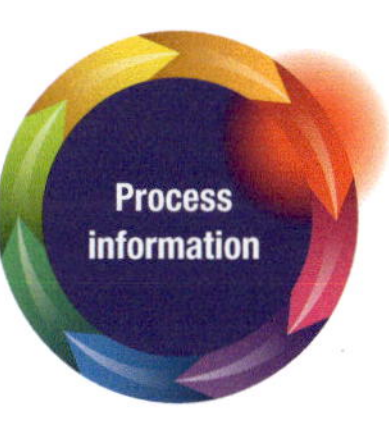

(a) Interpret

The next step in the clinical reasoning cycle is to interpret the data that you have collected about Haley.

National Safety and Quality Health Service (NSQHS) Standards

Recognising and responding to acute deterioration

This stage of the clinical reasoning cycle aligns with the NSQHS Standards which emphasise the need for systems and processes to effectively recognise when a patient's condition is deteriorating, and respond appropriately (ACSQHC, 2021).

Q1 Which of the following are within normal parameters for Haley?

- a Temperature: 38.4°C (tympanic)
- b Pulse rate: 140
- c Blood pressure: 80/50 mmHg
- d Respiratory rate: 32 (regular and deep)
- e BGL: 30 mmol/L
- f SpO_2: 100% on room air
- g U/A: large glucose and large ketones
- h Sleepy and difficult to rouse
- i Sweet-smelling breath
- j Poor capillary refill

Q2 The pathology report reveals the following. Which of these are not within normal limits for Haley?

- a WBC: 18.9 × 10^9/L
- b Haemoglobin (Hb): 125 g/L
- c Urea: 6.3 mmol/L
- d Blood ketones: 4.2.2 mmol/L
- e Serum potassium (K^+): 3.8 mmol/L
- f Serum sodium (Na^+): 140 mmol/L
- g pH: 7.18
- h CO_2: 44 mmHg
- i HCO_3: 16
- j pO_2: 92 mmHg

(b) Discriminate

Q From the following list, identify the clinical indicators that are of greatest importance.

- a Temperature
- b Pulse rate
- c BP
- d Respiratory rate and depth
- e Smell of sweet breath
- f Capillary refill
- g pH
- h CO_2
- i BGL
- j Ketones

k K^+
l Urea
m Condition of oral mucosa
n WBC
o Sleepy, requiring loud stimuli to wake her

(c) Relate and (d) Infer

It is now time to cluster the cues together, identify relationships between them and begin to make inferences about Haley's current condition.

Q Which of the following statements are true?

a Haley's sweet-smelling breath could be related to something she has eaten.
b Haley's sweet-smelling breath is related to ketone production in the liver.
c Haley's temperature and tachycardia may mean she has an infection.
d Haley's pH and CO_2 could indicate respiratory acidosis.
e The condition of Haley's oral mucosa is related to her fluid status.
f Haley's pH and CO_2 indicate metabolic alkalosis.
g Haley's respiratory rate and depth is how the body maintains a normal pH in metabolic acidosis.
h Haley's rapid respirations have no association with DKA.
i Haley's elevated WBC could be linked to an infection which is altering her blood glucose levels.
j Haley's pH and CO_2 indicate metabolic acidosis.
k Because Haley has an elevated BGL, her pancreas must be working effectively.

(e) Predict

Q If you do not take the appropriate actions at this time, what could happen to Haley? (Select three correct answers.)

a Haley could go into a diabetic coma and die.
b Haley's condition will continue to deteriorate.
c Haley's condition will gradually improve over the next few days.
d Haley could experience cerebral oedema.
e Haley could experience a hypoglycaemic episode.
f Haley could experience a cerebral vascular accident.

(f) Match

Q Have you ever seen someone with the same signs and symptoms as Haley? If so, what was done to manage the situation?

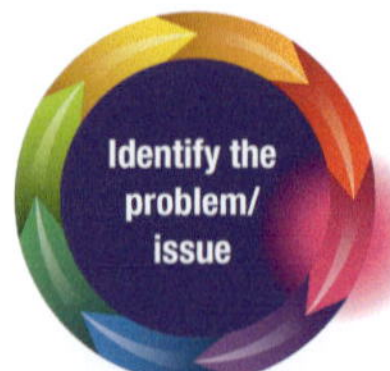

4. IDENTIFY THE PROBLEM/ISSUE

Q1 Complete the following nursing diagnoses for Haley.

a Dehydration related to _______________ diuresis and vomiting, evidenced by glycosuria, poor capillary refill, dry mucous membranes and hypotension.
b Ineffective breathing pattern related to metabolic acidosis, as evidenced by _______________ pH, CO_2 and HCO_3.
c Risk of electrolyte imbalance caused by a shift of _______________ from the intracellular to the extracellular space in an exchange with hydrogen ions that accumulate as a result of acidosis, and increased extraction of potassium via urine due to osmotic diuresis.
d Risk of coma related to _______________ and cellular dehydration.

Q2 Identify four factors that could have led to Haley's deterioration.

5. ESTABLISH GOALS

Q Identify four immediate goals for Haley's management at this time. Identify what you want to happen and when.

6. TAKE ACTION

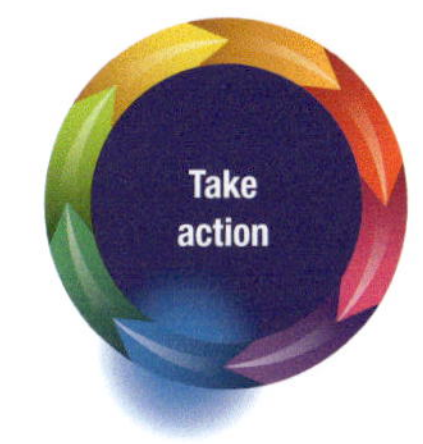

This stage of the clinical reasoning cycle includes all that you do as a nurse in delivering care: practical skills, intellectual activities and effective communication skills. However, you are aware that you cannot do everything at once and that Haley's condition is serious. As Haley's paediatrician has not replied to your phone message, you decide to notify the paediatric medical team and using ISBAR request an immediate review of Haley.

National Safety and Quality Health Service (NSQHS) Standards

Communicating for safety standard

The NSQHS Standards highlight the importance of effective and timely communication between patients, carers and families, and multi-disciplinary teams to promote patient safety (ACSQHC, 2021).

Q1 What are the six priority issues for Haley at this time?

- a Diuretic therapy
- b Resolving acidosis
- c Antihypertensive therapy
- d Fluid replacement
- e Electrolyte replacement
- f Anticoagulation therapy
- g Management of hyperglycaemia
- h Maintenance of airway
- i Monitoring for cerebral oedema

Q2 Haley is reviewed and transferred to ICU. Match the appropriate rationales to the medical orders in the three tables below.

Airway and breathing

Rationale

- To ensure adequate oxygen delivery
- To monitor respiratory and acid–base balance
- To ensure adequate oxygenation

Medical order	Rationale
Provide oxygen therapy via Hudson mask	
Check oxygen saturation level hourly	
Repeat ABGs in 2 hours	

Circulation

Rationale

- Hyperkalaemia may cause cardiac dysrhythmias
- To determine hydration status and enable administration of appropriate IV fluids
- To correct fluid and electrolyte imbalances

Medical order	Rationale
Maintain cardiac monitoring	
IV with N/Saline 0.9% with 20 mmol KCL	
Monitor fluid status	

Disability

Rationale

- To identify changes in Hayley's cognitive state
- To enable the titration of insulin and IV dextrose and maintain BGL at 5–10 mmol/L
- To monitor Hayley's response to insulin treatment

For further information about the management of DKA, refer to guidelines from *International Society for Pediatric and Adolescent Diabetes*, Chapter 11: Diabetic ketoacidosis and hyperglycemic hyperosmolar state by Wolfsdorf et al. (2018): https://www.ispad.org/page/ISPADGuidelines2018

Medical order	Rationale
Check neurological status hourly	
Check capillary BGL hourly	
Prepare insulin and 5% dextrose infusions	

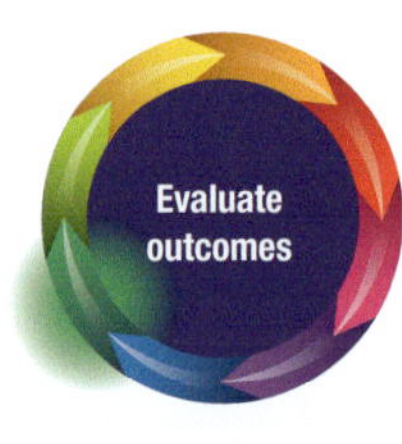

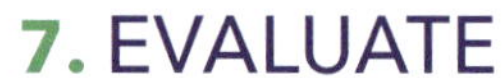

7. EVALUATE

Q1 List seven signs and symptoms that would indicate that Haley's condition has improved.

Q2 List five potential complications of DKA that you will closely monitor for in Haley.

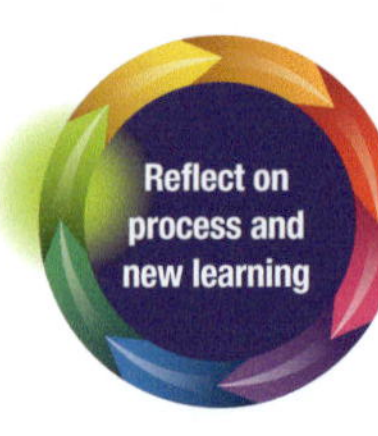

8. REFLECT

Q1 What actions will you take in clinical practice as a result of your learning from this scenario?

Q2 How do you think that your own beliefs, values and assumptions influence your ability to provide culturally safe care for Aboriginal and Torres Strait Islander peoples?

EPILOGUE

Haley was transferred to ICU and her condition remained serious for some time. An arterial line was inserted to enable painless blood sampling and regular analysis of her electrolyte and acid–base status. Two large-bore IV lines were inserted to enable delivery of fluids, electrolytes and IV insulin. Haley remained on neurological observations until her condition stabilised, but she did not develop cerebral oedema. She was transferred to the paediatric ward two days later.

Haley and her family had continuing education about the management of her diabetes and, in particular, about the appropriate action to take if she became ill. A plan of 'sick-day rules' was developed which included an alternative regime of how much extra insulin to take when blood glucose levels were uncontrolled, advice on appropriate foods and fluids, methods of managing fever or infection, and emergency contact numbers (Laffel et al., 2018).

Haley recently celebrated her 10th birthday and has been able to manage her condition with no further episodes of hyperglycaemia. She is attending school and has returned to playing soccer. Haley continues to travel to the regional hospital for consultation with her paediatrician bi-monthly and has a teleconference on alternate months. The family has made contact with a local diabetes educator via a GP care plan. Together with Haley and her family, the GP and diabetes educator have developed a plan to give Haley necessary background education so that she can start using an insulin pump within the next three months.

FURTHER READING

Ambler, G. & Cameron, F. (2010). *Caring for Diabetes in Children and Adolescents* (3rd edn). Australia: Blue Star Print Group. Retrieved from: www.rch.org.au/uploadedFiles/Main/Content/diabetes/diabetes-manual.pdf

Craig, M. E., Twigg, S. M., Donaghue, K. C., Cheung, N. W., Cameron, F. J., Conn, J., … & Silink, M. (2016). For the Australian Type 1 Diabetes Guidelines Expert Advisory Group. *National Evidence-Based Clinical Care Guidelines for Type 1 Diabetes in Children, Adolescents and Adults.* Australian Government Department of Health and Ageing. Canberra. 2011. Retrieved from: http://diabetessociety.com.au/documents/Type1guidelines14Nov2011.pdf

Danne, T., Phillip, M., Buckingham, B. A., Jarosz-Chobot, P., Saboo, B., Urakami, T., … & Codner, E. (2018). *ISPAD Clinical Practice Consensus Guidelines 2018: Insulin treatment in children and adolescents with diabetes.* Retrieved from: https://www.ispad.org/page/ispadguidelines2018

Hockenberry, M. J., Wilson D. & C. C. Rogers. (2019). *WONG'S Nursing Care of Infants and Children* (pp. 1192–1206). St. Louis, Missouri: C.V. Mosby Publishing Company.

REFERENCES

Australian Commission on Safety and Quality in Health Care (ACSQHC). (2021). *National Safety and Quality Health Service Standards* (2nd edn). Sydney, Australia.

Australian Institute of Health and Welfare. (2011). *The Health and Welfare of Australia's Aboriginal and Torres Strait Islander People: An Overview 2011.* Canberra: AIHW.

Australian Institute of Health and Welfare. (2019). *Australian Burden of Disease Study: Impact and Causes of Illness and Death in Australia 2015.* Australian Burden of Disease series no. 19. Cat. no. BOD 22. Canberra: AIHW.

Australian Institute of Health and Welfare. (2020). *Australia's Children*. Cat. no. CWS 69. Canberra: AIHW.

Bullock, S. & Hales, M. (2018). *Principles of Pathophysiology.* Melbourne: Pearson Australia.

Craig, M. E., Jefferies, C., Dabelea, D., Balde, N., Seth, A. & Donaghue, K. C. (2014). Definition, epidemiology, and classification of diabetes in children and adolescents. *Pediatric Diabetes*, *15*(Suppl 20), 4–17.

Diabetes Australia. (2017). *Diabetes in Australia*. Retrieved from: www.diabetessa.com.au/type-1/newly-diagnosed.html

Douglas, M. K., Rosenkoetter, M., Pacquiao, D. F., Callister, L. C., Hattar-Pollara, M., Lauderdale, J., . . . Purnell, L. (2014). Guidelines for implementing culturally competent nursing care. *Journal of Transcultural Nursing, 25*(2), 109–21. doi: 10.1177/1043659614520998

Karges, B., Schwandt, A., Heidtmann, B., Kordonouri, O., Binder, E., Schierloh, U., … & Holl, R. W. (2017). Association of insulin pump therapy vs insulin injection therapy with severe hypoglycemia, ketoacidosis, and glycemic control among children, adolescents, and young adults with type 1 diabetes. *Jama*, *318*(14), 1358–66.

Laffel, L., Limbert, C., Phelan, H., Virmani, A., Wood, J. & Hofer, S. (2018). ISPAD Clinical Practice Consensus Guidelines 2018: Sick day management in children and adolescents with diabetes. *Pediatr Diabetes.* doi: 10.1111/pedi.12741

LeMone, P., Burke, K., Levett-Jones, T., Dwyer, T., Moxham, L., Reid-Searl, K., … & Raymond, D. (2019). *Medical-Surgical Nursing: Critical Thinking for Person-Centred Care* (4th edn). Melbourne: Pearson.

Levett-Jones, T., Dwyer, T., Reid-Searl, K., Heaton, L., Flenady, T., Applegarth, J., Guinea, S. & Andersen, P. (2017). *The Patient Safety Competency Framework (PSCF) for Nursing Students*. Sydney, NSW. Retrieved from: http://psframework.wpengine.com/wp-content/uploads/2018/01/PSCF_Brochure_UTS-version_FA2-Screen.pdf

London, M., Ladewig, P., Ball, J., Bindler. C. & Cowen, K. J. (2016). *Maternal and Child Nursing Care* (5th edn, Chapter 55, pp. 1621–39). New Jersey: Pearson.

Mould, J., Rudd, C. & Wilkinson, A. (2014). Communicating with children and families. In T. Levett-Jones (Ed.), *Critical Conversations for Patient Safety: An Essential Guide for Health Professionals*. Sydney: Pearson.

Nursing and Midwifery Board of Australia (NMBA). (2016). *Registered Nurse Standards for Practice*. Retrieved from: www.nursingmidwiferyboard.gov.au/Codes-Guidelines-Statements/Professional-standards.aspx

Parrish, T. (2017). Nursing care of people with diabetes mellitis. In P. LeMone, K. Burke, G. Bauldoff, P. Gubrud-Howe, T. Levett-Jones, M. Hales, … K. Reid-Searl (Eds.), (2017). *Medical–Surgical Nursing: Critical Thinking for Person-Centred Care* (Australian edn). Sydney: Pearson.

Rewers, M., Pillay, K., De Beaufort, C., Craig, M., Hanas, R., Acerini, C. & Maahs, D. (2014). Assessment and monitoring of glycemic control in children and adolescents with diabetes. *Pediatric Diabetes*, *15*, 102–14.

Walton, M. K. (2014). Person and family-centred care. *British Journal of Nursing*, *23*(17), 949. doi:10.12968/bjon.2014.23.17.949

Wolfsdorf, J., Glaser, N., Agus, M., Fritsch, M., Hanas, R., Rewers, R., Sperling, M. & Codner, E. (2018). ISPAD Clinical Practice Consensus Guidelines 2018: Diabetic ketoacidosis and the hyperglycemic hyperosmolar state. *Pediatr Diabetes.* 19(27):155–177. doi: 10.1111/pedi.12701

Chapter 6

Caring for a person experiencing respiratory distress and hypoxia

AMANDA WILSON and TYSON PERRIN

LEARNING OUTCOMES

Completion of the activities in this chapter will enable you to:

- explain why an understanding of ventilation, respiration, hypoxia and oxygenation is essential to competent practice (**recall** and **application**)
- identify the clinical signs of respiratory distress and hypoxia that guide the collection and interpretation of cues (**gather, review, interpret, discriminate, relate** and **infer**)
- identify risk factors for respiratory distress (**match** and **predict**)
- use clinical information to identify the main nursing diagnoses for a person with respiratory distress and hypoxia (**synthesise**)
- describe the priorities of care for a person with respiratory distress and hypoxia (**goal setting** and **taking action**)
- identify clinical criteria for determining the effectiveness of nursing actions taken to manage respiratory distress and hypoxia (**evaluate**)
- apply what you have learnt about respiratory distress and hypoxia to clinical situations (**reflection** and **translation**).

INTRODUCTION

This chapter focuses on the care of Mr Trent Fulton, a 35-year-old man with a history of asthma who is diagnosed with community-acquired pneumonia. Chronic respiratory conditions affect almost a third of all Australians and contribute significantly to the disease burden in the population (Australian Institute of Health and Welfare [AIHW], 2020). Influenza and pneumonia were the 9th leading cause of death in Australia in 2019 (Australian Bureau of Statistics [ABS], 2020) and around 2.7 million Australians were diagnosed with asthma in 2017–18 (AIHW, 2020).

People with asthma can experience reduced quality of life and require a wide range of health services, from primary and tertiary care consultations to emergency department visits and hospital inpatient care. Symptoms of asthma are usually reversible with treatment; however, severe exacerbations, or 'flare ups', of the disease can result in death. While death rates from asthma in Australia have fallen slightly over the past decade, they are still considered high by international standards and many asthma-related deaths are avoidable. Mortality rates due to asthma are higher among people in low socioeconomic areas and those living outside major cities and inner regional areas. Because of racism, historical injustice and social determinants of health as drivers of illness, Aboriginal and Torres Strait Islander peoples experience 2.2 times higher asthma mortality rates than non-Indigenous Australians (AIHW, 2020).

Clinical reasoning skills are imperative to prevent deterioration, adverse patient outcomes and death resulting from respiratory diseases such as asthma. This chapter will help you to develop the clinical reasoning skills you need to respond effectively to hypoxia and respiratory distress.

KEY CONCEPTS

asthma
community-acquired pneumonia
hypoxia
oxygenation
respiratory distress

SUGGESTED READINGS

P. LeMone, G. Bauldoff, P. Gubrud-Howe, M.-A. Carno, T. Levett-Jones, . . . D. Stanley (Eds). (2020). *LeMone and Burke's Medical–Surgical Nursing: Critical Thinking in Person-Centred Care* (4th edn). Melbourne: Pearson Australia.

Chapter 33: A person-centred approach to assessing the respiratory system

Chapter 34: Assessing clients with upper respiratory disorders

Chapter 35: Nursing care of clients with ventilation disorders

Chapter 36: Nursing care of clients with gas exchange disorders

SCENARIO 6.1 Caring for a person with hypoxia and hypoxaemia

SETTING THE SCENE

Mr Trent Fulton, a fit and healthy 35-year-old gym instructor, saw his general practitioner (GP) about ongoing shortness of breath, fever, headaches and a productive cough over the past week. Trent tested negative for COVID and his GP diagnosed a respiratory tract infection, prescribing roxithromycin (Rulide) 150 mg BD. After taking the antibiotic for two days, Trent returned to his GP feeling much worse. A chest X-ray showed bilateral pneumonia and Trent was admitted to hospital via the emergency department (ED).

Trent was diagnosed with asthma when he was 8 years old. While he is usually symptom free, exercise can cause wheezing and Trent takes salbutamol (Ventolin) via a metred dose inhaler (MDI) for symptom relief. Over the past few months, Trent and his partner Ian have been converting an old warehouse into a gym. During this time, both of them developed flu-like symptoms, sore throats and chest infections; both have had multiple negative COVID results. He is immunocompetent and has not recently travelled to tropical Australia or overseas. When Trent arrives at the hospital with Ian, he is anxious and breathless.

Trent and Ian at their gym

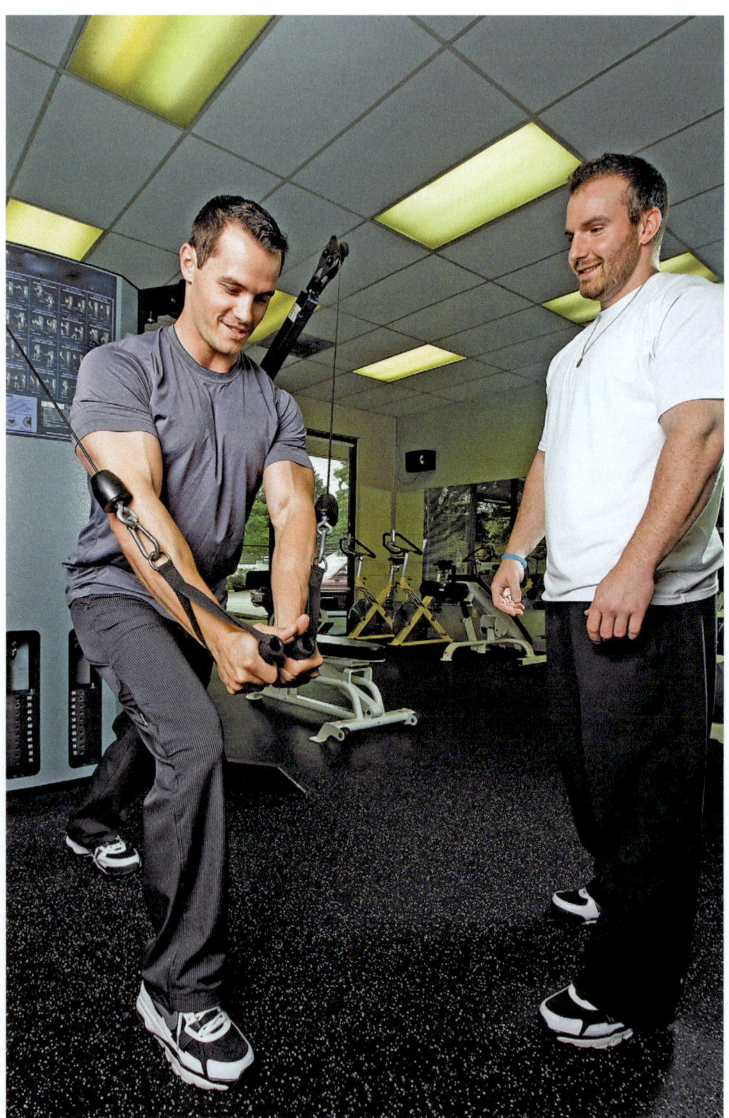

Patient Safety Competency Framework (PSCF)

Domain 8—Infection prevention and control

The PSCF specifies that nurses must know (a) the principles of standard and transmission-based precautions and (b) the principles of antimicrobial stewardship.

Source: *The Patient Safety Competency Framework for Nursing Students*, https://patientsafetyfornursingstudents.org

The epidemiology of pneumonia and asthma

In Australia, each year over 4,000 people die from pneumonia, often as a complication of another respiratory disease. Aboriginal and Torres Strait Islander peoples, the elderly and people who are immunocompromised are more likely to die as a result of this disease (AIHW, 2018).

Australia has one of the highest rates of asthma in the world, with approximately 11 per cent of people affected. Rates of asthma are higher in Aboriginal and Torres Strait Islander peoples and people from lower socioeconomic areas (AIHW, 2018).

National Safety and Quality Health Service (NSQH) Standards

Preventing and controlling infections standard

The NSQHS Standards emphasise the importance of preventing, managing or controlling healthcare-associated infections and antimicrobial resistance, to reduce harm and achieve good health outcomes for patients (ACSQHC, 2021).

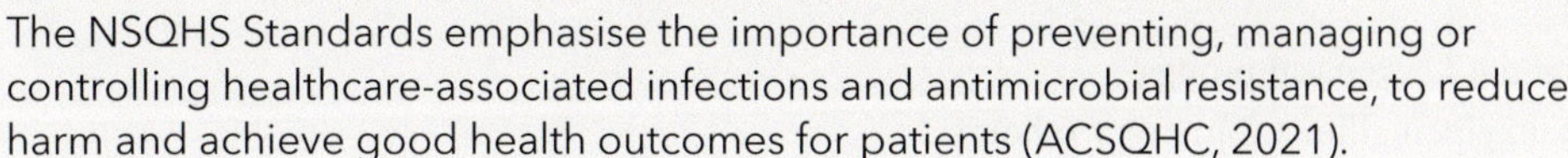

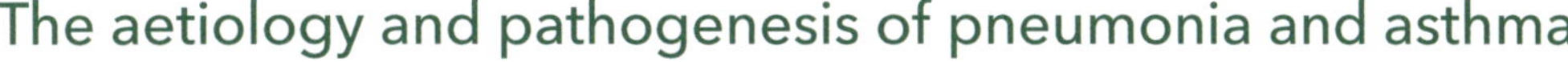

The aetiology and pathogenesis of pneumonia and asthma

Pneumonia is defined as inflammation of the lung parenchyma resulting from either infectious or non-infectious causes. Non-infectious causes include aspiration of gastric contents and inhalation of toxic gases (Kloehs & Hales, 2020). Infectious organisms include bacteria, viruses, fungi and protozoa. When infectious organisms colonise the alveoli of the lungs, inflammatory and immune responses occur. This in turn leads to vascular congestion and oedema as well as accumulation of infectious debris. Ventilation and gas exchange are impaired resulting in breathlessness and hypoxia. Pneumonia can be classified as either community-acquired or hospital-acquired (nosocomial).

Access the NSW Agency for Clinical Innovation clinical resource on pneumonia diagnosis and management at: https://www.aci.health.nsw.gov.au/networks/eci/clinical/clinical-resources/clinical-tools/respiratory/pneumonia

Asthma is a chronic inflammatory disorder of the airways characterised by variable episodes of wheezing, breathlessness, chest tightness and coughing, together with variable expiratory airflow limitation. These symptoms and the degree of airflow limitation usually vary in intensity and over time. Symptoms can reverse either spontaneously or with treatment (Kloehs & Hales, 2020); however, in some cases, particularly those complicated by infections and respiratory failure, acute asthma can result in death.

In asthma, airway narrowing can occur after a trigger initiates an inflammatory response leading to excess mucus production, bronchial oedema and airway hyper-responsiveness with broncho-constriction. Common triggers for asthma include household dust and allergens; environmental pollutants such as tobacco smoke, noxious gases and chemicals; respiratory infections; exercise; and emotional stress. Medications such as aspirin, non-steroidal anti-inflammatory drugs and beta-blockers can also trigger asthma (Kloehs & Hales, 2020).

Admission to the emergency department

On admission to the ED, Trent is sweating (diaphoretic) and flushed. He is alert and orientated but very breathless. He has chest pain which he rates as 2 out of 10 on the numerical pain scale. Trent has a productive cough with green and malodorous sputum. The doctor examines Trent and notes decreased air entry and breath sounds and coarse rales (crackles) on the left side. His chest X-ray (CXR) shows consolidation in the middle left lobe but no pleural effusion. Trent says he has never smoked and drinks only socially. He is admitted to the medical ward accompanied by Ian, who helps him settle in and then goes home to look after their two dogs.

Admission observations

Temperature	38.8°C
Pulse rate	128 beats/min
Respiratory rate	31 breaths/min
Blood pressure	100/60 mmHg
SpO_2	92% on room air
ABGs	PaO_2 55, $PaCO_2$ 32, pH 7.48, bicarbonate 24 mEq/L

Co-morbidities

Asthma

Medical orders

- Sputum cultures and sensitivities
- Blood cultures
- Serum for mycoplasma IgM
- Influenza PCR nose and throat swab samples
- MSU
- Oxygen 4 L via nasal prongs
- IV benzylpenicillin 1.2 g, every 6 hours
- Oral doxycycline 200 µg day 1, then 100 µg daily for 5 days
- Salbutamol (ventolin) via nebuliser, 5 mg in 1 mL normal saline (NS)
- Chest physiotherapy

Q The decision to admit Trent was based on which parameters? (Select the three correct answers.)

a Temperature: 38.8°C
b Urine output: 40 mL/hr
c Pain level: 2 out of 10
d Blood pressure: 100/60 mmHg
e Respiratory rate: 31 breaths/min
f Pulse rate: 128 beats/min
g Mental status: alert and orientated

Access the following resource and calculate Trent's risk of pneumonia using one of the pneumonia risk scores provided: https://aci.health.nsw.gov.au/networks/eci/clinical/clinical-resources/clinical-tools/respiratory/pneumonia/pneumonia-scores

Person-centred care

Trent was born in the regional town of Tamworth in NSW, Australia, where his parents and sister still live. At school, Trent excelled academically and in sport, despite having exercise-induced asthma. He moved to Sydney when he was 18 to undertake an accountancy degree. Ten years later, Trent completed a Certificate IV in fitness and qualified as a master trainer. With Ian, his partner of many years, he is now establishing his own gym. Trent has been working long hours and has also been training for an upcoming marathon.

1. CONSIDER THE PATIENT SITUATION

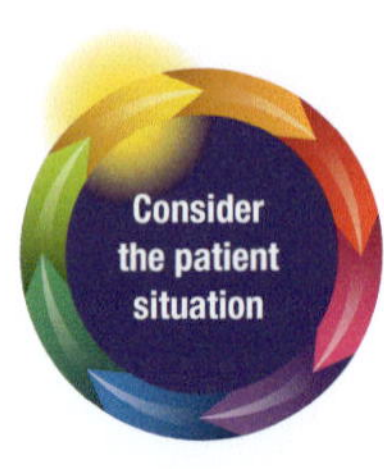

Morning handover report

Trent had a very unsettled evening after his partner left. At 2000 hours, we found him out of bed with his nasal prongs still in place but the tubing detached from the oxygen outlet. He was confused and disorientated, and it took 25 minutes to settle him down. We eventually got him back to bed and put his oxygen on but he was reluctant to lie down. At 0200 hours, his temperature was 39°C and his respirations were 33 per minute. It was difficult to monitor his saturations as he kept removing his finger probe but they varied between 80 and 92 per cent, so I changed him to a Hudson mask at 6 L/min.

After handover, you read through Trent's admission notes before going to his room.

Quick Quiz!

The admission notes and the handover report use a number of abbreviations and terminologies that you should be familiar with.

Q1 Match the term to the correct definition.

Term

- Haemoptysis
- Tachypnoeic
- Cyanosis
- AGBs
- Coarse rales
- Stats

Term	Definition
	Increased respiratory rate
	A test of the oxygen-saturated haemoglobin
	A test of gases and pH in arterial blood
	A series of short low popping sounds, also called 'crackles'
	Coughing bloody sputum
	Bluish tinge of skin, nail beds and mucus membranes due to lack of oxygen in blood

Q2 Trent's oxygen flow rate with the Hudson mask was 6 L/min. What FiO_2% or percentage of oxygen was being delivered?

a 22%
b 44%
c 66%
d 88%

Q3 Pneumonia affects gas exchange in which of the following structures of the lungs?

a Pleural space
b Alveoli
c Bronchi and bronchioles
d Trachea

2. COLLECT CUES/INFORMATION

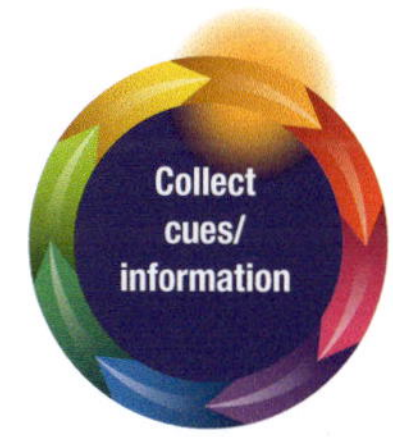

(a) Review current information

While you are thinking about Trent's care, you look at his CXR.

Q A healthy person would have areas of lung consolidation on a chest X-ray.

a True
b False

(b) Gather new information

To help with this question, access: www.patient.info/doctor/chest-x-ray-systematic-approach

You enter Trent's room and he appears to be settled. His oxygen mask is in place. You do another set of observations, with the following results:

Temperature	38.8°C
Pulse rate	110 beats/min
Respiratory rate	33 breaths/min
Blood pressure	100/55 mmHg
SpO_2	90%

You then repeat Trent's ABGs.

Q1 Which of the following would you not include in an assessment for someone with suspected pneumonia?

- a Urine output
- b White cell count
- c ECG
- d Urinalysis
- e Mental status
- f Full blood count and serum electrolytes
- g Breath sounds

To revise your knowledge of respiration and ventilation, access these web-based activities:

https://www.getbodysmart.com/respiratory-system

http://www.khanacademy.org/science/health-and-medicine/respiratory-system-diseases

Q2 A person with pneumonia is likely to have rales (crackles) on auscultation.

- a True
- b False

Q3 A person with pneumonia is likely to have hyper-resonance on percussion.

- a True
- b False

Q4 Which two of the following is an abnormal finding on chest inspection?

- a Respiratory rate of 12–20 breaths/min in an adult
- b Abdominal movement
- c Mouth breathing
- d Inspiration lasting approximately twice as long as expiration

Q5 The body's respiratory centre is primarily stimulated by:

- a An increase in heart rate
- b A rise in blood carbon dioxide
- c A decrease in blood oxygen
- d All of the options

Q6 Inflammation in the lungs can result in changes to:

- a Pulmonary circulation
- b Diffusion of gases
- c Effort of breathing
- d Regulation of breathing

Q7 A person experiencing respiratory difficulties may be able to speak only one or two words between breaths.

- a True
- b False

Q8 When gathering information from a person who is very breathless, it is important to ask _______________ ended questions.

(c) Recall knowledge

Care of a patient experiencing respiratory difficulties can be challenging because it requires analysis of the properties of gases and gaseous exchange, lung volumes and the mechanics of breathing, and the ability to apply this knowledge to clinical situations that are often complex and quickly changing.

Access these guidelines for acute oxygen use in adults: doi.org/10.1111/resp.12620

Quick Quiz!

Test yourself with the following questions about pneumonia and hypoxia.

Q1 Which groups of people are most likely to be affected by pneumonia? (Choose four.)

a Older people
b Sportspeople
c People with alcohol addiction issues
d Immunocompromised people
e First Nations People
f People with a chronic illness
g People with cancer

Q2 Match the following definitions to the correct description.

Definitions

- Dyspnoea
- Bacteremia or septicaemia
- Pleural effusion
- Mucus production
- Secondary infection

Description	Definition
Sputum material coughed up from the lungs	
Pockets of pus that form in the lung tissue	
Secondary bacterial lung infection after a viral infection	
Bacteria in the bloodstream or throughout the body	
Clinical sign of hypoxia, manifested by a feeling of breathlessness	

Nursing and Midwifery Board of Australia (NMBA) *Registered Nurse Standards for Practice* Registered nurses require highly developed skills in patient assessment and, according to the NMBA's *Registered Nurse Standards for Practice* (2016), must use 'a range of assessment techniques to systematically collect relevant and accurate information and data to inform practice'.

3. PROCESS INFORMATION

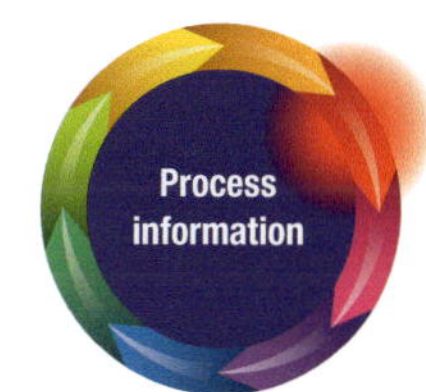

(a) Interpret

You review and interpret all the information you have about Trent's respiratory condition.

Q1 Trent's respiratory rate is 33 breaths/min. Is this described as tachypnoea or orthopnoea?

Q2 You review Trent's current ABGs. His PaO_2 is 50 mmHg. The normal PaO_2 for a healthy male of Trent's age would be between:

a 0 and 20
b 20 and 40

c 40 and 60
d 80 and 100

Q3 Trent's $PaCO_2$ is 33. A normal $PaCO_2$ for Trent would be between:
a 5 and 15
b 15 and 25
c 25 and 45
d 35 and 45

Access further information on arterial blood gases at: http://patient.info/doctor/arterial-blood-gases-indications-and-interpretation

Q4 Trent's $PaCO_2$ is low and his pH of 7.45 indicates alkalosis. The most likely reason for this would be which of the following:
a Trent's respiratory rate is raised due to hypoxaemia and a low PaO_2, and he is retaining CO_2 which has raised his pH.
b Trent's respiratory rate is raised as he is hypoxic, he has a low PaO_2, and his rapid respiratory rate has caused him to 'blow off' CO_2 and raise his pH.
c Trent's respiratory rate is decreased, so he is retaining CO_2 and his pH is consequently raised.
d Trent's respiratory rate is faster and the low PaO_2 is causing a raised pH.

(b) Discriminate

From the cues and information you now have, you need to narrow down the information to what is most important.

Q1 Select four cues that you believe are *most relevant* to the assessment of Trent's hypoxia.
a Blood pressure: 100/55 mmHg
b Respiratory rate: 33 breaths/min
c Temperature: 38.8°C
d Headache
e SpO_2: 90% on room air
f ABGs: PaO_2 50 mmHg, $PaCO_2$ 33 mmHg, pH 7.45
g Urine output: 40 mL/hr

To help you answer this question, access the Clinical Excellence Commission's *Between the Flags: Standard Calling Criteria:* https://www.cec.health.nsw.gov.au/keep-patients-safe/deteriorating-patient-program/between-the-flags/standard-calling-criteria

Q2 When Trent complained of chest pain during his initial assessment in the ED, the nurse asked him to describe the pain and whether it was travelling to his jaw or to his left arm. The nurse's question was asked to determine whether the chest pain could be due to:
a Myocardial infarction
b Congestive heart failure
c Bronchitis
d Pneumonia

(c) Relate

It is important to cluster the cues together and identify relationships between them (based on the information you have collected so far).

Q1 Which of the following statements are *true*?
a Trent is tachypnoeic due to a high fever.
b Trent is hypoxic, as mucus is partially blocking his airways and impeding gas exchange.
c Trent's pulse is faster as a compensatory mechanism to increase gas exchange.

Q2 Select the most important cue cluster for a patient with pneumonia.
a Purulent sputum, clubbing of the fingers, cyanosis, cough, hyper-resonance, excessive thirst
b Cough, low oxygen saturation, an elevated blood glucose level (BGL), fluid retention as shown by weight gain, hypo-resonance, tactile fremitus

c Tachypnoea, fever, purulent sputum, cough, coarse rales, oxygen saturation lower than normal
d Weight loss over recent weeks, fatigue, low oxygen saturations, frothy blood-tinged sputum

(d) Infer

Think about the cues you have collected regarding Trent and make inferences based on your analysis and interpretation of those cues.

Q1 In your opinion, and from what you know of Trent's history, signs and symptoms, Trent is (select two from the following list):

- a Afebrile and tachypnoeic
- b Tachypnoeic and tachycardic
- c Hypertensive and afebrile
- d Hypoxic and febrile
- e Hypotensive and afebrile

Q2 Which two of the following are not early signs of hypoxia?

- a Tachypnoea or bradypnoea
- b Dyspnoea
- c Tachycardia or bradycardia
- d Hypotension
- e Fatigue
- f Cardiac arrhythmias
- g Confusion

Q3 Trent's SpO_2 and PaO_2 are both abnormal, indicating hypoxia. What factors do you think have contributed to his hypoxia? (Select two.)

- a Age
- b Partial obstruction of his airways by mucus
- c History of smoking
- d Poor gas exchange due to mucus and fluid in the alveoli
- e History of asthma

(e) Predict

Q1 If you do not take the appropriate actions at this time, what could happen to Trent if his hypoxia is not corrected? (Select two.)

- a He will gradually improve over the next few days.
- b He may become even more febrile and develop delirium.
- c His chest pain could worsen leading to a cardiac arrest.
- d His hypoxia will worsen and may lead to a respiratory arrest.

Q2 From the following list, choose the clinical indicator *most* indicative of impending respiratory arrest.

- a Blood pressure: 100/55 mmHg
- b Respiratory rate: 33 breaths/min
- c Urine output: 40 mL/hr
- d ABGs: PaO_2 50 mmHg, $PaCO_2$ 33 mmHg, pH 7.45

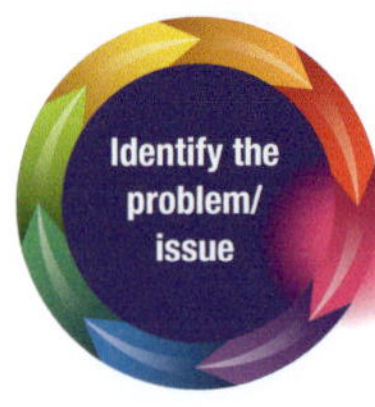

4. IDENTIFY THE PROBLEM/ISSUE

Q Now bring together (synthesise) all of the facts you've collected and inferences you've made to identify the *most correct* nursing diagnosis for Trent.

a Risk of hypoxia due to confusion, low SpO_2 level, tachypnoea and abnormal ABGs

b Hypoxia related to ineffective breathing pattern, as evidenced by confusion, low SpO_2, tachypnoea and abnormal ABGs

c Impaired gas exchange related to airway obstruction due to excessive secretions, bronchospasm and alveoli destruction

d Risk of oxygen toxicity related to the provision of high concentrations of oxygen over a prolonged period of time

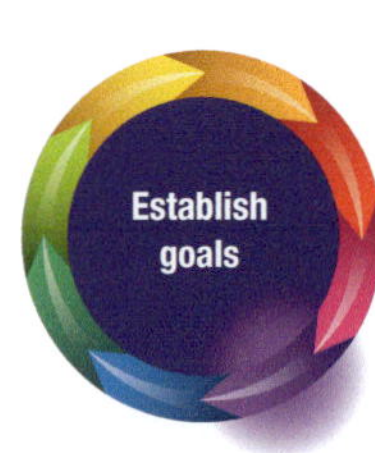

5. ESTABLISH GOALS

Before implementing any actions to improve Trent's condition, it is important to clearly specify what you want to happen and when.

Q From the list below, choose the most important short-term goal for Trent's management at this time.

a For Trent to be afebrile and to have no pain within 20 minutes

b For Trent's infection to be resolved within 3–5 days

c For Trent to have a normal respiratory rate and an oxygen saturation level of >94%

d For Trent to be normotensive and euvolaemic

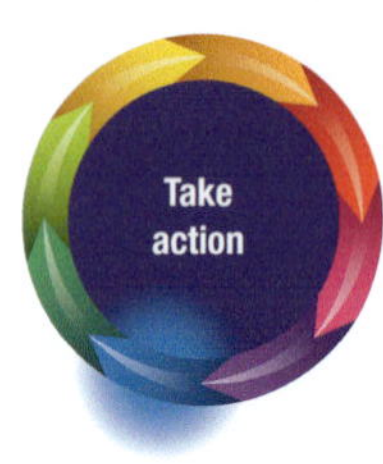

6. TAKE ACTION

Now that you have a nursing diagnosis and short-term goals for Trent, you need to identify appropriate nursing actions.

Q1 In the table below, match the rationales for care to the corresponding nursing action.

Rationale

- Anxiety and restlessness may indicate worsening hypoxia
- To increase partial pressure of oxygen in alveoli and increase diffusion into capillaries
- To help loosen secretions
- Changes may indicate worsening hypoxia
- To aid in removal of secretions
- To reduce oxygen demand

Nursing action	Rationale
Monitor oxygen saturations and ABGs regularly	
Check cognitive status regularly	
Place in semi or high Fowler's position	
Teach patient deep breathing and coughing	
Keep patient well hydrated	
Maintain oxygen therapy via nasal prongs or Hudson mask	

Respiratory conditions can change rapidly. When you check on Trent 15 minutes later, you find him collapsed on the floor with his oxygen disconnected. He is cyanotic and does not answer your questions. You note that he now has stridor. You do another set of observations with the following results:

Respiratory rate	Irregular and 5 breaths/min
Pulse rate	38 beats/min
Blood pressure	75/60 mmHg
SpO_2	85%

Members of the rapid response team typically include:

ICU resident or registrar

ICU ALS-accredited RN

Cardiology registrar or medical registrar.

Q2 Identify three priority nursing actions from the list below.

- a Reassure patient.
- b Run to find another nurse to help you.
- c Initiate a rapid response or medical emergency team (MET) call.
- d Reconnect the oxygen.
- e Get ready to start CPR (cardiopulmonary resuscitation).
- f Check that Trent's fluids are running.

Q3 Identify three factors that may have caused deterioration in Trent's respiratory status, leading to severe hypoxia and acute respiratory failure.

- a Trent was given too much to drink as well as IV fluids, leading to fluid overload and pulmonary oedema.
- b The increase in Trent's mucus secretions led to decreased gas exchange.
- c Increasing confusion and continual removal of the oxygen mask led to increasing hypoxia.
- d Decreased neurological status due to administering the central nervous system (CNS) depressant morphine, which affected the brain stem and reduced breathing rate.
- e Failure of the ward nurses to recognise Trent's increasing respiratory distress, as evidenced by his increasing confusion and low SpO_2.

While waiting for the rapid response team/MET to arrive, a senior nurse comes to help and changes Trent's Hudson mask to a non-rebreather mask with a flow rate of 12 L/min. You are confused as you thought that nurses are only allowed to initiate oxygen using nasal prongs at 2 L/min. Access and read the article in the margin note, and decide what you would do in a similar situation.

For further information, access J. Cousins, P. Wark, S. Hiles & V. McDonald (2020). Understanding clinicians' perceived barriers and facilitators to optimal use of acute oxygen therapy in adults. *International Journal of Chronic Obstructive Pulmonary Disease, 15*, 2275–87. doi. 10.2147/COPD.S263696

Patient Safety Competency Framework (PSCF)

Domain 7–Preventing, minimising and responding to adverse events

The PSCF specifies that nurses must conduct regular and appropriate risk assessments; recognise particular risks associated with vulnerable individuals and groups, and initiate actions to prevent adverse outcomes.

Source: *The Patient Safety Competency Framework for Nursing Students*, https://patientsafetyfornursingstudents.org

Q4 Match the oxygen delivery devices to the appropriate flow rate and FiO_2.

Oxygen delivery device

- Nasal prongs
- Non-rebreather mask
- Hudson mask

Oxygen delivery device	Flow rate	FiO_2
	2-4 L/min	0.24-0.36
	6-15 L/min	0.4-0.6
	10-15 L/min	0.6-0.9

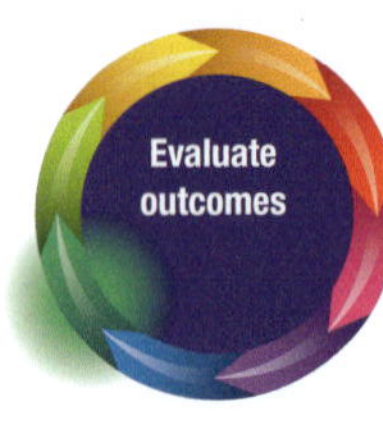

7. EVALUATE

Q1 With the correct treatment, you would expect Trent's SpO_2 to increase to ~97% and his respiratory rate increase to between 12 and 18 if his condition resolves.

a True

b False

Q2 Match the expected outcome measures with the appropriate interventions.

Outcomes

- Changes in condition are identified early
- SpO_2 increases from 94% to 97%
- Trent is able to expectorate secretions effectively
- Trent reports adequate sleep and rest

Interventions	Outcomes
Change Hudson mask to a non-rebreather mask to improve oxygenation	
Position Trent in a high Fowler's to assist lung expansion	
Monitor Trent's vital signs hourly	
Promote adequate rest	

Q3 What nursing actions may have prevented Trent's deterioration? (Choose three from the list below.)

a A sedative should have been administered to help Trent settle.

b More frequent observations of pulse oximetry and vital signs should have been conducted.

c The significance of his ABGs should have been recognised.

d A medical review should have been requested earlier.

e Trent's fluids should have been increased.

f Trent should have received more antibiotics to treat his infection.

Q4 Review Trent's observations since his admission and identify which of the following statements is most correct.

Observations

On admission	0700 hours	Now
Temperature 38.8°C	Temperature 38.8°C	Temperature 39°C
Pulse 128	Pulse 110	Pulse 38
Respiratory rate 31	Respiratory rate 33	Respiratory rate 5; stridor and cyanosis present
SpO_2 92% on room air	SpO_2 90% on 6 L/min via Hudson mask	SpO_2 85% on 6 L/min via Hudson mask
Blood pressure 100/60 mmHg	Blood pressure 100/55 mmHg	Blood pressure 78/60 mmHg

a Since admission, Trent's vital signs have significantly improved and he now is experiencing tachycardia, tachypnoea, hypoxia and hypertension.
b Since admission, Trent's vital signs have significantly worsened and he now is experiencing bradycardia, bradypnoea, hypoxia and hypotension.
c Since admission, Trent's vital signs have remained stable and his observations are all normal.
d Since admission, Trent's vital signs have significantly worsened and he now is afebrile, hypertensive and hypoxic.

The rapid response team/MET quickly respond to your call. Trent is ventilated and transferred to the intensive care unit (ICU) for further care. He remains in ICU for the next few days, until his condition improves and he returns to the ward.

The rapid response team uses the mnemonic DRSABCD to assess and manage Trent (Craig et al., 2020):
Danger
Response
Send
Airway
Breathing
Circulation
Defibrillation (not required)

8. REFLECT

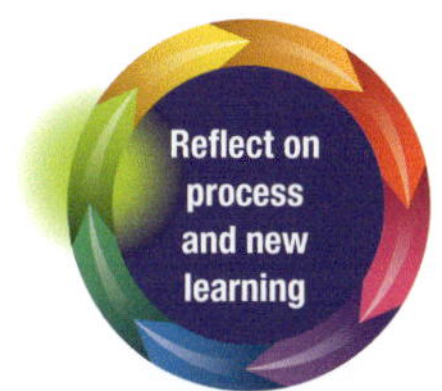

Reflect on your learning from this scenario and consider the following questions.

Q1 What factors led to Trent's deterioration? Were they preventable?
Q2 What are three of the most important things that you have learnt from this scenario?
Q3 What actions will you take in clinical practice as a result of your learning from this scenario?

SCENARIO 6.2 Caring for a person with respiratory distress

CHANGING THE SCENE

1. CONSIDER THE PATIENT SITUATION

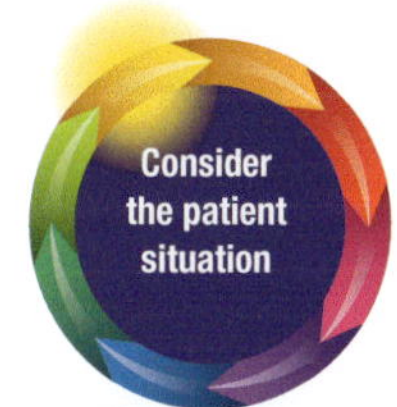

Trent responds well to his treatment and, although he has been spiking temperatures during the last few days, he is now afebrile. Although he still feels fatigued at times, Trent wants to go home as the opening date for the gym is fast approaching and he and Ian need to finish the renovations. However, Trent confides in you that he is feeling anxious as he has had increasing episodes of what he describes as 'chest tightness' over the last two days.

In preparation for this scenario, access the *Australian Asthma Handbook* at www.nationalasthma.org.au/health-professionals/australian-asthma-handbook

Q1 Label the following as either *objective* or *subjective* clinical data.
a Increased pulse rate
b A nurse's assessment of a patient's temperature
c A patient's report of breathlessness
d Trent's complaint of chest tightness

Q2 To further understand Trent's 'chest tightness', you would collect information about which of the following? (Select all you consider to be appropriate.)
a Circulation
b Respiration
c Skin
d Pain
e Sleep/rest pattern
f Coping strategies
g Musculoskeletal system

Q3 Which communication strategy would be most effective when assessing Trent's 'chest tightness'? (Select three correct responses.)
a Using a calm tone of voice
b Observing Trent's behaviours and respiratory effort
c Assessing Trent's concerns while at the same time attending to other tasks and patients
d Open-ended questions
e Closed questions

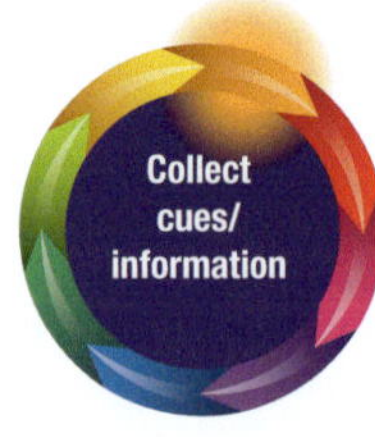

2. COLLECT CUES/INFORMATION

(a) Review current information

You review Trent's charts and note the following:

Temperature	37°C
Pulse rate	110 beats/min
Respiratory rate	26 breaths/min
Blood pressure	140/85 mmHg
SpO_2	94% on room air
Hourly urine output (average)	40 mL/hr
Breath sounds	Wheezing on auscultation
BGL	6.2 mmol/L

Q1 Which of these observations are not within normal limits?

Q2 While you are talking with Trent, he tells you that he had a vision where an angel came and watched over him. From the following list, choose how you would respond.

- a This probably occurred because you were hypoxic.
- b You were very ill at the time; it must be comforting to believe that someone was looking after you.
- c It was probably one of the nurses as angels don't exist.
- d Only a Catholic could believe that they saw an angel.

(b) Gather new information

Q You note that Trent is dyspnoeic. What respiratory assessments are required at this stage?

(c) Recall knowledge

Quick Quiz!

Q1 A wheeze is caused by:

- a Collapsed alveoli
- b Fluid in the alveoli
- c Narrowed airways
- d Collapsed lungs

Q2 An asthma exacerbation can be caused by substances released from mast cells which cause:

- a Smooth muscle dilation
- b Bronchodilation and capillary permeability
- c Broncho-constriction and inflammation
- d Decreased capillary permeability and fluid leakage

Q3 FEV_1 can be defined as:

- a The rate of gas exchange in the alveoli during normal respiration
- b The maximum amount of air a person is capable of blowing in one second
- c The amount of air left in the lungs at the end of maximal forced expiration
- d The amount of air that is breathed in and out during a single respiratory cycle

Q4 Expiration occurs when:

- a The intercostal muscles and diaphragm relax
- b The intercostal muscles and diaphragm contract
- c The diaphragm rises and the ribs move upward and outward
- d The air pressure inside the thorax decreases and becomes less than external air pressure

3. PROCESS INFORMATION

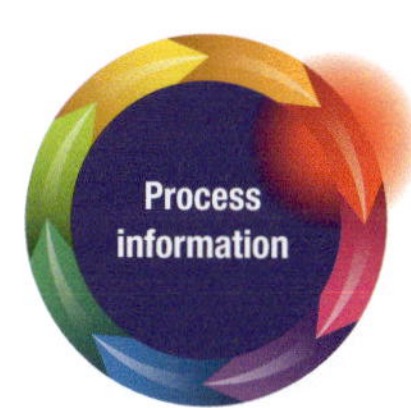

(a) Interpret, (b) Discriminate and (c) Relate

Q1 Which of the following is the *most* characteristic alteration in lung volume caused by air trapping in asthma?

- a Tidal volume
- b Inspiratory reserve volume
- c Expiratory reserve volume
- d Functional residual capacity

Q2 Which of the following is *necessary* to diagnose asthma?

- a Reversibility of airflow limitation
- b Reduced FEV_1
- c Reduced FVC
- d Irreversibility of airflow limitation

Q3 Which of the following is *not* suggestive of asthma?

- a Chest tightness that recurs
- b Cough that becomes worse at night
- c Stridor
- d Wheezing

Q4 Which of the following are characteristic of asthma? (Select three.)

- a Clubbing of the fingers
- b Cough
- c Chest tightness
- d Barrel chest
- e Chest pain
- f Wheeze

(d) Infer

Q Which of the following factors might indicate asthma? (Select all that you consider appropriate.)

- a Presence of coarse rales (crackles)
- b Worsening symptoms after taking aspirin or beta-blockers
- c Worsening signs and symptoms after exposure to an identified allergy trigger
- d A previous allergic reaction of any kind

(e) Predict

Q Identify two factors from the following list that would *not* put Trent at an increased risk of deterioration.

- a Previous ICU admissions
- b Infrequent, mild asthma attacks
- c Asthma requiring use of a reliever occasionally (once a month)
- d Current or recent use of oral corticosteroids
- e Previous severe exacerbations requiring hospitalisation

(f) Match

Q Have you seen someone with the same signs and symptoms as Trent? If so, what was done to manage the situation?

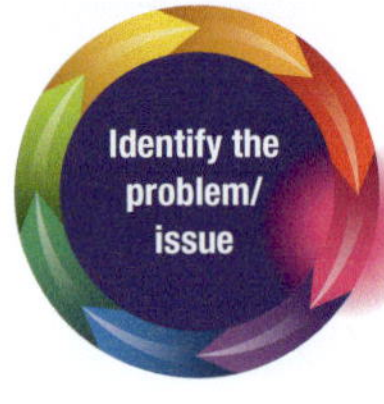

4. IDENTIFY THE PROBLEM/ISSUE

The current information that you have collected about Trent includes:

Temperature	37°C
Pulse rate	120
Respiratory rate	26
Blood pressure	140/85
Oxygen saturation level	93% on room air
Hourly urine output (average)	40 mL/hr
BGL	6.2 mmol/L
Breath sounds	Wheezing on auscultation
Cough	Productive
Spirometry	Airflow limitation
Chest tightness	
Fatigue	

Q Use the information collected to complete the following nursing diagnoses for Trent.

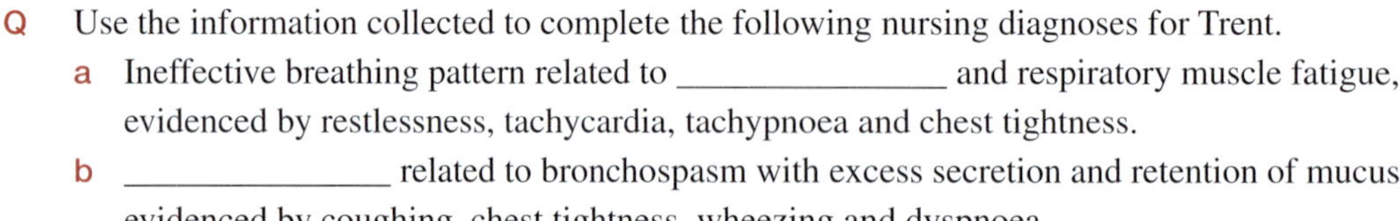

- a Ineffective breathing pattern related to _______________ and respiratory muscle fatigue, evidenced by restlessness, tachycardia, tachypnoea and chest tightness.
- b _______________ related to bronchospasm with excess secretion and retention of mucus, evidenced by coughing, chest tightness, wheezing and dyspnoea.

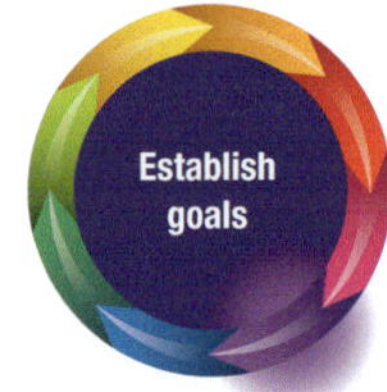

5. ESTABLISH GOALS

Q1 In relation to the nursing identified diagnoses, what are the two *most* appropriate short-term goals of management for Trent?

- a For Trent to have clear lung sounds and a reduced amount of secretions
- b For Trent to be able to resume his normal exercise regime
- c For Trent to have effective gas exchange, without dyspnoea or tachypnoea and with normal SpO_2 level
- d For Trent to have normal food and fluid intake

Q2 Side effects of bronchodilators that Trent may experience are:

- a Insomnia and restless legs
- b Dry mouth and furry tongue
- c Palpitations, tachycardia and tremors
- d Eye-watering and runny nose

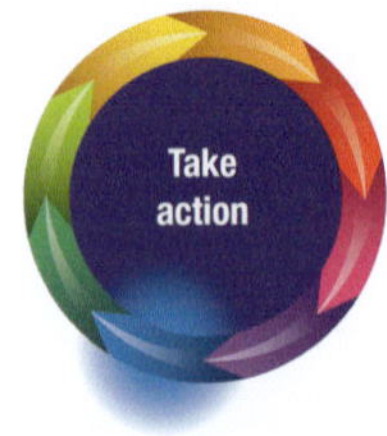

6. TAKE ACTION

Q In the table below, match the nursing action you would take to the appropriate rationale, in order to achieve appropriate short-term goals.

Rationale

- To promote self-management
- To aid in bronchodilation
- To conserve energy and reduce fatigue
- To detect increasing respiratory distress
- To reduce hypoxaemia
- To increase lung expansion

Nursing action	Rationale
Place in high Fowler's position	
Administer oxygen	
Administer nebuliser/spacer as ordered	
Assess level of understanding of asthma management	
Monitor vital signs	
Assist with ADLs as needed	

Trent is reviewed by the doctor who starts him on a preventer medication—fluticasone and salmeterol (Seretide), an inhaled corticosteroid—with a spacer, and long-acting β_2-agonist combination therapy. He is continued on the short-acting β_2-agonist, salbutamol (Ventolin), as a reliever therapy and commenced on home monitoring of his peak expiratory flow rate. He is also referred to the asthma physician and educator for review of his asthma management plan in preparation for discharge.

Patient Safety Competency Framework (PSCF)

Domain 9–Medication safety

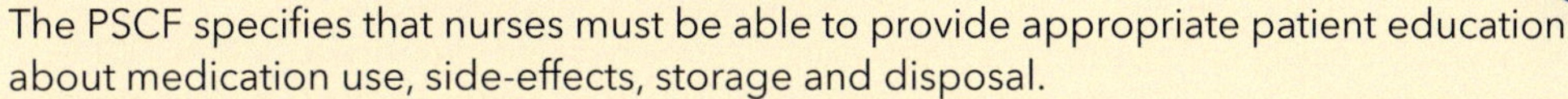

The PSCF specifies that nurses must be able to provide appropriate patient education about medication use, side-effects, storage and disposal.

Source: *The Patient Safety Competency Framework for Nursing Students*, https://patientsafetyfornursingstudents.org

7. EVALUATE

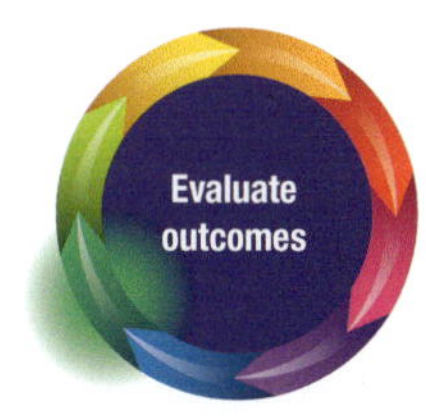

Q Which of the following signs and symptoms would indicate that, following clinical review and initiation of appropriate actions, Trent's condition has improved?

a Oxygen saturations > than 95%

b Respiratory rate >20

c Heart rate 60–100

d BP > 150/90

e Signs of anxiety absent or decreased

8. REFLECT

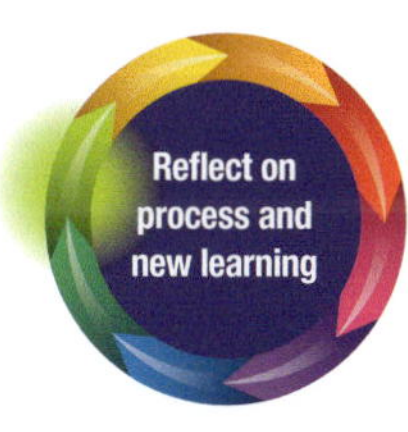

Reflect on what happened to Trent and the care he received. Answer the following questions.

Q1 How could Trent's deterioration have been prevented?

Q2 What have you learnt from the scenario that you can apply to your future practice?

Q3 Based on what you have learnt from this scenario, what advice would you give to people with asthma?

EPILOGUE

The gym opening had to be delayed for a few weeks while Trent recovered, but it was successfully launched two months later. Trent remained well with no further respiratory infections. He visited his GP, respiratory physician and asthma educator and, with their help, developed a written asthma management plan and optimised his asthma management knowledge and skills (National Asthma Council Australia, 2021). He continues to take his preventer medication as prescribed and regularly monitors his peak flow rate. He has also made some changes to his lifestyle, including spending more time warming up before running and taking his reliever before exercising. He decided not to participate in the marathon but plans to compete in next year's City to Surf race. Trent has his asthma reviewed by his GP every six months and whenever his symptoms start to flare up.

FURTHER READING

Reddel, H., FitzGerald, J., Bateman, E., Bacharier, L., Becker, A., Brusselle, . . . Boulet, L. (2019). GINA 2019: A fundamental change in asthma management: Treatment of asthma with short-acting bronchodilators alone is no longer recommended for adults and adolescents. *European Respiratory Journal, 53*(6), 1901046, doi: 10.1183/13993003.01046–2019

Rolfe S. (2019). The importance of respiratory rate monitoring. *British Journal of Nursing, 28*(8), 504–08, doi: 10.12968/bjon.2019.28.8.504

Winders, T. A., Wilson, A. M., Fletcher, M. J., McGuinness, A., Price, D. B. (2019). A patient-centered description of severe asthma: Patient understanding leading to assessment for a severe asthma referral (PULSAR). *Patient, 12*(5): 539–49, doi: 10.1007/s40271-019-00371-0

REFERENCES

Australian Bureau of Statistics (ABS). (2020). *Causes of Death, Australia 2019*. Retrieved from: https://www.abs.gov.au/statistics/health/causes-death/causes-death-australia/2019

Australian Commission on Safety and Quality in Health Care (ACSQHC). (2021). *National Safety and Quality Health Service Standards* (2nd edn), Sydney, Australia. Retrieved from: https://www.safetyandquality.gov.au/publications-and-resources/resource-library/national-safety-and-quality-health-service-standards-second-edition

Australian Institute of Health and Welfare (AIHW). (2018). *Asthma 2017–18 Financial Year*. Retrieved from: https://www.abs.gov.au/statistics/health/health-conditions-and-risks/asthma/2017-18

Australian Institute of Health and Welfare (AIHW). (2020). *Australia's Health 2020*. Australia's health snapshots 2020. Retrieved from: https://www.aihw.gov.au/reports-data/australias-health/australias-health-snapshots

Craig, S., Cubitt, M., Jaison, A., Troupakis, S., Hood, N., Fong, C., . . . Cameron, P. (2020). Management of adult cardiac arrest in the COVID–19 era: Consensus statement from the Australasian College for Emergency Medicine. *Medical Journal of Australia*, *213*(3), 126–33. doi.org/10.5694/mja2.50699

Kloehs, A. & Hales, M. (2020). A person-centred approach to assessing the respiratory system. In P. LeMone, G. Bauldoff, P. Gubrud-Howe, M.-A. Carno, T. Levett-Jones, . . . D. Stanley (Eds), *LeMone and Burke's Medical–Surgical Nursing: Critical Thinking for Person-Centred Care* (4th edn). Melbourne: Pearson.

Levett-Jones, T., Dwyer, T., Reid-Searl, K., Heaton, L., Flenady, T., Applegarth, J., Guinea, S. & Andersen, P. (2017). *Patient Safety Competency Framework (PSCF) for Nursing Students*. Retrieved from: http://psframework.wpengine.com/wp-content/uploads/2018/01/PSCF_Brochure_UTS-version_FA2-Screen.pdf

National Asthma Council Australia. (2021). *Asthma Action Plan*. Retrieved from: www.nationalasthma.org.au/health-professionals/asthma-action-plans

Nursing and Midwifery Board of Australia (NMBA). (2016). *Registered Nurse Standards for Practice*. Retrieved from: www.nursingmidwiferyboard.gov.au/Codes-Guidelines-Statements/Professional-standards.aspx

Chapter 7

Caring for a person with a cardiac condition

SAMANTHA JAKIMOWICZ and BELINDA CAUSBY

LEARNING OUTCOMES

Completion of the activities in this chapter will enable you to:

- explain why an understanding of ischaemia and arrhythmias is essential to competent practice (**recall** and **application**)
- identify the clinical manifestations of chest pain that will guide the collection and interpretation of cues (**gather, review, interpret, discriminate, relate** and **infer**)
- identify risk factors for cardiac conditions (**match** and **predict**)
- review clinical information to identify the main nursing diagnoses for a person with cardiac conditions (**synthesise**)
- describe the priorities of care for a person with a cardiac condition (**goal setting** and **taking action**)
- identify clinical criteria for determining the effectiveness of nursing actions when managing chest pain and arrhythmias (**evaluate**)
- apply what you have learnt about cardiac conditions and ischaemia to new clinical situations with different patients (**reflection** and **translation**).

INTRODUCTION

This chapter focuses on the care of Mr David Parker, a 55-year-old man who experiences a prolonged episode of chest pain and is admitted to the regional hospital near where he lives. Accurate assessment of a person presenting with chest pain requires well-developed clinical reasoning skills and a sound knowledge base.

Early presentation to health services in the event of chest pain is a key factor that can influence positive clinical outcomes (Chew et al., 2016). Although 66 per cent of people who present to hospital with chest pain are admitted, only 15 per cent are confirmed to have had an acute myocardial infarction (AMI). However, rates of mortality for those who *are not* admitted are up to four times higher than those who *are* admitted, as up to 5 per cent of those not admitted will have had a missed AMI (Yan et al., 2020). Geographical location also impacts clinical outcomes, with mortality rates following AMI significantly worse for those in remote areas (Beck et al., 2016). Consequently, coronary heart disease is the leading cause of death in remote areas of Australia (Australian Institute for Health and Wellbeing [AIHW], 2020). In addition to geographical location, outcomes from acute cardiac events are influenced by delayed presentation to hospital, the capabilities of the rural or remote health services and knowledge of the person experiencing the cardiac event (Beck et al., 2016).

KEY CONCEPTS

chest pain
arrhythmias
ischaemia
cardiac arrest
heart failure
rehabilitation

SUGGESTED READINGS

P. LeMone, G. Bauldoff, P. Gubrud-Howe, M.-A. Carno, T. Levett-Jones, . . . D. Stanley (Eds). (2020). *LeMone and Burke's Medical–Surgical Nursing: Critical Thinking in Person-Centred Care* (4th edn). Melbourne: Pearson Australia.

Chapter 28: A person-centred approach to assessing the cardiac and lymphatic systems

Chapter 29: Nursing care of people with coronary heart disease

Chapter 30: Nursing care of people with cardiac disorders

SCENARIO 7.1 Caring for a person with ischaemic chest pain

SETTING THE SCENE

You are a registered nurse (RN) working in the emergency department (ED) of a regional hospital in the Snowy Mountains area when David Parker, a middle-aged man, is brought in by ambulance. His wife, Sophie, arrives at the same time through the main entrance. The man is sitting upright on the ambulance trolley with an oxygen mask over his ashen-grey face. He is diaphoretic and gripping the trolley with his right hand while his left hand is held close to his body holding an emesis bowl. He looks frightened. His wife rushes forward, telling him, 'Everything will be alright. You'll be fine.' She turns to you and asks, 'Won't he?'

The ambulance officer tells you that David was repairing fences on his property and the chest pain started when lifting heavy fence posts. He returned to the farmhouse and took some antacids but the pain continued. He had about two hours of central chest pain prior to his collapse at 1200 hours. He did not lose consciousness. Sophie called the ambulance against his wishes as he had 'a lot of things to do'. The ambulance officer estimated the chest pain started at 1000 hours and it took the ambulance 90 minutes to get to the property and back. David's chest pain is centrally located and described as crushing. The pain is radiating to his left arm, neck and teeth. He is anxious and worried about his farm where he runs large mobs of merino sheep. David is tachycardic and hypertensive. He has a history of hypertension but it is usually well controlled.

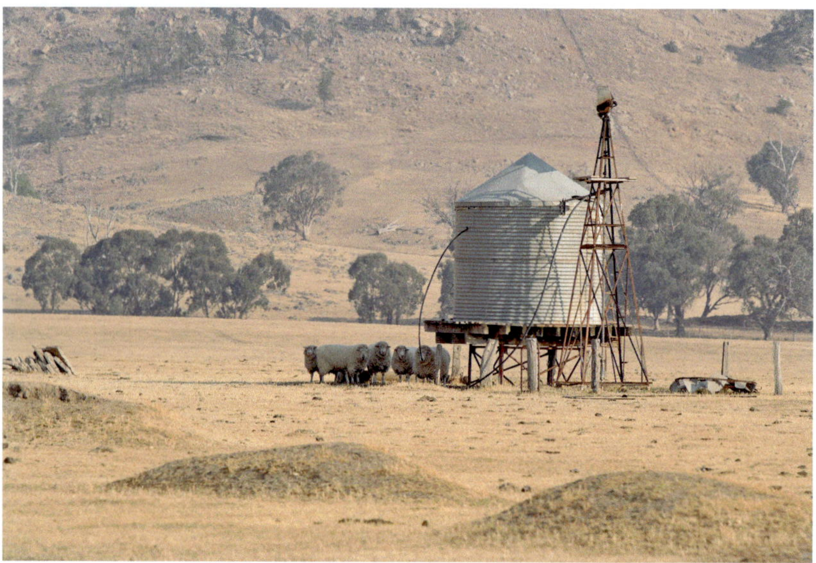

David Parker's farm in the Snowy Mountains, New South Wales

The epidemiology of ischaemic chest pain and heart failure

View this website for cardiovascular disease mortality and trends at different ages: https://www.aihw.gov.au/reports/heart-stroke-vascular-diseases/cardiovascular-health-compendium/contents/deaths-from-cardiovascular-disease

The most common form of cardiovascular disease (CVD) is coronary heart disease (CHD), also known as ischaemic heart disease (IHD). There are two major clinical forms of CHD:

1. 'Heart attack', clinically known as acute myocardial infarction (AMI)
2. Angina.

The AIHW (2020) report CHD as being responsible for 11 per cent of all deaths in Australia. In 2018, over 17,500 deaths were attributed to CHD—more than any other single disease—and of these, 42 per cent were from an acute AMI (AIHW, 2020). Death rates from CHD have fallen steadily since the 1970s, not because there are fewer heart attacks but because of better survival rates (AIHW, 2020). CHD occurs more frequently in older people (1.1% in those aged 45–54, rising to 13.9% in Australians aged 75 years or over [AIHW, 2020]). Men are twice as likely to experience CHD as women, and CHD is 2.6 times more common in Aboriginal and Torres Strait Islander people than in non-Indigenous Australians (AIHW, 2020).

The aetiology and pathogenesis of ischaemic chest pain and heart failure

The main cause of CHD is atherosclerosis, where lipids accumulate in the arteries forming a build-up called plaque. Blood flow through the coronary arteries becomes impaired by plaque as it reduces the lumen of these vessels. Plaque lesions may ulcerate, leading to clot (thrombus) formation that may completely block or occlude the vessel. The manifestations of CHD are angina pectoris, acute coronary syndrome and/or myocardial infarction. Chest pain precipitated by exercise (which increases oxygen demand) and relieved by rest (when oxygen meets myocardial demand) is the main characteristic of angina (LeMone et al., 2019).

More information on risk prevention for CVD can be obtained from: www.heartfoundation.org.au/heart-health-education/are-you-at-risk-of-heart-disease.

If a coronary artery becomes completely occluded, blood supply to the myocardium is interrupted and the affected muscle tissue becomes ischaemic (acute coronary syndrome). These ischaemic tissues will eventually die if blood supply is not restored (myocardial infarction). Risk factors for CHD may be modifiable or non-modifiable and include age, heredity, hypertension, high serum cholesterol, diabetes mellitus and lifestyle factors, such as smoking, obesity and lack of exercise. Some of these risk factors are more common in Aboriginal and Torres Strait Islander people, with diabetes being four times higher, and smoking and obesity twice as common in this population.

Heart failure is the most common disorder of cardiac function. It occurs as a result of impaired myocardial contraction. The heart cannot fill or contract with sufficient strength, so its ability to act as a pump is compromised. This 'pump failure' means there is less blood leaving the heart (cardiac output) and less oxygen reaching the body tissues (tissue perfusion). Hypertension is the leading cause of heart failure and the most common risk factor is CHD.

The best treatment option for an AMI is percutaneous coronary intervention (PCI), provided an angiography laboratory is available. When this is not available, thrombolytic treatment is used to try to dissolve the clot. For more information, access the *Acute Coronary Syndrome Clinical Care Standard* at: https://safetyandquality.gov.au/wp-content/uploads/2014/12/Acute-Coronary-Syndromes-Clinical-Care-Standard.pdf

Admission to the emergency department

On admission to the ED, David is diaphoretic and pale. He is alert and orientated but very anxious with central chest pain. The doctor examines him and orders a stat dose of IV morphine. David's ECG is attended and shows ischaemic injury (ST elevation) in the anterior leads. As ST elevation indicates a coronary artery blockage, treatment is aimed at unblocking the vessel.

The doctor asks David if he has any history of head injuries, malignancies, stroke or gastric bleeding to ensure there are no contraindications for thrombolytic treatment. No risk factors are identified and David is given thrombolytic therapy.

Nurse-administered thrombolysis (NAT) is a model of care for rural and remote hospitals that do not have 24-hour onsite doctors. The fact sheet for NAT (Agency for Clinical Innovation [ACI], 2016) can be accessed at: www.aci.health.nsw.gov.au/__data/assets/pdf_file/0011/319196/NAT-clinican.pdf

Admission observations

Temperature	36.8°C
Pulse rate	108 beats/min
Respiratory rate	24 breaths/min
Blood pressure	150/90 mmHg
SpO_2	95% on room air
BGL	14.1 mmol/L
Pain score	8
GCS	15

Co-morbidities

- Osteoarthritis
- Hypertension
- Hyperlipidaemia
- Type 2 diabetes mellitus

Medical orders

- Full blood count (FBC)
- Urea, electrolytes and creatinine (UECs)
- Arterial blood gases (ABGs)
- Troponin levels

- Start GTN infusion and titrate to blood pressure and pain; maintain diastolic >60 mmHg
- Morphine 2.5 mg IV PRN
- Start rTPA

Quick Quiz!

Q1 The __________ has the thickest walls as it pumps blood to __________. Choose the correct responses from the options below.

a Right atrium, systemic circulation
b Right ventricle, pulmonary circulation
c Left atrium, pulmonary circulation
d Left ventricle, systemic circulation

Q2 Freshly oxygenated blood enters the heart through the __________, and is pumped out into the __________. Choose the correct responses from the options below.

a Right atrium, aorta
b Left atrium, aorta
c Right ventricle, pulmonary arteries
d Left ventricle, pulmonary arteries

Q3 Why do you think the ambulance officer was so precise in his estimation of times in David's admission story?

Person-centred care

Awareness of David's life story will assist you in understanding his responses to his situation, and in providing person-centred care. David is an Aboriginal man who was part of the 'stolen generation'. He was raised in a foster home in the region where he now lives. His childhood and adolescent life were difficult, although he managed to complete his schooling. He has no contact with any biological family members and does not know his family or medical history. He believes that the past should remain 'where it can't hurt'.

David's foster family had a large property where he developed skills in animal husbandry, including breeding fine wool merino sheep. After school, he worked as a farm hand and, later, as a manager on the property where he now lives. David has a very strong work ethic and sense of responsibility. He married a local woman, Sophie, who is a teacher at the local high school, and they have two teenage children. David's family describe him as 'driven' and as having difficulty relaxing. David smokes but he drinks alcohol only occasionally.

At this stage, if you were the RN caring for David, would you refer him to the Aboriginal Liaison Officer?

Patient Safety Competency Framework (PSCF)

Domain 3–Cultural competence

The importance of cultural competence is clearly articulated in the PSCF. Cultural competence encompasses 'the willingness to adapt practice to meet the needs of people from diverse cultures, and the ability to interact with persons from cultures and/or belief systems different to one's own'.

Source: *The Patient Safety Competency Framework for Nursing Students*, https://patientsafetyfornursingstudents.org

Cultural competence

Hospitals and healthcare settings are sometimes feared by Aboriginal and Torres Strait Islander people as they may have previously experienced insensitivity to their culture, racism or mistreatment. David's cultural background must be considered in order to provide person-centred, culturally safe care. Most healthcare services offer specific resources to support Aboriginal and Torres Strait Islander peoples and a referral to an Aboriginal Liaison Officer should also be made. The person in this role is usually an Aboriginal health worker who provides non-clinical services such as advocacy and support during the person's hospital stay (NSW Health, 2018).

National Safety and Quality Health Service (NSQH) Standards

Communicating for safety standard

The NSQHS Standards specify that *health service organisations* must provide a 'timely, purpose-driven and effective communication and documentation (strategy) that supports continuous, coordinated and safe care for patients' (ACSQHC, 2021). The criteria included in the *Communicating for safety* standard include partnering with consumers, structured clinical handover and communication of critical information, especially at a time of risk; for example, during an in-hospital cardiac arrest. It is vitally important for multi-disciplinary teams to use specific communication frameworks (e.g., the ISBAR handover tool) to ensure a global understanding of what is being conveyed (ACSQHC, 2021).

1. CONSIDER THE PATIENT SITUATION

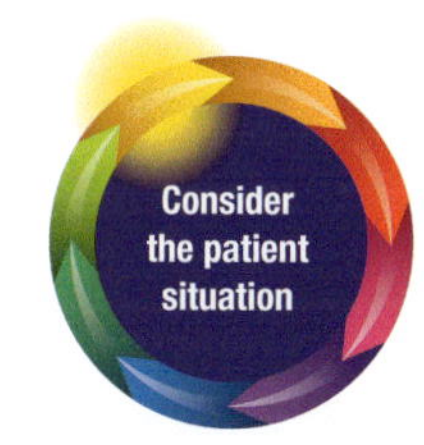

David has been admitted to the coronary care unit. It is now eight hours since David's acute myocardial infarction (AMI) was confirmed. He has been increasingly agitated since his admission, wanting to call the farm and check with his employees as it is lambing season. He has been rudely ordering his wife, Sophie, to bring his mobile phone and he has been increasingly abrupt with the staff.

1400 hours—Handover report

This is David Parker, a 55-year-old man with ACS, brought in by ambulance earlier today with chest pain. He's a type 2 diabetic, diet controlled, and his hypertension and cholesterol are managed and monitored by his GP. On admission, his pain was 7/10, central with some radiation into his jaw, associated with nausea and breathlessness. He was initially treated in ED with anginine and morphine, but the IV GTN is continuing to manage his pain. He's a STEMI and had rTPA in ED. He was supposed to have had a cardiology review last month but couldn't get away from work to attend. He manages a sheep farm and his wife works here in town. His troponin's back and it's pretty high at 0.25 µg/L. I'm a bit worried. He's been anxious this afternoon. I would have asked his wife and children to leave, however it is important to consider his cultural background. I have contacted the Aboriginal Liaison Officer who may be able to offer some support. I don't think he's being honest about his pain as all he wants to do is get back to work.

Quick Quiz!

Test your understanding of abbreviations and terminologies used in this handover report by selecting the correct response for each of the following.

Q1 What does ACS mean?

- a Acute cardiac syndrome
- b Actual coronary sickness
- c Acute coronary syndrome
- d Acute cardiac sickness

Q2 What does GTN mean?

- a Glycerol trinitrate
- b Glycerine tartrate
- c Glycerol tartrate
- d Glycerine trinitrate

Q3 What are the two signs of a myocardial infarction that may be seen on an ECG?

- a ST depression
- b ST elevation
- c Abnormal Q-wave development
- d Abnormal P-wave development

Q4 What does STEMI mean?

- a Standard total emergency myocardial infarction
- b ST elevation myocardial infarction
- c ST emergency myocardial infarction
- d Standard total evolving myocardial infarction

Q5 Normal troponin T level is less than 0.14 µg/L.

- a True
- b False

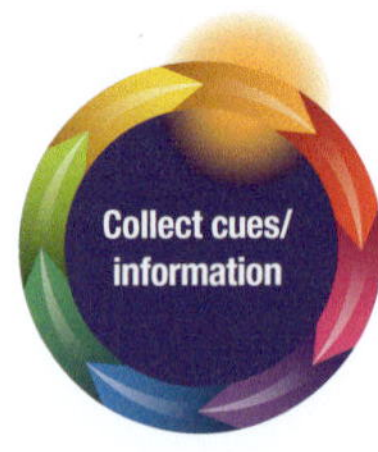

2. COLLECT CUES/INFORMATION

Access the National Heart Foundation (2021) site to review 'Are you at risk of heart disease?': www.heartfoundation.org.au/heart-health-education/are-you-at-risk-of-heart-disease

Q1 From the list below, identify the cue that is *not* relevant to your assessment of David at this time.

a 12-lead ECG
b Potassium level
c Blood pressure
d Sodium level
e Pain score
f Alcohol withdrawal score

Q2 As soon as David is stable, you plan to collect the following information to complete your assessment of his risk factors. Which cue will you *not* be able to collect?

a Weight
b Smoking history
c Alcohol consumption history
d Family history of cardiac conditions
e History of depression

Q3 The normal ST segment on an ECG is usually iso-electric.

a True
b False

(a) Review current information

Towards the end of the day, you are outside David's room preparing his medications and you hear him speaking to his wife Sophie, saying, 'Where is my mobile phone? I told you to bring it hours ago. Why are the kids here? They don't need a day off school just because I'm stuck in here! I'm alright, I tell you. Why is everyone carrying on so much?' David pauses and then Sophie calls out, 'David? Nurse! Quickly! Something's wrong with David!' You enter the room to find him slumped in the bed with the following heart rhythm on the continuous cardiac monitor:

Visit this resource for assistance in understanding cardiac rhythms: https://www.practicalclinicalskills.com/ekg

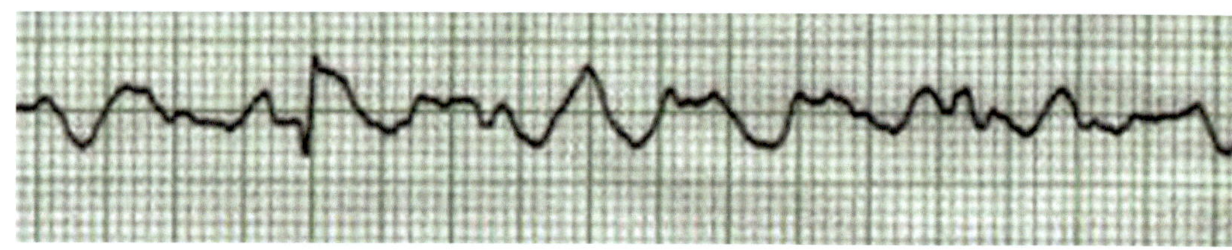

(b) Gather new information

Q1 What does the T wave on the ECG indicate is happening in the heart?

a The atria have depolarised.
b The ventricles are depolarising.
c The ventricles have repolarised.
d The atria are repolarising.

Q2 Cardiac output is calculated by:

a Heart rate minus stroke volume
b Stroke volume divided by heart rate
c Heart rate plus stroke volume
d Heart rate multiplied by stroke volume.

Q3 David is in cardiopulmonary arrest.

a True
b False

(c) Recall knowledge

Caring for patients with coronary conditions requires knowledge and understanding of cardiac physiology, pathophysiology, pharmacology, epidemiology and therapeutics.

The chart at the following link provides information on managing coronary conditions: www.heartfoundation.org.au/getmedia/669ddeab-205e-4974-b591-8bff0e6ee31d/Assessment_protocol_for_suspected_ACS_using_point-of-care_assay-2016.pdf

Quick Quiz!

Test your understanding of risk factors for coronary conditions by answering the following question.

Q Select from the following list, the five groups of people most likely to be affected by coronary disease.

a People over 55 years of age
b Sportsmen/women
c Alcoholics
d Men
e Obese people
f Healthy middle-aged women
g Aboriginal and Torres Strait Islander people
h People with diabetes mellitus
i People with cancer

3. PROCESS INFORMATION

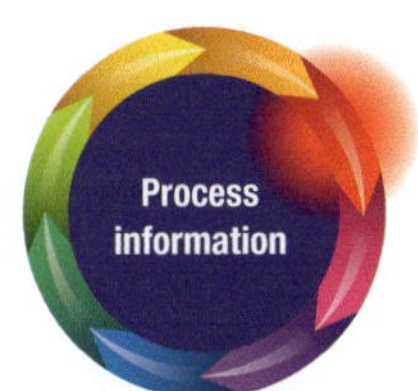

(a) Interpret

You review and interpret all the information you have about David's condition.

Q1 The monitor is showing ventricular fibrillation.

a True
b False

Q2 What is the most likely cause for this rhythm?

a He is experiencing a reperfusion arrhythmia due to the GTN infusion.
b He is experiencing an allergic reaction to repeated doses of morphine.
c He is experiencing a reperfusion arrhythmia following the dose of rTPA.
d He is experiencing an arrhythmia due to hypoxia from his AMI.

When calling the rapid response team, the RN caring for David would use ISBAR to provide handover to ensure effective communication in accordance with the *Communicating for safety* standard (ACSQHC, 2017). Adhering to this safety standard will provide the safest care possible for David during a time of high risk.

Q3 The rapid response team arrives and takes over the CPR that you have started. Place the following actions in the correct order.

Actions

- Check monitor and assess rhythm as shockable or non-shockable
- Deliver shock
- Attach defibrillator pads
- Continue CPR

Order	Action
1	
2	
3	
4	

Access *ARC Guideline 11.1—Introduction to and Principles of In-hospital Resuscitation* in the Australian Resuscitation Council guidelines for help in answering this question: https://resus.org.au/guidelines

Q4 The ratio of breaths to compressions in basic life support is:

a 15:1

b 15:2

c 30:2

d 40:2

Q5 Which of the following rhythms is a 'shockable' rhythm?

a Asystole

b Ventricular tachycardia with a pulse

c Ventricular tachycardia without a pulse

d Pulseless electrical activity

(b) Discriminate

From the cues and information you now have, you need to narrow down the information to what is most important.

Q1 What information do you think is *not* particularly important at this time?

a Impaired cardiac conduction due to a reperfusion arrhythmia

b Hypoxia due to impaired circulation

c Impaired cardiac output

d Impaired glucose metabolism

Q2 In the list in Q1, what is the *most* important information at this time?

a Impaired cardiac conduction due to a reperfusion arrhythmia

b Hypoxia due to impaired circulation

c Impaired cardiac output

d Impaired glucose metabolism

(c) Relate

It is important to understand and cluster the cues you have collected so far.

Q1 Label the following statements *true* or *false*.

a Ventricular fibrillation causes ineffective quivering of the ventricles.

b Ventricular fibrillation has a regular pattern.

c Ventricular fibrillation has a rate exceeding 300 beats/min.

d Ventricular fibrillation has identifiable R waves.

Q2 Select the *most* important cue cluster for a patient with ventricular fibrillation.

a Audible heartbeat, no palpable pulse, normal respirations, non-responsiveness

b No audible heartbeat, a weak thready pulse, no respirations, diminishing responsiveness

c No audible heartbeat, no palpable pulse, no respirations, normal responsiveness

d No audible heartbeat, no palpable pulse, no respirations, non-responsiveness

(d) Infer

Think about all the cues that you have collected about David's condition and make inferences based on your analysis and interpretation of those cues.

Q Consider the following two statements and choose the one that is *most* correct.

a David is experiencing a cardiac arrest and will be defibrillated to deliver an electric current to the left ventricle so that it can re-establish the heart's pumping action and increase cardiac output.

b David is experiencing a cardiac arrest and will be defibrillated to deliver an electric current to depolarise a critical mass of cardiac cells so that, when the cells repolarise, the sinus node can recapture its role as the heart's pacemaker.

David is successfully defibrillated and his rhythm is re-established as sinus rhythm. You obtain another set of observations with the following results:

Pulse rate	65 beats/min
Respiratory rate	24 breaths/min
Blood pressure	100/60 mmHg
SpO_2	100% on 15 L/m with a non-rebreather mask

The rapid response team hand over care to the treating medical team and leave. You go with the doctor to speak to Mrs Parker. The doctor tells her that David is now stable. Initially, he had ischaemic changes in his anterior leads on ECG, indicating a blockage in his left anterior descending artery. This has damaged his heart muscle, as indicated by the troponin level. It appears the thrombolytic has unblocked this; however, this treatment may also have caused the change in his heart rhythm. You explain that more time is needed to determine the extent of damage to the heart.

(e) Predict and (f) Match

At this stage, you need to consider the potential outcomes for David, as this will guide your actions.

Q David may experience a number of healthcare issues as a result of the AMI and episode of ventricular fibrillation. In the following table, match the potential condition to the outcome.

Condition

- ... unless his family can identify a management strategy to address his concerns.
- ... if his myocardial demand can be reduced through oxygen supply, medication and bed rest.
- ... if he experiences no further arrhythmias.
- ... if there is myocardial damage and the pumping ability of the left ventricle is compromised.

Outcome	Condition
David's condition may gradually improve and he may have no adverse effects	
David's vital signs may continue within normal parameters	
David may experience signs of heart failure	
David may experience more chest pain as a result of his anxiety	

4. IDENTIFY THE PROBLEM/ISSUE

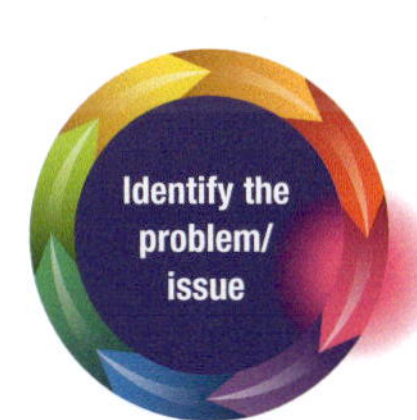

Q Now bring together (synthesise) all of the facts you've collected and inferences you've made to determine David's nursing diagnoses. Which of the following are correct nursing diagnoses for David at this time?

a Chronic pain related to tissue ischemia, evidenced by facial grimacing, restlessness, changes in level of consciousness, changes in pulse rate and/or blood pressure

b Acute pain related to tissue ischemia, evidenced by further reports of chest pain with or without radiation, facial grimacing, restlessness, changes in level of consciousness, changes in pulse rate and/or blood pressure

c Risk of fluid volume deficit (hypovolaemia) related to decreased sodium/water retention

d Risk of fluid volume excess (hypervolaemia) related to increased sodium/water retention

e Risk of decreased cardiac output related to changes in rate, rhythm and electrical conduction

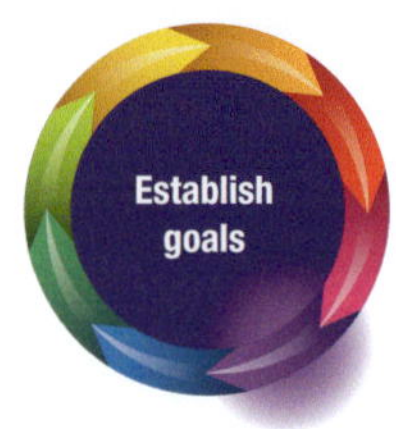

5. ESTABLISH GOALS

Before implementing any actions to improve David's condition, it is important to clearly specify what you want to happen and when.

Q From the following list of goals for David's management, choose the five most important *short-term* goals.

- a For David to have no chest pain within 20 minutes
- b For David's daily fluid restriction to be maintained during his admission
- c For David to have no evidence of impaired gas exchange within one hour
- d For David to participate in education and adhere to a self-care program following discharge
- e For David to be normotensive and have a pulse rate in acceptable parameters within two hours
- f For David to be free from anxiety by using stress reduction techniques within five days
- g For David's next ECG to show no signs of ischaemia
- h For David to understand the reason for each of his medications prior to discharge

Nursing and Midwifery Board of Australia (NMBA) *Registered Nurse Standards for Practice* Effective communication is central to person-centred care and effective therapeutic relationships. The NMBA's *Registered Nurse Standards for Practice* (2016) state that registered nurses must provide support and direct people to resources to optimise their health-related decisions.

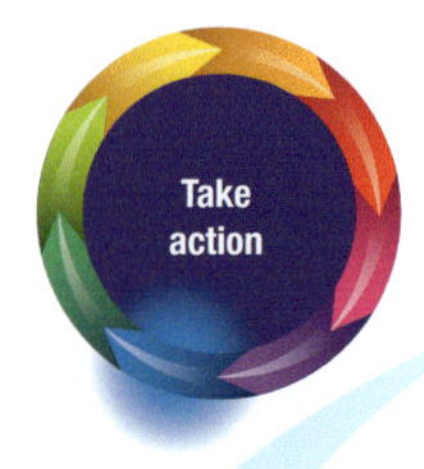

6. TAKE ACTION

You now need to decide which nursing actions take priority and who should be notified, when.

Q Create a care plan for David using the tables below by placing the *short-term nursing goals* into the correct order and matching the nursing actions to the corresponding goals.

You may find this resource helpful in answering this question: www.heartfoundation.org.au/Conditions/FP-ACS-Guidelines

	Short-term nursing goals
1	BP and HR within normal range within two hours
2	No chest pain within 20 minutes
3	No evidence of impaired gas exchange within one hour
4	No evidence of impaired gas exchange within one hour

Nursing actions
Continue antihypertensive therapies
SaO_2 >95%, RR <20 bpm on exertion and <16 bpm at rest
Administer morphine as required
Monitor vital signs continuously
Monitor rhythm continuously; conduct 12-lead ECG during any symptomatic event
Administer oxygen as per protocol
Assess for pain using a visual analogue scale (1 to 10)

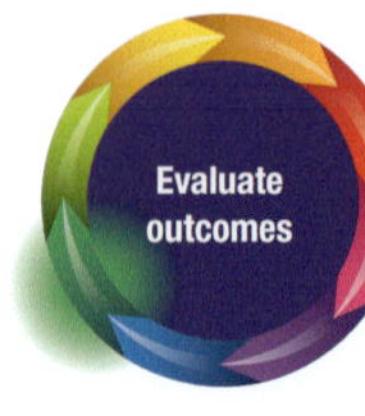

7. EVALUATE

Q Using the following table, identify the trends in David's signs and symptoms that would indicate clinical improvement by matching the appropriate observations to the signs and symptoms.

Desired observation

- Normal range
- 0.5 to 1.0 mL/kg/hr
- 60 bpm and <100 bpm

- <20 on exertion and <16 at rest
- 95%
- Nil
- Within normal range with no postural drop

Sign or symptom	Desired observation
Blood pressure	
Pulse	
Respirations	
Temperature	
Oxygen saturations	
Chest pain level	
Urine output	

8. REFLECT

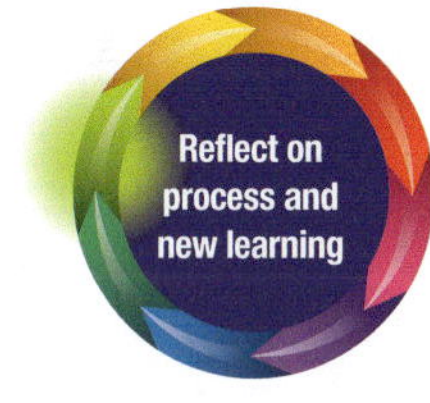

Reflect on your learning from this scenario and consider the following questions.

Q1 What factors led to David's deterioration? Were they predictable and preventable?

Q2 What are three important things you have learnt from this scenario?

SCENARIO 7.2 Caring for a person with heart failure

CHANGING THE SCENE

1. CONSIDER THE PATIENT SITUATION

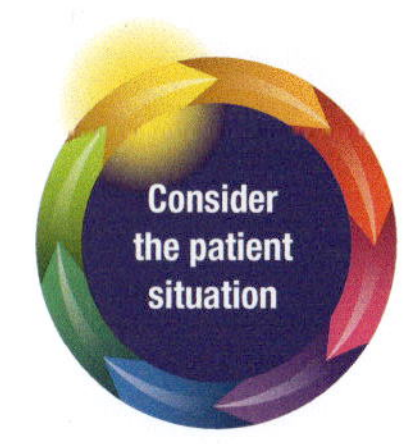

David Parker recovered and was discharged with referrals to an outpatient cardiac rehabilitation program, his general practitioner (GP), a cardiologist and the Aboriginal Liaison Officer. After returning home, David recommenced working on the farm almost immediately as lambing season had begun. He did not attend the cardiac rehabilitation program, saying that driving all the way into town and back would take up too much time. David soon began to experience breathlessness which was worse when lying down and not relieved by rest. He also developed a cough and increasing fatigue.

National Safety and Quality Health Service (NSQH) Standards

Comprehensive care standard

The NSQHS Standards highlight the importance of comprehensive and coordinated healthcare that is aligned with an individual's expressed goals of care and healthcare needs, considers the impact of health issues on their life and wellbeing, and is clinically appropriate (ACSQHC, 2021).

Visit the following resource to learn more about how ejection fractions are determined: www.hrsonline.org/Patient-Resources/The-Normal-Heart/Ejection-Fraction

David made an appointment with the cardiologist who organised an echocardiogram, 12-lead ECG, chest X-ray, full blood count, urea, creatinine and electrolytes. The echocardiogram identified that his left ventricular ejection fraction was 38 per cent. The cardiologist diagnosed heart failure and started David on a number of new medications. He emphasised that David should attend the cardiac rehabilitation program so that he could learn to manage his heart failure as independently as possible.

Quick Quiz!

Q1 Remembering the difference between a sign and a symptom, which of the following is a sign of heart failure?

- a The person says he or she feels breathless.
- b The nurse notes the person's weight has increased by 2 kg.
- c The person says he or she has swollen lower legs in the evening.
- d The person feels increasingly tired.

Q2 Which of the following is *not true* of heart failure?

- a Myocardial failure leads to an increase in circulating volume.
- b Ischaemic heart disease and hypertension are common causes of heart failure.
- c One of the compensatory mechanisms activated in heart failure is the rennin-angiotensin system.
- d Ventricular remodelling can occur as the myocardium adapts to increases in fluid volume and pressure.

Q3 Left ventricular ejection fraction is best described as the fraction of blood pumped out of the left ventricle during each heartbeat and it is equal to the stroke volume divided by the end-diastolic volume.

- a True
- b False

To learn more about heart failure, access: https://www.heartfoundation.org.au/health-professional-tools/the-heart-failure-toolkit

Q4 A normal left ventricular ejection fraction is an ejection fraction >50%.

- a True
- b False

Q5 The most informative test in determining heart failure is:

- a Chest X-ray
- b Blood tests
- c Echocardiogram
- d Electrocardiogram

Q6 Identify all of the statements below that are *true*.

- a Heart failure often develops at an earlier age in Aboriginal and Torres Strait Islander people.
- b Mortality from heart failure is higher in Aboriginal and Torres Strait Islander people.
- c Heart failure progresses more rapidly in Aboriginal and Torres Strait Islander people.
- d Aboriginal and Torres Strait Islander people generally have fewer hospital visits from heart failure than non-Indigenous people.
- e People living in remote and rural areas have less access to cardiac rehabilitation services.
- f Aboriginal and Torres Strait Islander people may feel more comfortable if an Aboriginal Liaison Officer accompanies them to cardiac rehabilitation.

Read the six steps to cardiac recovery: https://www.heartfoundation.org.au/recovery-and-support/FP-cardiac-rehabilitation-patient-resources

On his first visit to cardiac rehabilitation where you work, David is subdued and contemplative. He tells you that being diagnosed with heart failure has been a big shock, but he wants to improve his condition so he can get back to running the farm as quickly as possible.

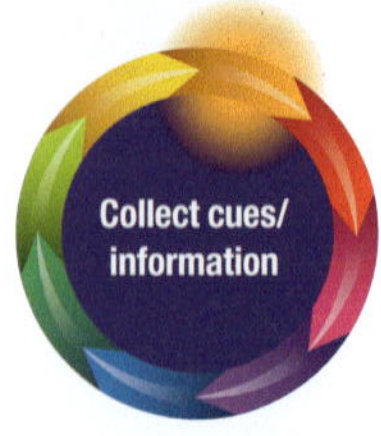

2. COLLECT CUES/INFORMATION

(a) Review current information

Q Review David's previous history and identify from the following list the three risk factors he has for heart failure.

- a Aged over 65
- b History of hypertension
- c Previous myocardial infarction
- d Damaged heart valves
- e History of a heart murmur
- f An enlarged heart
- g Family history of enlarged heart
- h Diabetes type 2

Visit this National Heart Foundation site for information on heart failure: www.heartfoundation.org.au/conditions/heart-failure

David's visit to his cardiologist and subsequent tests revealed the following:

Temperature	37°C
Pulse rate	68 beats/min
Respiratory rate	24 breaths/min

Blood pressure	140/85 mmHg
SpO_2	95% on room air
BGL	14.1 mmol/L
Breath sounds	Inspiratory crackles (rales) on auscultation
Left ventricular ejection fraction	38%
Chest X-ray	Some diffuse pulmonary infiltrates
Haemoglobin	150 g/L
White cell count	9.2×10^9
Urea	5 mmol/L
Creatinine	0.7 mg/dL
Potassium	4.0 mmol/L
Sodium	128 mmol/L

Medical orders

- Ramipril 10 mg daily
- Metoprolol 12.5 mg twice daily
- Frusemide 40 mg mane
- Aspirin 150 mg daily
- Simvastatin 40 mg daily
- Daily fluid restriction of 1500 mL
- Yearly influenza and pneumococcal vaccination

Visit the following Heart Foundation site for a reference guide on the diagnosis and management of heart failure: https://www.heartfoundation.org.au/conditions/fp-heart-failure-clinical-information

(b) Gather new information

On presentation to the outpatient cardiac rehabilitation unit, David is assessed prior to commencing the program.

Q1 Which of the following components are important to a comprehensive cardiac rehabilitation assessment?

a Medical and surgical history
b Psychosocial history
c Risk of heart failure decompensation
d Observations and vital signs during activity
e All options are correct

Q2 It is important to conduct a full neurological examination.

a True
b False

Access the *National Heart Foundation of Australia and Cardiac Society of Australia and New Zealand: Guidelines for the Prevention, Detection, and Management of Heart Failure in Australia 2018* at: doi.org/10.1016/j.hlc.2018.06.1042

(c) Recall knowledge

Quick Quiz!

Q1 People who have heart failure may think they have the 'flu' because:

a They have a fever
b They have a cough
c They have a headache
d They are sweating and nauseated

Q2 Congestive cardiac failure is a condition where excessive fluid builds up in the lungs due to inadequate pumping of the heart.

a True
b False

Q3 Pulmonary oedema is more likely to occur with:

a Hypotension
b Right-sided heart failure
c Atrial fibrillation
d Left-sided heart failure

Q4 Systemic oedema is more likely with:

a Hypotension
b Right-sided heart failure
c Atrial fibrillation
d Left-sided heart failure

Quick Quiz! continued

Q5 Which of these statements are *true* regarding heart failure?

a It causes simultaneous depolarisation.
b It is caused mainly by obesity.
c Failure of the left ventricle can lead to failure of the right ventricle.
d Defibrillation is necessary when the patient in heart failure becomes more breathless.

Q6 Cardiac rehabilitation programs are an important part of recovery as they:

a Provide education for the first few days
b Help the person return to an active and satisfying life
c Make people comply with treatments
d All of the options

Q7 In left-sided heart failure, pressure builds up in the ______________.

Q8 In right-sided heart failure, pressure builds up in the ______________.

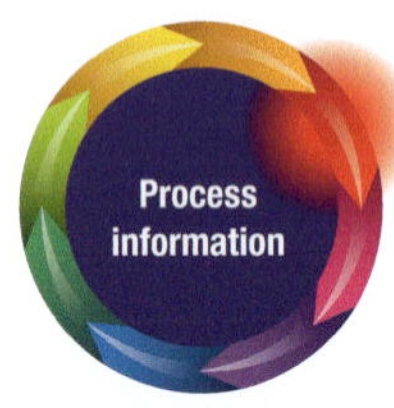

3. PROCESS INFORMATION

During his assessment by the multi-disciplinary team at the nurse-led Cardiac Rehabilitation Unit, it is identified that David is cognitively competent and has good support from his wife. However, he has continued to smoke, as he says it helps relieve the stress associated with running of the farm and financial issues. He has the occasional alcoholic drink, usually on Friday night at the 'local' with friends. His knowledge of the correct dietary management of his diabetes and heart disease is low, and he says that Sophie does all the cooking and buying of food. He does not do any particular exercise, as he says running the farm is exercise enough. David states he is not depressed and that he is motivated to improve his health, as 'the farm does not look after itself'. His knowledge of his medications is limited and he is not aware of what he should do if his condition worsens. David says that he finds it hard to stick to his fluid restriction, especially when he is working out in the fields, and he admits to having problems with his sexual function.

(a) Interpret, (b) Discriminate and (c) Relate

Q1 It is most likely that David did not attend the cardiac rehabilitation program initially as:

a He was busy with the farm and had little or no time.
b He did not realise the seriousness of his condition and the possibility of it worsening.
c The cardiac rehabilitation unit was too far from his home.
d All of the options.

Q2 From the following list, identify the signs and symptoms you would expect if David developed subsequent right-sided heart failure.

a Orthopnoea
b Distended neck veins
c Dependent area oedema
d Cyanosis
e Nausea and anorexia
f Right upper quadrant pain from liver engorgement
g Nocturia
h Crackles on auscultation

Q3 David is taking ramipril, an ACE inhibitor. Because of this, he needs to have blood tests regularly to monitor his:

a INR
b Potassium levels and renal function
c White cell count
d Blood sugar level and glycosylated haemoglobin

Q4 David should be taught which of the following in relation to his diet and lifestyle?

a To make sure that he eats fatty foods to help put on weight
b To ensure that he continues to smoke cigarettes as it will help to relax him
c To ensure he reduces his salt intake
d That engaging in high-intensity aerobic exercise is not advised for him

Q5 David should be taught to check his ____________ daily to be able to detect fluid retention and help prevent further deterioration.

Q6 Infection can lead to a worsening of David's heart failure. He should therefore be taught the signs and symptoms of infection. Which *three* from the following list apply.

a Increased temperature
b Increased weight gain
c Swollen ankles
d Pain on urination
e Sore throat and cough
f Reduced bowel sounds

(d) Infer

Q David's heart failure may have been exacerbated by not adhering to which elements of his cardiac rehabilitation program?

a Cessation of smoking
b Maintenance of a low-salt diet
c Appropriate activity and rest periods
d A decrease in stress through stress management programs
e Compliance with diabetic and healthy heart diet

(e) Predict

Q Select three signs or symptoms that David would need to recognise in order to pre-empt a deterioration in his condition.

a New and increasing chest pain
b Improvement in activity tolerance
c Slow and steady weight loss
d Increasing shortness of breath
e Rapid weight gain

(f) Match

Q Have you ever seen someone with the same signs and symptoms as David? If so, what was done to manage the situation and what was the outcome?

4. IDENTIFY THE PROBLEM/ISSUE

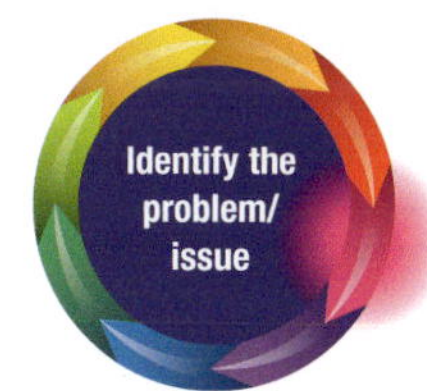

Q Re-examine the information you have about David in both his medical examination and test results, as well as the cardiac rehabilitation assessment. From this information, identify three *correct* nursing diagnoses for David.

a Risk of impaired health maintenance due to lack of knowledge about diet, exercise and medications
b Risk of hyperglycaemia related to impaired kidney function

c Anxiety related to changing health status, resulting in inability to manage feelings of uncertainty and apprehension regarding the lifestyle changes
d Fluid volume deficit (hypovolaemia) related to increased cardiac output and glomerular filtration rate, evidenced by peripheral and pulmonary oedema
e Excess fluid volume (hypervolaemia) related to decreased cardiac output and reduced glomerular filtration rate, evidenced by peripheral and pulmonary oedema
f Activity intolerance related to muscular degeneration

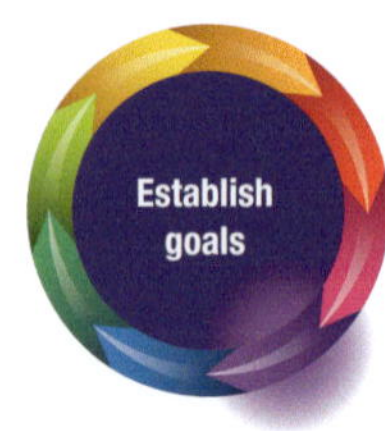

5. ESTABLISH GOALS

Q With reference to the nursing diagnoses identified earlier, select three *long-term* goals for David from the following list.
a For David to maintain his daily fluid restriction
b For David to have no evidence of impaired gas exchange
c For David to be back working long days on the farm
d For David to participate in education and adhere to a self-care program
e For David to manage his anxiety, using stress reduction techniques
f For David to be eating and drinking what he enjoyed before he became unwell
g For David to access community support for his condition

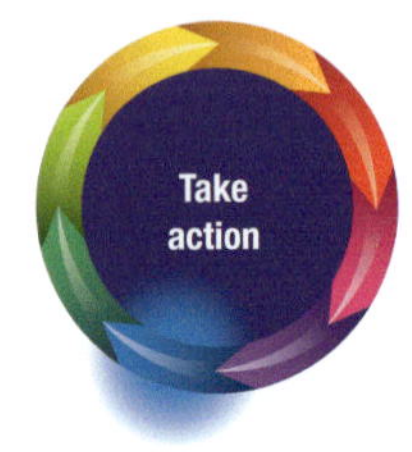

6. TAKE ACTION

Q Create a care plan for David. Using the table below, construct your care plan by matching the long-term nursing goal to the nursing action.

Nursing actions

- Provide information on cardiac rehabilitation programs and support groups
- Provide information for stress management programs
- Commence a nutrition education program
- Continue daily weight

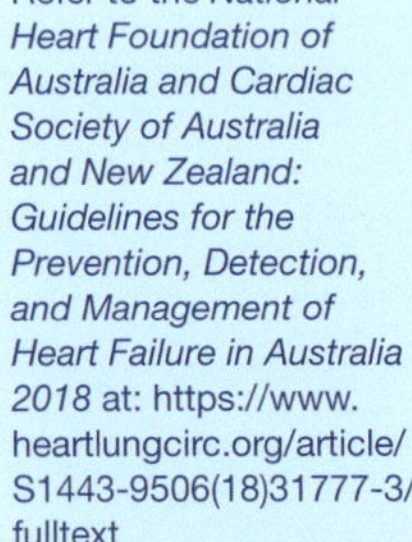
Refer to the *National Heart Foundation of Australia and Cardiac Society of Australia and New Zealand: Guidelines for the Prevention, Detection, and Management of Heart Failure in Australia 2018* at: https://www.heartlungcirc.org/article/S1443-9506(18)31777-3/fulltext

Long-term nursing goal	Nursing action
David to obtain support from the community	
David to adhere to a self-care program	
David to manage anxiety	
David to maintain his daily fluid restriction	

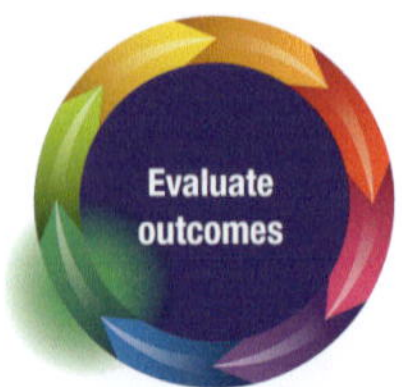

7. EVALUATE

Q If David's cardiac rehabilitation is successful, what would you expect to observe?
a Maintenance of fluids through adherence to fluid restriction
b Managed level of stress
c Controlled diabetes—maintaining glucose levels between 4 and 8 mmol/L
d Maintenance of healthy heart diet and exercise program
e All of the options

8. REFLECT

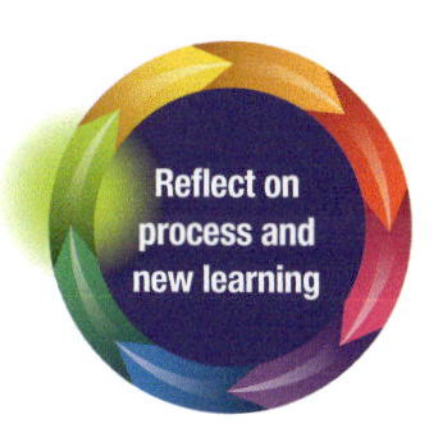

Reflect on what happened to David and the care that he received by considering the following questions.

Q1 What factors influence the success of discharge education and planning for someone who has had a heart attack?

Q2 How could David's deterioration after his heart attack have been prevented?

Q3 What have you learnt from the scenario that you can apply to your future practice?

Q4 What factors influence how people adapt to chronic and life-limiting conditions?

Q5 What strategies would you use to provide culturally safe care to people who are finding their chronic illness journey particularly challenging?

EPILOGUE

David continued to recover from his heart attack and learnt to manage his heart failure with support from his family. During a visit to his GP, he expressed his gratitude at having the opportunity to re-evaluate his life and his priorities. He feels in the right frame of mind to find out more about his heritage and has stayed in contact with the Aboriginal Liaison Officer who is helping him to make inquiries about how to trace members of his family. He has become a member of the local 'heart support' group and helps out by visiting other farmers who are hospitalised with a cardiac condition, including other Aboriginal men. Although he delegates many of the heavier tasks in managing the farm to his employees, he continues with his sheep-breeding program and recently won the major title for a fine wool merino ram at the Royal Easter Show.

FURTHER READING

Australian Commission on Safety and Quality in Health Care. (2019). *Acute Coronary Syndromes Clinical Care Standards*. Sydney: ACSQHC.

Disler, R., Glenister, K. & Wright, J. (2020). Rural chronic disease research patterns in the United Kingdom, United States, Canada, Australia and New Zealand: A systematic integrative review. *BMC Public Health, 20*(1), 770. doi:10.1186/s12889-020-08912-1

Heart Foundation. (2021). *Heart Failure Clinical Resources*. Retrieved from: https://www.heartfoundation.org.au/conditions/fp-heart-failure-clinical-information

NSW Health. (2018). *Aboriginal Health Worker Guidelines*. Sydney, NSW: Retrieved from: https://www.health.nsw.gov.au/workforce/aboriginal/Publications/aboriginal-health-worker-guidelines.pdf

REFERENCES

Agency for Clinical Innovation (ACI). (2016). *Nurse Administered Thrombolysis (NAT) for ST Elevation Myocardial Infarction (STEMI)*. Clinical Fact Sheet. Retrieved from: www.aci.health.nsw.gov.au/__data/assets/pdf_file/0011/319196/NAT-clinican.pdf

Australian Commission on Safety and Quality in Health Care (ACSQHC). (2021). *National Safety and Quality Health Service Standards* (2nd edn). Sydney, Australia.

Australian Institute of Health and Welfare (AIHW). (2020). *Cardiovascular Disease.* Retrieved from: www.aihw.gov.au/reports/heart-stroke-vascular-diseases/cardiovascular-health-compendium

Beck, B., Bray, J. E., Smith, K., Walker, T., Grantham, H., Hein, C., ... Finn, J. (2016). Description of the ambulance services participating in the Aus-ROC Australian and New Zealand out-of-hospital cardiac arrest Epistry. *Emergency Medicine Australasia*, *28*(6), 673–83. doi:10.1111/1742-6723.12690

Chew, D. P., Scott, I. A., Cullen, L., French, J. K., Briffa, T. G., Tideman, P. A., . . . Aylward, P. E. G. (2016). National Heart Foundation of Australia & Cardiac Society of Australia and New Zealand: Australian Clinical Guidelines for the Management of Acute Coronary Syndromes. *Heart, Lung and Circulation*, *25*, 895–951.

LeMone, P., Burke, K., Bauldoff, G., Gubrud-Howe, P., Levett-Jones, T., Dwyer, T., ... Raymond, D. (Eds). (2019). *Medical–Surgical Nursing: Critical Thinking in Person-Centred Care* (4th edn). Melbourne: Pearson.

Levett-Jones, T., Dwyer, T., Reid-Searl, K., Heaton, L., Flenady, T., Applegarth, J., Guinea, S. & Andersen, P. (2017). *The Patient Safety Competency Framework (PSCF) for Nursing Students*. Retrieved from: http://psframework.wpengine.com/wp-content/uploads/2018/01/PSCF_Brochure_UTS-version_FA2-Screen.pdf

National Heart Foundation of Australia. (2021). *Are You At Risk of Heart Disease?* Retrieved from: www.heartfoundation.org.au/heart-health-education/are-you-at-risk-of-heart-disease

NSW Health. (2018). *Aboriginal Health Worker Guidelines*. Sydney, NSW. Retrieved from: https://www.health.nsw.gov.au/workforce/aboriginal/Publications/aboriginal-health-worker-guidelines.pdf

Nursing and Midwifery Board of Australia (NMBA). (2016). *Registered Nurse Standards for Practice*. Retrieved from: www.nursingmidwiferyboard.gov.au/Codes-Guidelines-Statements/Professional-standards.aspx

Yan, S., Gan, Y., Jiang, N., Wang, R., Chen, Y., Luo, Z., . . . Lv, C. (2020). The global survival rate among adult out-of-hospital cardiac arrest patients who received cardiopulmonary resuscitation: A systematic review and meta-analysis. *Critical Care*, *24*(1), 61. doi:10.1186/s13054-020-2773-2

Chapter 8

Caring for a person with an acquired brain injury

JACQUI PICH and ROCHELLE FIRTH

LEARNING OUTCOMES

Completion of the activities in this chapter will enable you to:

- explain why an understanding of neurological deterioration is essential to competent practice (**recall** and **application**)
- identify the clinical manifestations of altered level of consciousness and deteriorating neurological status that will guide the collection and interpretation of cues (**gather, review, interpret, discriminate, relate** and **infer**)
- identify patients at risk of increasing intracranial pressure (**match** and **predict**)
- review clinical information to identify the main nursing diagnoses for a patient with an acquired brain injury, altered consciousness and disability (**synthesise**)
- describe the priorities of care for a patient with an acquired brain injury, altered consciousness and disability (**goal setting** and **taking action**)
- identify clinical criteria for determining the effectiveness of nursing actions taken to manage an acquired brain injury, altered consciousness and disability (**evaluate**)
- apply what you have learnt about acquired brain injury, altered level of consciousness and disability to new situations involving different patients (**reflection** and **translation**).

INTRODUCTION

This chapter focuses on the care of a person who experiences a stroke. You will meet Mr Iosefa Apulu and follow his healthcare journey through acute care and into rehabilitation. Stroke is a medical emergency; therefore, recognition of the signs and symptoms, and early presentation to acute care are critical (Stroke Foundation, 2020). Neurological deterioration following a stroke can occur rapidly and lead to serious complications; however, early intervention may prevent mortality and reduce the severity of long-term disability (Stroke Foundation, 2020). Well-developed clinical reasoning skills will help you to recognise and manage people at risk of neurological deterioration, thus preventing or reducing adverse patient outcomes.

KEY CONCEPTS

stroke
acquired brain injury
altered level of consciousness
neurological deterioration
raised intracranial pressure
disability
transient ischaemic attack
cerebrovascular accident

SUGGESTED READINGS

P. LeMone, G. Bauldoff, P. Gubrud-Howe, M.-A. Carno, T. Levett-Jones, . . . D. Stanley (Eds). (2020). *LeMone and Burke's Medical–Surgical Nursing: Critical Thinking in Person-Centred Care* (4th edn). Melbourne: Pearson Australia.

Unit 11: Responses to altered neurological function

SCENARIO 8.1 Caring for a person with an acquired brain injury and altered level of consciousness

SETTING THE SCENE

Mr Iosefa Apulu
D. Smith/Travel-Images.com

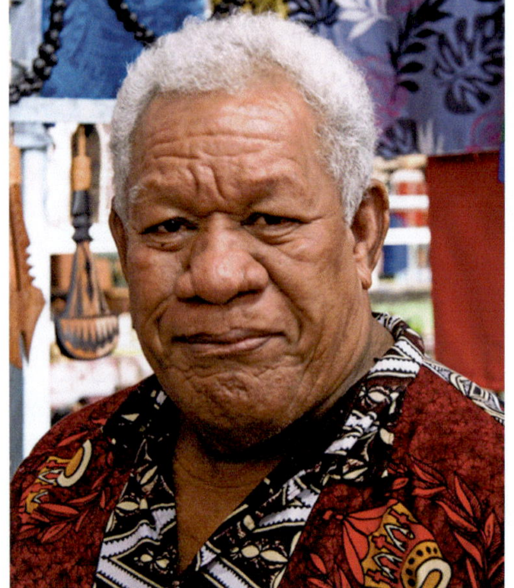

Mr Iosefa Apulu is a 52-year-old Samoan man who presented to his general practitioner (GP) with dizziness and headaches. After clinical review, a CT brain scan was ordered. The results were normal but the GP told Mr Apulu that he had suffered a transient ischaemic attack (TIA). Mr Apulu was started on Cardiprin (aspirin), 100 mg once daily and atorvastatin, 40 mg daily. However, his dizziness persisted and he was started on Prochlorperazine (Stemetil). Because of his history of high blood pressure and obesity, the GP also prescribed Coversyl (perindopril arginine) tablets 10 mg once daily and Lipitor (atorvastatin) tablets 40 mg once daily.

A week after his review by the GP, Mr Apulu rose early to help his sons get ready for work. By 0500 he had developed a left-sided headache and by 1100 it was severe and intolerable so his son drove him to the emergency department (ED) at his local hospital.

On admission to the ED, Mr Apulu's pain score was 8/10 and he had some transient weakness of his left side, face and arm. He stated that he had intermittent double vision, felt like he was spinning, but had no nausea or vomiting.

A neurological assessment identified that Mr Apulu had left upper limb severe weakness and decreased tone. He was observed to have dysarthria, vertigo and ataxia. He was opening his eyes to speech, confused to time, able to obey commands and his Glasgow Coma Score was 13. A posterior circulation stroke was suspected and a CT brain angiography was ordered.

The epidemiology of stroke

The acronym FAST has been introduced to educate the public on recognition of symptoms of stroke and the importance of timely access to care. It stands for:

Face—Has their mouth drooped?

Arms—Can they lift both arms?

Speech—Is their speech slurred? Do they understand you?

Time—Is critical. If you see any of these signs, call 000 straight away.

Stroke death rates fell by 75 per cent between 1980 and 2018; however, as of 2018, strokes still accounted for 5.3 per cent of all deaths in Australia (Australian Institute of Health and Welfare [AIHW], 2020). Older Australians are more likely to have a stroke, with 72 per cent of patients aged over 65 (AIHW, 2018). More women than men die from strokes, and Aboriginal and Torres Strait Islander people are 1.5 times more likely to die from a stroke than non-Indigenous Australians (AIHW, 2018).

More people are now surviving stroke, and disability caused by stroke declined from 45 per cent to 35 per cent in the period from 1998 to 2009 (AIHW, 2013). However, many survivors still experience significant health issues that impact their quality of life. One in three people who have a stroke will have a resulting disability that interferes with everyday activities, and will require ongoing care and assistance (AIHW, 2020). Many stroke survivors with disability return home and the burden of care often falls on family members.

The aetiology and pathogenesis of stroke

Refer to this blog for an overview of what strokes are and the signs and symptoms: https://strokefoundation.org.au/Blog/2016/09/12/A-stroke-is-a-medical-emergency-the-facts

Stroke (also known as cerebrovascular accident [CVA]) is an acquired brain injury that occurs when the blood supply to the brain is suddenly disrupted by either a blocked artery (ischaemic stroke) or haemorrhage (haemorrhagic stroke). Disruption of blood supply to the brain starves brain cells of oxygen and glucose, resulting in ischaemia and infarction (Stroke Foundation, 2021).

An ischaemic stroke can be caused by either an emboli or a thrombus and accounts for approximately 80 to 85 per cent of strokes. Haemorrhagic strokes occur when blood vessels rupture, often as a result of long-standing hypertension (Stroke Foundation, 2021).

Risk factors for developing a stroke include hypertension, hypercholesterolaemia, previous strokes, atrial fibrillation, diabetes, fibromuscular dysplasia, age, family history, smoking, obesity, alcohol and lack of exercise (Stroke Foundation, 2021).

On admission to the stroke unit

Mr Apulu was transferred from the interventional neuroradiology unit to the stroke unit under the care of a neurologist. The CT brain angiography showed a right vertebral artery occlusion with a thrombus present and large amounts of viable tissue noted. There was no evidence of a haemorrhage.

Mr Apulu was not a candidate for intravenous thrombolysis such as tPA as he had presented to the ED more than 4.5 hours after symptom onset. However, given his high level of independence prior to admission and identification of vessel occlusion and salvageable tissue, he was assessed as a suitable candidate for endovascular clot retrieval (ECR)/thrombectomy. He therefore underwent successful revascularisation and was transferred to the stroke unit.

Endovascular clot retrieval is the standard of care in the treatment of acute stroke patients with large vessel occlusion. It has been shown to have major benefits in selected patients up to 24 hours following the stroke; however, earlier treatment is linked to greater benefits. This presents logistical challenges in Australia as this treatment is only offered in a limited number of metropolitan centres.

On admission to the stroke unit, Mr Apulu's observations were:

Temperature	36.5°C
Pulse rate	73, regular
Respiratory rate	15 breaths/min
Blood pressure	170/90
SpO_2	94% on room air
BSL	6.5 mmol/L
Pupil reaction to light	Brisk and equal in both left and right pupil
Pupil size	3 mm left and right pupil
Limbs	Left arm and leg severe weakness, right arm and leg normal power
Glasgow Coma Score	13: eyes open = 3 (to speech); best verbal response = 4 (confused); best motor response = 6 (obeys commands)
National Institutes of Health Stroke Scale (NIHSS)	10 (moderate severity of stroke)
BMI	35 kg/m^2

His comorbidities were:

- Type 2 diabetes (diet controlled)
- Hypertension
- Recurrent cellulitis right leg (currently no cellulitis present)
- Smoking
- Obesity (weight 110 kg), height 1.70 m, BMI 35 kg/m^2
- Osteoarthritis (Mr Apulu takes over-the-counter (OTC) paracetamol PRN)

An ECG showed that Mr Apulu was in normal sinus rhythm and a series of blood tests were taken with the following results:

Cholesterol	5.9 mmol/L
Triglycerides	1.35 mmol/L
PT	14 secs
APPT	29 secs
INR	1.0
Hb	170 g/L
Urea	8.7 mmol/L
eGFR	86 mmol/L
Potassium	4.0 mmol/L
Sodium	139 mmol/L
ABGs	PaO_2 = 75, $PaCO_2$ = 37, pH = 7.38

Access *Stroke and its management in Australia: an update* (AIHW, 2013) for further information on the epidemiology of stroke in Australia: https://www.aihw.gov.au/reports/heart-stroke-vascular-diseases/stroke-management-australia-update/summary

For a brief overview of stroke, access: https://www.aihw.gov.au/reports/australias-health/stroke

For more about endovascular clot retrieval in rural areas, access the Agency for Clinical Innovation's *Eligibility for endovascular clot retrieval* (2019) at: https://aci.health.nsw.gov.au/resources/charts and Gangadharan et al. (2020) at: doi.org/10.3389/fneur.2020.00628

For more information about stroke management, access the following: https://app.magicapp.org/#/guideline/QnoKGn/section/EaWDdL and https://informme.org.au/Guidelines/Clinical-Guidelines-for-Stroke-Management

For further information, access the *Adult Neurological Observation Chart—Education Package* on the NSW Agency for Clinical Innovation website: www.aci.health.nsw.gov.au and the National Institute of Health's Stroke Scale (NIHSS): https://www.stroke.nih.gov/resources/scale.htm

Medical orders that followed were:

- Maintain systolic blood pressure between 160 and 180
- Oxygen therapy to maintain SpO_2 above 95%
- Continue aspirin
- 2/24 neurological observations
- Nil by mouth
- IV fluids normal saline, 1 litre over 12 hours
- For review by speech pathologist

Q Review Mr Apulu's health history and identify five risk factors that he had for the development of an ischaemic stroke from the list below.

a Age over 65
b History of hypertension
c Previous TIAs
d Smoking
e Family history of stroke
f Cardiac arrhythmias, AF (atrial fibrillation)
g Diabetes
h Obesity

Person-centred care

Mr Apulu was born in the independent state of Samoa. He moved to Auckland, New Zealand, with his family when he was a boy and came to Australia in his late teens to work on a construction site. He has worked in construction, mainly in Sydney, ever since. He married Susan, an Australian girl that he met at a local church group, 26 years ago and became an Australian citizen. Susan died two years ago after suffering with multiple sclerosis for many years. Mr Apulu now lives with his two sons, Jonah and Joshua, who also work in construction. Due to his recent illness, he has been on sick leave but still cares for his two 'boys', getting them up for work and cooking and cleaning for them. His wife's mother helps out when she can but she is 76 and not in good health. Mr Apulu and his sons have a 'tinnie' which they often take out on the weekends for fishing. He has a large extended family and a strong and supportive network of friends from church. Mr Apulu asks people to call him Joe, as he says most 'Aussies' have trouble pronouncing his Samoan name.

Patient Safety Competency Framework (PSCF)

Domain 1–Person-centred care

Person-centred care is the central tenet underpinning the delivery of safe and effective nursing care. It is a holistic approach that is grounded in a philosophy of personhood. Person-centred care means treating each person as an individual, protecting their dignity, respecting their rights and preferences, and developing a therapeutic relationship that is built on mutual trust and empathic understandings.

Source: *The Patient Safety Competency Framework for Nursing Students,* https://patientsafetyfornursingstudents.org

Something to think about ...

People from culturally and linguistically diverse (CALD) backgrounds experience a higher incidence of medication errors, misdiagnosis, incorrect treatment and poor pain management than English-speaking people, with misunderstandings and miscommunication frequently reported (Gilligan, Outram & Buchanan, 2020). CALD patients often describe feelings of powerlessness, vulnerability, loneliness and fear when undergoing healthcare (Garrett et al., 2008).

Nursing and Midwifery Board of Australia (NMBA) *Registered Nurse Standards for Practice* Standard 2 of the *Registered Nurse Standards for Practice* (2016) states that registered nurses must communicate effectively and be respectful of each person's dignity, culture, values, beliefs and rights.

Patient Safety Competency Framework (PSCF)

Domain 3–Cultural competence

Cultural competence refers to the willingness to adapt practice to meet the needs of people from diverse cultures, and the ability to interact with persons from cultures and/or belief systems different to one's own.

Source: *The Patient Safety Competency Framework for Nursing Students*, https://patientsafetyfornursingstudents.org

Patients with suspected stroke can be screened for swallowing difficulties using the ASSIST—Acute Screening of Swallow in Stroke/TIA (ACI, 2016) tool available at: https://www.acu.edu.au//media/qasc-download/assist_screening_tool.pdf

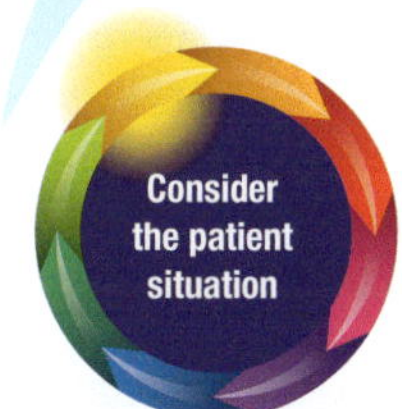

1. CONSIDER THE PATIENT SITUATION

Mr Apulu has been on the stroke ward for 48 hours. You have just begun your shift and receive the following handover report:

We have Mr 'Joe' Apulu in room 10. He's 52 years old. He has had a right vertebral artery stroke and is under Dr Isaacs. He has left-sided weakness and is NBM. He has had a speech pathology review that diagnosed dysphagia and he is for nasogastric feeds, waiting on a dietitian review.

Mr Apulu is a type 2 diabetic, diet controlled. He currently has an IV, normal saline at 84 mL/hr. He slept on and off overnight but seemed restless. He was a little confused when woken for 0600 observations; I am not sure if that is new or he was just sleepy. He has oxygen therapy at 4 L via nasal prongs and his sats are around 96%. His BGLs yesterday were stable and his 0600 BGL was 6.5 mmol/L. His obs are due again at 0800. He lives with his two sons; they will probably be in later today. His wife passed away a couple of years ago. He is due for an MRI of the brain today.

Strokes from a vertebral artery occlusion are not as common as strokes involving the middle cerebral artery. For information on the signs and symptoms of a vertebral artery stroke, see http://patient.info/doctor/vertebrobasilar-occlusion-and-vertebral-artery-syndrome

Quick Quiz!

Q1 The National Institutes of Health's Stroke Scale (NIHSS) is used to assess:

- a Stroke risk factors
- b Stroke severity
- c The number of strokes someone has suffered
- d Recovery of stroke

Q2 A normal Glasgow Coma Score (GCS) would be:

- a 10
- b 12
- c 13
- d 15

Q3 Stroke should be considered a medical emergency, as:

- a Multi-disciplinary assessments need to be carried out within three hours of onset of symptoms to ensure the best chance of recovery.
- b Families are very distressed when a patient has a stroke and early attention to the stroke patient can relieve their distress.
- c Diagnosis and treatment with tPA needs to occur within four and a half hours from the onset of symptoms.
- d Stroke patients often deteriorate very rapidly and will need cardiopulmonary resuscitation.

Q4 A thrombus which has broken loose and is moving with the blood flow is called:

- a A thrombosis
- b An embolism
- c An occlusion
- d A clot

Q5 Atheroma is:

- a The blockage of a vein due to a clot
- b The blockage of an artery due to a clot
- c A weakness in an artery wall causing it to burst
- d Fatty plaque on the wall of an artery

Q6 Which of the following statements are *not true* regarding a TIA or 'mini stroke'?

- a A TIA is a stroke whose symptoms are milder and harder to detect.
- b A TIA is a brief period of localised ischaemia lasting less than 24 hours.
- c TIAs are often warning signs of an impending ischaemic stroke.
- d During a TIA, a person may experience signs and symptoms similar to a stroke.

Quick Quiz! continued

Q7 A stroke-in-evolution is a thrombotic stroke that occurs rapidly but then progresses slowly over two to three days.

a True
b False

Q8 The immediate treatment for a stroke includes:

a Taking an aspirin and calling an ambulance
b Cardiopulmonary resuscitation
c Receiving a thrombolytic in the ED once a CT brain scan has been done
d All of the options

Q9 A patient who opens his or her eyes in response to pain, localises to pain and has incomprehensible speech has a GCS of:

a 7
b 9
c 11
d 15

Q10 In relation to obesity, mark each statement below as *true* or *false*.

a A body mass index of <30 kg/m^2 is considered as class 1 obesity.
b Obesity increases the likelihood of diseases such as diabetes, cardiac disease, sleep apnoea, cancer and osteoporosis.
c Obesity is one of the leading preventable diseases worldwide.
d People with central obesity (apple shape) have a greater risk of complications such as diabetes and heart disease.
e Peripheral obesity is more common in men.

Q11 The term 'cerebrovascular accident' (CVA) is currently less commonly used in relation to stroke. The term 'brain attack' has been adopted. Select the correct statements from the following list in relation to the reason for the adoption of the term 'brain attack'.

i A stroke is not really an 'accident'.
ii 'Cerebrovascular accident' is too long and hard to remember.
iii The term 'brain attack' stresses the urgency of a stroke, as does the term 'heart attack', and encourages people to access care quickly.

a i and ii
b i and iii
c ii and iii
d i, ii and iii

Q12 Which is the most important goal in the immediate phase of acute stroke care?

a Ensure the patient is comfortable and aware of what is happening.
b Maximise oxygen delivery to the patient and minimise oxygen demand.
c Test for a gag and cough reflex and instigate appropriate precautions.
d Minimise damage to the penumbra and re-establish perfusion as quickly as possible.

Q13 Why may tPA medication be given for both a myocardial infarction and an ischaemic stroke?

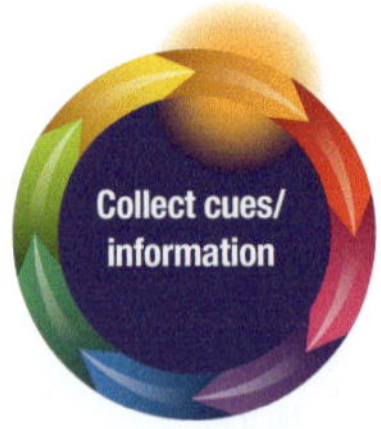

2. COLLECT CUES/INFORMATION

(a) Review current information

You go in to say good morning to Mr Apulu, who you had cared for the previous evening, and find that his confusion has worsened. You are concerned so immediately take his vital signs and neurological observations:

Temperature	36.8°C
Pulse rate	68, regular
Respiratory rate	13
Blood pressure	175/85
SpO_2	97% on 4 L oxygen via nasal prongs
BGL	6.5 mmol/L
Pupil reaction to light	sluggish in left pupil
Pupil size	5 mm left pupil
Limbs	left arm and leg severe weakness, right arm and leg normal strength
GCS	11: eyes open = 3 (to speech); best verbal response = 3 (inappropriate word responses); best motor response = 5 (localises to pain)
NIHSS	15

National Safety and Quality Health Service (NSQH) Standards

Recognising and responding to acute deterioration standard

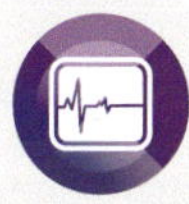

The NSQHS Standards emphasise that acute deterioration must be recognised promptly and appropriate action taken. Acute deterioration includes physiological changes as well as acute changes in cognition and mental state (ACSQHC, 2021).

Q1 The difference between the systolic and diastolic pressures is called the:
- a Mean arterial blood pressure
- b Blood pressure
- c Pulse pressure
- d End-ventricular pressure

Q2 Mr Apulu's pulse pressure on admission was:
- a 60
- b 70
- c 80
- d 90

Q3 Mr Apulu's pulse pressure is now:
- a 60
- b 70
- c 80
- d 90

Q4 Mr Apulu's GCS has changed by ________ points.

Q5 What other changes have occurred since Mr Apulu's admission?

(b) Gather new information

Something to think about . . .

Mr Apulu is from Samoa. A body of evidence has identified that healthcare professionals who do not acknowledge and address cultural factors contribute significantly to adverse patient outcomes and health inequality. A practical strategy for enhancing cultural competence is to take a cultural assessment. Access this site to explore the ABCD mnemonic for taking a quick and easy cultural assessment: https://ethnomed.org/resource/cultural-relevance-in-end-of-life-care/

Q From the list below, identify the three cues that you believe are *most relevant* to your assessment of Mr Apulu at this time (that have not already been assessed).
- a Pattern of breathing
- b Temperature
- c Condition of oral mucosa
- d Headache
- e Nausea/vomiting
- f Colour
- g Increasing contra-lateral limb weakness

(c) Recall knowledge

Quick Quiz!

To ensure that you have a good understanding of the key concepts related to stroke and deteriorating neurological status, test yourself with the following questions.

Q1 Cushing's triad is associated with:
- a Tension pneumothorax
- b Cardiac tamponade
- c Massive haemothorax
- d Raised intracranial pressure

Q2 Identify three parameters from the following list that form Cushing's triad.
- a Raised temperature
- b Raised pulse pressure
- c Lowered pulse pressure
- d Decreased pulse
- e Normal breathing pattern
- f Abnormal breathing pattern

Quick Quiz! continued

Q3 Mannitol is an osmotic diuretic. It would most likely be given for:

a Cerebral oedema
b Peripheral oedema
c Pulmonary oedema
d None of the options

Q4 The rigid cranial cavity contains three non-compressible elements, the _______ (80%), _______ (8%) and _______ (12%).

Q5 If the volume of any of these components increases, the volume of the others must decrease to maintain equilibrium. This is known as the _______ hypothesis.

Q6 Normal intracranial pressure is:

a 0–3 mmHg
b 0–5 mmHg
c 0–10 mmHg
d 0–20 mmHg

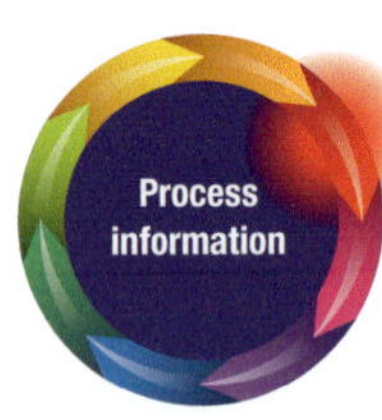

3. PROCESS INFORMATION

(a) Interpret

Q1 Which of the following is not considered to be within normal parameters for Mr Apulu?

a Temperature: 36.8°C
b Pulse rate: 68 beats/min, regular
c Respiratory rate: 13 breaths/min
d GCS: 11
e SpO_2: 97% on 4 L oxygen
f BGL: 6.5 mmol/L

Q2 Mr Apulu appears to be hypertensive; however, his medical orders are to maintain his blood pressure at 160–180 systolic. Why might the medical team have decided to keep his blood pressure higher than normal?

Q3 The GCS is an important neurological observation. If a patient's GCS drops by more than two points, what action should a nurse take?

a Lie the patient flat and raise their feet.
b Sit the patient in a semi-Fowler's position.
c Immediately contact the medical officer.
d Continue monitoring GCS until it drops further.

(b) Discriminate

Q From the list below, select three cues that are *least relevant* to Mr Apulu's neurological status *at this time*.

a Blood pressure
b Respiratory rate
c Temperature
d Pulse
e Oxygen saturation
f Condition of oral mucosa
g Level of consciousness
h Pupil size and reaction

(c) Relate

Mr Apulu's stroke is most likely to have been caused by atherosclerosis, which led to a thrombus in the vertebral artery.

Q Which of the following is *not* a risk factor for developing atherosclerosis?

a Male gender
b Diabetes
c Smoking
d High HDL level
e High dietary fat intake

(d) Infer

Q1 Early warning signs of an altered level of consciousness include which *four* of the following?
- a Increasing pulse pressure
- b GCS <12
- c A drop of GCS by 2 points
- d Unresponsiveness to verbal commands
- e BGL 1–2.9 mmol/L
- f Decreasing blood pressure
- g Any seizure

Q2 Late warning signs of an altered consciousness state are:
- a Increasing pulse pressure
- b GCS ≤8
- c Unresponsive to verbal command
- d Incomprehensible speech
- e Respiratory rate <9
- f BGL <1 mmol/L

Q3 Of most concern for Mr Apulu currently is the fact that:
- a He is afebrile and normotensive.
- b He is hypertensive and afebrile.
- c He has a decreasing GCS and pupillary changes.
- d He is hypertensive with a normal heart rate.

(e) Predict

Q If you do not take the appropriate actions at this time, what might happen if Mr Apulu's altered level of consciousness is not addressed?

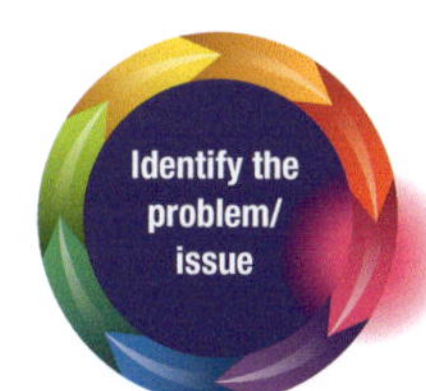

4. IDENTIFY THE PROBLEM/ISSUE

Something to think about ...

Mr Apulu's altered level of consciousness may be a warning sign that he is developing raised intracranial pressure (ICP) subsequent to cerebral oedema from his stroke. Cerebral oedema is an excess accumulation of fluid in the intra- or extracellular spaces of the brain. Strokes can cause cerebral ischaemia, resulting in cerebral oedema and raised ICP. If not attended to, rising intracranial pressure can have very serious consequences (including death) as pressure is exerted downward on the brainstem (Mellish, 2020).

Bring together (synthesise) all of the facts you've collected and inferences you've made to come to your nursing diagnoses.

Q The nursing diagnoses below are all correct. From this list, identify the three *priority* nursing diagnoses for Mr Apulu at this time.
- a Risk of impaired nutrition, related to increased metabolic demands and inadequate intake
- b Risk of ineffective cerebral tissue perfusion, related to increased ICP
- c Risk of ineffective airway clearance, related to altered level of consciousness and diminished protective reflexes (cough, gag)
- d Risk of impaired skin integrity, related to bed rest and hemiparesis
- e Risk of disturbed thought processes, related to raised ICP and confusion
- f Risk of seizures, related to increased ICP and hypoxaemia

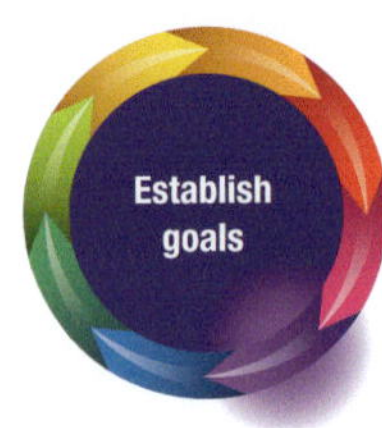

5. ESTABLISH GOALS

Q From the following list, choose the three most important *short-term* goals for Mr Apulu's management at this time.

a For Mr Apulu's GCS to improve within the next 24 hours
b For Mr Apulu to be normovolaemic within the next 24 hours
c For Mr Apulu's confusion to begin to resolve within 24 hours
d For Mr Apulu to be normotensive within the next 24 hours
e For Mr Apulu's pupil size to be 3 mm and reaction brisk within 24 hours
f For Mr Apulu's oxygen saturations to be >95% within half an hour

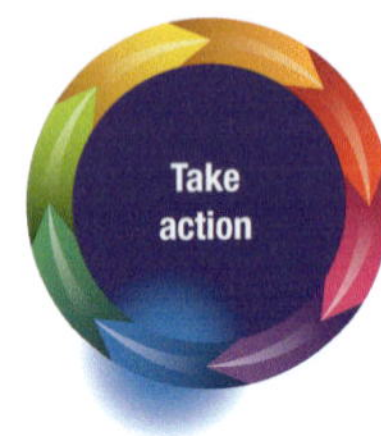

6. TAKE ACTION

The medical officer reviews Mr Apulu and orders an urgent CT brain scan. A diagnosis of cerebral oedema and consequent neurological deterioration is determined. The medical officer orders IV mannitol stat, and for Mr Apulu to be transferred to ICU for ventilation if he continues to deteriorate or his airway and breathing become compromised.

Q In the tables below, match the rationales for care to the corresponding nursing actions.

Airway and breathing

Rationale

- To ensure adequate oxygen delivery
- Sudden changes in vital signs can indicate deterioration

Nursing action	Rationale
Maintain oxygen therapy via nasal prongs or Hudson mask	
Monitor vital signs, oxygen saturation level and behaviour	

Circulation

Rationale

- Osmotic diuretic draws fluid out of the brain cells by increasing the osmolality of the blood
- To ensure patency and delivery of IV fluids
- Excess carbon dioxide and hypoxaemia can cause vasodilation and further raise ICP
- To ensure patient is not retaining fluid and/or becoming dehydrated after the osmotic diuretic

Nursing action	Rationale
Check that the IV cannula is not kinked or blocked	
Administer IV mannitol as ordered	
Monitor Mr Apulu's ABGs and electrolytes	
Strictly monitor Mr Apulu's input and output	

Disability

Rationale

- Facilitates venous drainage and prevents obstruction of the jugular veins
- Patients experiencing raised ICP can suffer from seizures and need to be kept safe from injury.

- Changes in LOC can indicate a rise in ICP and further deterioration.
- Severe headache can indicate worsening condition and can also cause anxiety, raising ICP.

Nursing action	Rationale
Monitor Mr Apulu's level of consciousness	
Monitor Mr Apulu's pain score	
Instigate seizure precautions	
Raise the head of Mr Apulu's bed to 30° and keep his head in midline	

7. EVALUATE

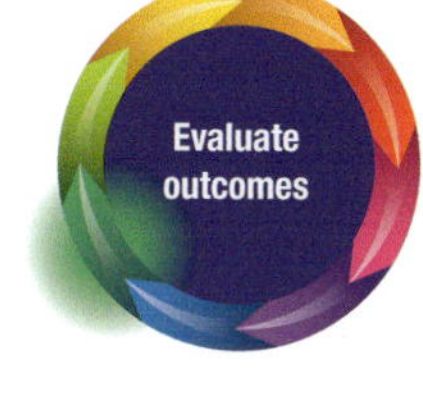

It is now two hours since Mr Apulu was given a mannitol infusion. Each of Mr Apulu's signs and symptoms provide you with data to make a determination of whether or not these interventions have been effective and whether his condition is improving.

Q Rate each of the following signs and symptoms as *unchanged, improving* or *deteriorating*.

a Cognitive status: patient confused and restless
b GCS: 13
c Pulse: 70
d Urine output: 60 mL/hr
e Left pupil size: 4 mm
f Pupil reaction: brisk both sides
g Blood pressure: 175/85
h Speech: inappropriate words
i Oxygen saturation level: 97% on 4 L

8. REFLECT

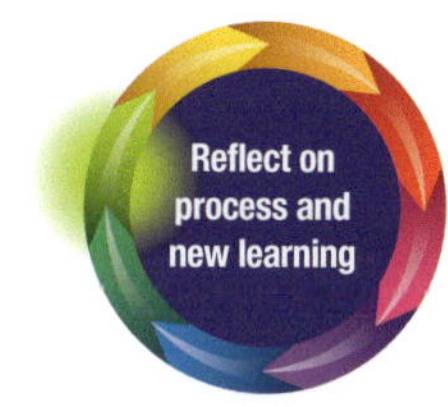

Reflect on your learning from this scenario and consider the following questions.

Q1 Might the outcome for Mr Apulu have been different if he and his family had been made aware of the early signs and symptoms of stroke? Why?

Q2 How could you promote understanding and use of the acronym FAST in your community?

Q3 What factors led to Mr Apulu's neurological deterioration following admission? Were they preventable?

Q4 What are three of the most important things that you have learnt from this scenario?

Q5 What actions will you take in clinical practice as a result of your learning from this scenario?

SCENARIO 8.2 Caring for a person recovering from a stroke

CHANGING THE SCENE

1. CONSIDER THE PATIENT SITUATION

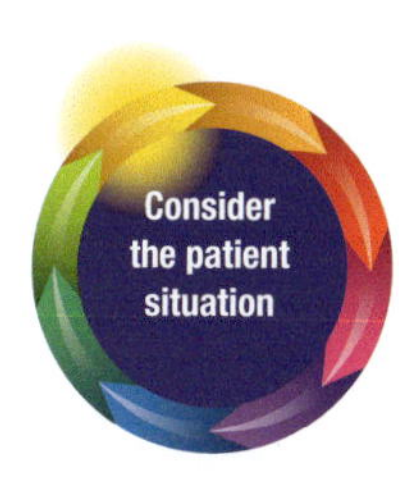

It is now 48 hours since Mr Apulu's condition deteriorated as a result of cerebral oedema and raised ICP. Although his condition is now stable, his swallowing remains impaired and he remains dysphagic, as well as having some limb weakness and visual problems. Mr Apulu has also been a little impulsive at times and had a fall when trying to stand unaided to go to the bathroom. His IV fluids have been discontinued but he continues on aspirin 100 mg daily via the nasogastric tube and is having diabetic nasogastric feeds.

Mr Apulu's sons think their father may be depressed as he cries easily and does not seem interested in what is happening to or around him. They are distressed that he had a fall and want to know what can be done to prevent further accidents from occurring. They are also concerned about how difficult it is to communicate with their father. Although Mr Apulu's sons helped look after their mother in the final stages of her illness, and have some understanding of what it is like to care for someone with a disability, they are not sure how they will manage their father's care at home.

Q What would you say to Mr Apulu's sons about their concerns? Who else might you bring into this discussion and why?

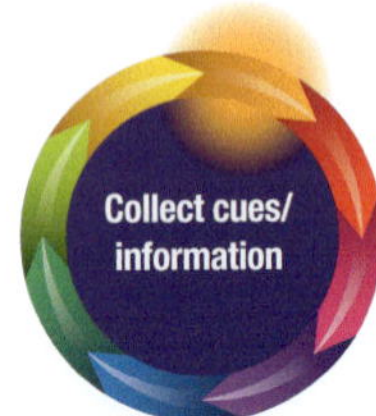

2. COLLECT CUES/INFORMATION

(a) Review current information

You review Mr Apulu's charts and identify the following:

Temperature	37°C
Pulse rate	67 (regular)
Respiratory rate	16
Blood pressure	150/95
Oxygen saturation level	96% on room air
GCS	13
NIHSS	10
Hourly urine output (average)	40–50 L/hr
BGL	6.1 mmol/L
Serum potassium	3.8 mmol/L
Serum sodium	130 mol/L

Q1 Stroke can affect many different body systems, leaving patients with a range of disabilities depending on which areas of the brain were damaged. The disabilities can be temporary but are more often permanent. Complete the table below by matching the term to the definition.

Term

- Dysarthria
- Unilateral neglect
- Hemiplegia
- Aphasia/dysphasia
- Dysphagia
- Diplopia

For further information about rehabilitation following a stroke, review Chapter 5 of the *Clinical Guidelines for Stroke Management:* https://app.magicapp.org/#/guideline/Kj2R8j

Term	Definition
	Paralysis of the left or right half of the body
	Difficulty speaking/incomprehensible speech or inability to understand speech
	Difficulty speaking/pronouncing words
	Unaware of and inattentive to one side of the body
	Unilateral or bilateral double vision
	Difficulty swallowing

You are caring for Mr Apulu on a busy morning shift and when you walk into his room you find him trying to stand on his own. He is agitated and when you ask him what he needs you have difficulty understanding his answer. The nurse who is making beds in the same room repeats your questions to Mr Apulu slowly and in a very loud voice. You motion to a urinary bottle and Mr Apulu nods his head.

Q2 What assumption(s) did the nurse who shouted at Mr Apulu make? Which clinical reasoning error is this an example of?

(b) Gather new information

Q From the following list, select the four assessments that are *least appropriate* at this stage.

a Glasgow Coma Scale: 13
b Pupillary response: PEARL (pupils equal and reactive to light)
c Falls risk (Ontario Modified Stratify): high
d Pain score: 1
e Waterlow score: high risk
f Mental health assessment: emotionally labile
g Bladder scan: residual 130 mL
h Temperature: 37°C
i Limb strength: severe weakness left side
j Mobility assessment: assist with two persons

(c) Recall knowledge

Quick Quiz!

Q1 A stroke patient is the most likely to develop a deep vein thrombosis (DVT) following a stroke when:
a He or she is a smoker or an ex-smoker
b He or she has hypertension
c He or she has decreased mobility
d He or she is overweight

Q2 When monitoring for thrombophlebitis, limbs should be assessed for:
a Decreased warmth, increased redness and decreased calf circumference
b Increased warmth, increased redness and decreased calf circumference
c Increased warmth, increased redness and increased calf circumference
d Decreased warmth, decreased redness and increased calf circumference

Q3 Hyperthermia may develop in a stroke patient due to damage to the hypothalamus.
a True
b False

Q4 Mr Apulu had continuous cardiac monitoring in the acute phase following a stroke for what reason?
a A stroke is likely to cause life-threatening ventricular fibrillation.
b A stroke may directly cause cardiac damage.
c A stroke may cause cardiac arrhythmias such as bradycardia and AV blocks.
d A stroke may cause cardiomegaly and consequent changes on the ECG.

Q5 A stroke patient who has weakness in their dominant side will find it easier to learn to accomplish tasks with their non-dominant side after the stroke.
a True
b False

Q6 Indicate whether the following statements are *true* or *false*.
a Supplemental oxygen should be given to all patients, even those who are not hypoxic.
b Early BGL monitoring should be instigated for all stroke patients and patients kept euglycaemic if they are a known diabetic.
c Antipyretics should routinely be used for stroke patients with a fever.
d Patients who have seizures after a stroke should not be given anti-convulsants.
e All stroke patients should be screened for swallowing ability before being given oral food, fluids or medications.
f The gag reflex is a valid screening tool for dysphagia.

Q7 When communicating with Mr Apulu, you should do all of the following *except*:
a Treat him as an adult
b Don't let him know that you do not understand him
c Use short simple sentences
d Try alternative methods of communication, including writing boards, picture boards and flash cards

Nursing and Midwifery Board of Australia (NMBA) *Registered Nurse Standards for Practice* The NMBA's *Registered Nurse Standards for Practice* (2016) state that RNs must communicate effectively, and be respectful of each person's dignity, culture, values, beliefs and rights.

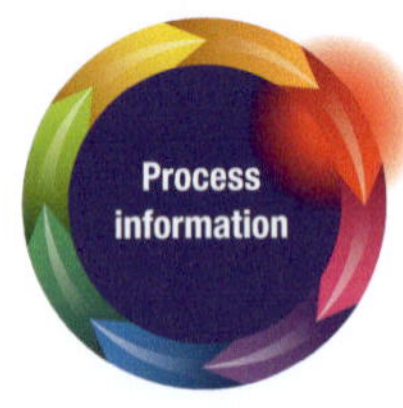

3. PROCESS INFORMATION

(a) Interpret

Q Indicate whether the following statements are *true* or *false*.

- a The deficits that Mr Apulu has have put him at risk of a fall.
- b Mr Apulu's loss of sensation and temperature in the affected limbs pose no risk of injury.
- c Mr Apulu's visual problems do not put him at risk of falls or injury.
- d Mr Apulu's limb weakness will make it difficult for him to mobilise.
- e It is common for patients post-stroke to display emotional lability.

(b) Discriminate, (c) Relate and (d) Infer

Q1 Mr Apulu's limb weakness makes him more prone to developing:

- a Joint dislocation
- b Foot drop
- c Sore feet
- d None of the options

Q2 Stroke patients who have dysphagia may become:

- a Overweight
- b Hungry
- c Malnourished
- d All of the options

National Safety and Quality Health Service (NSQH) Standards

Comprehensive care standard

The NSQHS Standards highlight the importance of minimising patient harm. This includes strategies designed to prevent pressure injuries, falls and malnutrition (ACSQHC, 2021).

Q3 Stroke patients who are incontinent should have an indwelling catheter if:

- a They have urge incontinence
- b They have urinary retention
- c They are frequently incontinent
- d None of the options

Q4 Which of the two cues that Mr Apulu is displaying may indicate a mood disturbance?

- a Anxiety
- b Emotional lability
- c Aggression
- d Anger
- e Irritability/agitation

(e) Predict

Q Mr Apulu, like many people who have had a stroke, is at risk of serious complications. In the table below, indicate which of the complications he is most at risk.

Complication	At risk	Not at risk
Shoulder dislocation		
Bleeding		
Aspiration pneumonia		
Seizures		
Pneumothorax		
DVT (deep vein thrombosis)		
Hepatic coma		
Pulmonary oedema		
Further stroke		

Something to think about . . .

People who have had a stroke are twice as likely to have a fall as other patients. They should be assessed for falls risk using a tool such as the Barthel's Index, and falls prevention should include exercises to strengthen muscles (Dean et al., 2011). Other interventions to prevent falls include easy access to the call bell, use of low-rise beds, avoidance of physical restraints, increased observation and surveillance, regular toileting, reduction of clutter, and observation when patients are walking and showering.

For more information on care planning and documentation of falls prevention strategies review the Falls Risk Assessment and Management Plan (FRAMP) *at: https://www.cec.health.nsw.gov.au/keep-patients-safe/older-persons-patient-safety-program/falls-prevention/hospitals/risk-screening*

(f) Match

Q Have you ever cared for someone with the same or similar post-stroke signs and symptoms as Mr Apulu? If so, what was done to manage the situation?

4. IDENTIFY THE PROBLEM/ISSUE

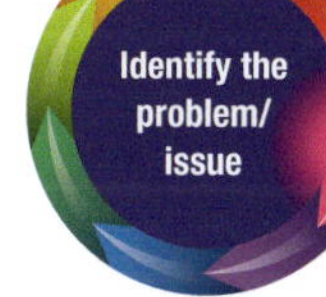

Q Complete the following nursing diagnoses for Mr Apulu.

a Impaired verbal communication related to neuromuscular impairment, evidenced by dysarthria and ________________.

b Impaired physical mobility related to, ________________ and unilateral neglect, evidenced by limb weakness, limited range of motion and decreased muscle strength/control.

c Risk of impaired swallowing related to ________________ and poor gag reflex.

d Risk of falls related to hemiplegia ________________ and hearing problems.

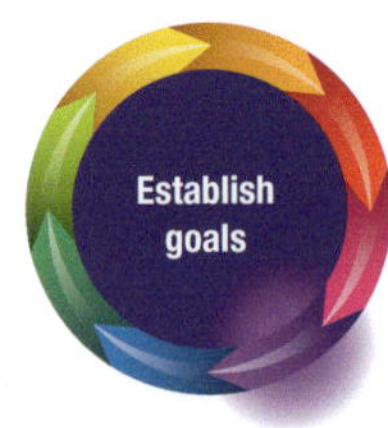

5. ESTABLISH GOALS

Q From the list below, choose the three most important *short-term* nursing goals for Mr Apulu's management at this time.

a For Mr Apulu to remain well nourished
b For Mr Apulu's GCS to improve within the next 24 hours
c For Mr Apulu to be able to communicate effectively
d For Mr Apulu to be continent of urine and to have no constipation
e For Mr Apulu to be hypotensive within the next 24 hours
f For Mr Apulu not to have any falls

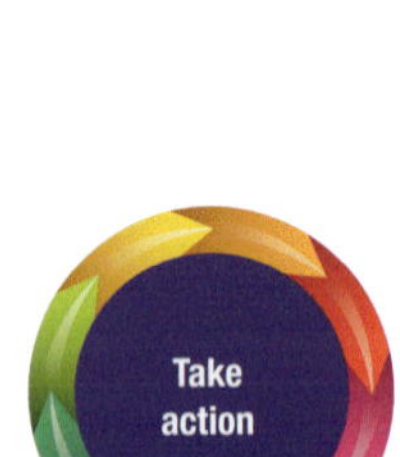

6. TAKE ACTION

Q1 In the following tables, match the nursing actions you would take in caring for Mr Apulu with the related rationales.

Airway and breathing

Nursing action

- Regular monitoring of vital signs and respiratory status
- Regular chest physiotherapy

Nursing action	Rationale
	To detect early developing complications such as pneumonia
	To prevent chest infections such as aspiration pneumonia

Circulation

Nursing action

- Assess for warmth, redness and increase in size of calves
- Anti-embolic stockings and early mobilisation

Nursing action	Rationale
	To monitor for development of thrombophlebitis
	To prevent thrombophlebitis and contractures

Disability

Nursing action

- Instigate range-of-motion exercises, and support joints and limbs at rest
- Assess for changes in neurological deficit

Nursing action	Rationale
	To identify early signs for further deterioration
	To maintain and improve muscle strength and joint flexibility

Exposure

Nursing action

- Mouth care, including suctioning on affected side
- Two-hourly position change

Nursing action	Rationale
	To keep mouth clean and prevent infections and aspiration pneumonia
	To prevent pressure areas developing

Holistic assessment

Nursing action

- Face patient, speak slowly and allow time for answers
- Use picture boards, gestures, writing boards and computers

Nursing action	Rationale
	To maintain patient's dignity and decrease frustration with communication
	To assist in communication

Key to quality care during the acute and rehabilitation phases for people who have experienced a stroke is timely referral to appropriate members of the multi-disciplinary healthcare team in the community. This requires you to be aware of the roles and responsibilities of team members, and to know when and how to coordinate referrals.

Q2 From the table below, match the allied health professionals to their role in the care of Mr Apulu.

Health professionals

- Speech pathologists
- Social workers
- Dieticians
- Occupational therapists
- Physiotherapists
- Physicians, neurologists, general practitioners

Health professional	Role and responsibilities
	Help patients with aphasia relearn how to communicate and assess ability to swallow
	Help patients retrain motor and sensory impairments, and assess strength and endurance
	Help patients organise such things as finances and referrals
	Responsible for managing and coordinating patient care
	Help determine right food choices for patients and also right food consistency
	Help improve motor skills and the ability to perform such things as grooming, meal preparation and house cleaning

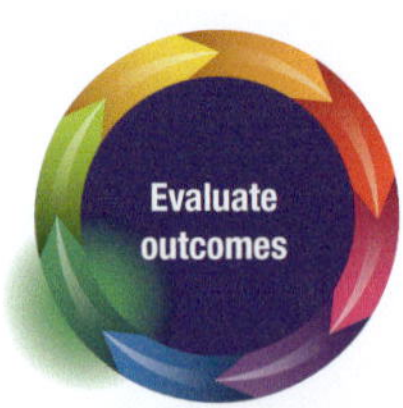

7. EVALUATE

Q Outline how you would determine the efficacy of your nursing actions in the prevention of complications for Mr Apulu.

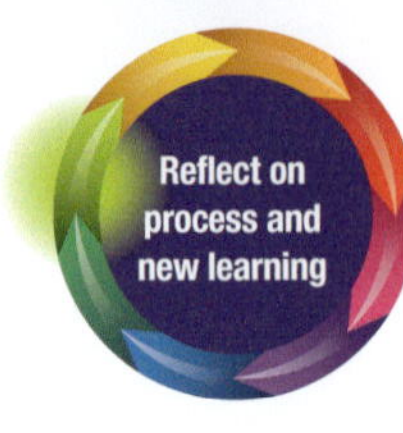

8. REFLECT

Reflect on your learning from this scenario and consider the following questions.

Q1 What are three of the most important things you have learnt from this scenario?

Q2 What actions will you take in clinical practice as a result of your learning from this scenario?

EPILOGUE

Mr Apulu remained on the acute stroke ward for two weeks, during which time he was assessed and managed by the multi-disciplinary stroke care team. He was then transferred to a rehabilitation unit.

While in rehabilitation, Mr Apulu's house was modified on the recommendation of the occupational therapist, and a raised toilet seat and shower chair were provided, along with equipment to help him with activities of daily living. Two months later, Mr Apulu was discharged into the care of his sons and an aunt from New Zealand who stayed with them for a few months. A community nurse helps shower Mr Apulu in the mornings and his sons assist with this on the weekends. Samoan friends from his church visit and help when they can.

Mr Apulu has mobilising splints for his arm and leg which his sons help him apply before they go to work so that he can mobilise independently if somewhat slowly. He still has some dysarthria, but his speech and comprehension have improved significantly. His vision problems remain, but he has learnt to cope with these and he borrows large-print books from the local library.

Mr Apulu now has a pureed diet and thickened fluids. He lost a lot of weight initially as he did not enjoy this diet; however, he understands that it is important for him to maintain adequate nutrition. He has stopped smoking and his BGLs remain stable. He has continued on aspirin daily, as well as his blood pressure medications and statins.

Mr Apulu goes to hydrotherapy once a week and attends a respite group where he enjoys participating in the activities. He is also a member of the local stroke support group and enjoys the outings they arrange. His friends pick him up on Friday nights to go to the local pub and, although he can no longer have a few beers, he enjoys getting out with his 'mates'. He has been fishing with his sons since his return home, but they now fish off the pier. Mr Apulu misses being able to go out in the 'tinnie', but it was too difficult for his sons to get him in and out of the small boat.

Mr Apulu still feels sad at the loss of his normal functioning but says he is learning to adapt to his disabilities. He has not been able to return to work and finds it hard that his sons now need to care for him, as he feels he should still be caring for them. However, he is immensely proud of his 'boys' and what they do for him.

FURTHER READING

Clinical Guidelines for Stroke Management. Retrieved from: https://app.magicapp.org/#/guideline/Kj2R8j

Gillespie, D. & Campbell, F. (2011). Effect of stroke on family carers and family relationships. *Nursing Standard,* 26(2), 39–46.

Stroke Foundation. (2020). *Stroke Is Always a Medical Emergency.* Retrieved from: https://strokefoundation.org.au/Media-Releases/2020/03/30/22/22/Stroke%20is%20always%20a%20medical%20emergency

Stroke Foundation. (2021). *What Is a Stroke?* Retrieved from: https://strokefoundation.org.au/About-Stroke/Learn/Types-of-stroke

REFERENCES

Australian Commission on Safety and Quality in Health Care (ACSQHC). (2021). *National Safety and Quality Health Service Standards* (2nd edn). Sydney, Australia.

Australian Institute of Health and Welfare (AIHW). (2013). *Stroke and Its Management in Australia: An Update*. Retrieved from: https://www.aihw.gov.au/reports/heart-stroke-vascular-diseases/stroke-management-australia-update/contents/table-of-contents

Australian Institute of Health and Welfare (AIHW). (2018). *Australia's Health 2018—Stroke.* Retrieved from: https://www.aihw.gov.au/getmedia/56bb591f-6c56-4397-b928-8de6872e2cdd/aihw-aus-221-chapter-3-7.pdf.aspx#:~:text=in%202016%2c%20there%20were%208%2c200,7.2)

Australian Institute of Health and Welfare (AIHW). (2020). *Australia's Health—Stroke.* Retrieved from: https://www.aihw.gov.au/reports/australias-health/stroke

Dean, C., Rissel, C., Sharkey, M., Sherrington, C., Cumming, R., Barker, R.,... Kirkman, C. (2011). *Exercise Intervention to Prevent Falls and Enhance Mobility in Community Dwellers After Stroke: A Protocol for a Randomised Controlled Trial.* Sydney: NSW Ministry of Health. Retrieved from: www.health.nsw.gov.au/research/Publications/2006-exercise-for-falls.pdf

Gangadharan, S., Lillicrap, T., Miteff, F., Garcia-Bermejo, P., Wellings, T., O'Brien, . . . Spratt, N. J. (2020). Air vs. road decision for endovascular clot retrieval in a rural telestroke network. *Frontiers in Neurology, 11*, 628. doi.org/10.3389/fneur.2020.00628

Garrett, P., Dickson, H., Young, L., Whelan, A. & Forero, R. (2008). What do non-English-speaking patients value in acute care? Cultural competency from the patient's perspective: A qualitative study. *Ethnicity and Health*, *13*(5), 479–96.

Gilligan, C., Outram, S. & Buchanan, H. (2020). Communicating with people from culturally and linguistically diverse backgrounds. In Levett-Jones, T. (Ed.), *Critical Conversations for Patient Safety: An Essential Guide for Health Professionals* (2nd edn). Sydney: Pearson.

Levett-Jones, T., Dwyer, T., Reid-Searl, K., Heaton, L., Flenady, T., Applegarth, J., Guinea, S. & Andersen, P. (2017). *The Patient Safety Competency Framework for Nursing Students*. Retrieved from: http://psframework.wpengine.com/wp-content/uploads/2018/01/PSCF_Brochure_UTS-version_FA2-Screen.pdf

Mellish, L. (2020). Nursing care of people with intracranial disorders. In P. LeMone, K. Burke, G. Bauldoff, P. Gubrud-Howe, T. Levett-Jones, T. Dwyer,... D. Raymond (Eds), *Medical–Surgical Nursing: Critical Thinking in Person-Centred Care* (4th edn). Melbourne: Pearson.

Nursing and Midwifery Board of Australia (NMBA). (2016). *Registered Nurse Standards for Practice.* Retrieved from: www.nursingmidwiferyboard.gov.au/Codes-Guidelines-Statements/Professional-standards.aspx

Stroke Foundation. (2020). *Stroke Is Always a Medical Emergency.* Retrieved from: https://strokefoundation.org.au/Media-Releases/2020/03/30/22/22/Stroke%20is%20always%20a%20medical%20emergency

Stroke Foundation. (2021). *What Is a Stroke?* Retrieved from: https://strokefoundation.org.au/About-Stroke/Learn/Types-of-stroke

Chapter 9

Caring for a person receiving blood component therapies

ELIZABETH NEWMAN and VIVIENNE CHAU

LEARNING OUTCOMES

Completion of the activities in this chapter will enable you to:

- explain why an understanding of blood components and their function is essential to competent practice (**recall** and **application**)
- identify the clinical manifestations of anaemia, leukopaenia, thrombocytopaenia and transfusion reactions that will guide the collection and interpretation of appropriate cues (**gather information, interpret** and **discriminate**)
- identify risk factors for patients receiving blood component therapies (**match** and **predict**)
- review clinical information to identify the main nursing diagnoses for a person experiencing a transfusion reaction (**analyse, synthesise** and **evaluate**)
- describe the priorities of care for a patient receiving blood component therapies and experiencing a transfusion reaction (**goal setting**)
- identify clinical criteria for determining the effectiveness of nursing actions taken to manage transfusion reactions (**evaluate**)
- apply what you have learnt to new situations (**reflection** and **translation**).

INTRODUCTION

In this chapter, you will follow the experiences of Mrs Hayma (meaning: Forest) Hlaing as she undergoes treatment, initially for haemorrhage and later for leukaemia, across time and in different healthcare contexts. Managing the transfusion of blood cells, which are in fact live human tissues with significant risks, requires a depth of knowledge and sound clinical reasoning skills. However, there is added complexity when caring for someone who requires a transfusion because of leukaemia, as the person's own blood cells are affected by the disease process (EdCaN, 2016a). Therefore, excellent clinical reasoning skills are needed in order for you to recognise and respond to actual or potential problems that may arise from both the disease and the therapies provided.

Prior to seeking asylum in Australia, Mrs Hlaing was exposed to prolonged periods of deprivation, human rights abuses, the loss of many members of her family and a perilous escape from her homeland. Learning about her story will help deepen your understanding of the importance of cultural empathy and cultural competence, and your role in promoting refugee health.

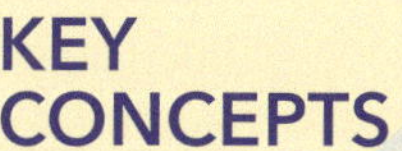

KEY CONCEPTS

blood component therapies
haematological diseases
transfusion reactions

SUGGESTED READINGS

P. LeMone, G. Bauldoff, P. Gubrud-Howe, M.-A. Carno, T. Levett-Jones, . . . D. Stanley (Eds). (2020). *LeMone and Burke's Medical-Surgical Nursing: Critical Thinking in Person-Centred Care* (4th edn). Melbourne: Pearson Australia.

Chapter 11: Nursing care of people with infection

Chapter 12: Nursing care of people with altered immunity

Chapter 13: Nursing care of people with cancer

Chapter 32: Nursing care of people with haematological disorders

T. Levett-Jones (Ed.), (2019). *Critical Conversations for Patient Safety: An Essential Guide for Health Professionals* (2nd edn). Sydney: Pearson.

Chapter 17: Communicating with people from culturally and linguistically diverse backgrounds

SCENARIO 9.1 Caring for a person requiring an emergency transfusion of packed red blood cells

SETTING THE SCENE

Mrs Hayma Hlaing, her husband and their 5-year-old daughter had travelled from Rohingya by foot into Thailand, which they used as a transit country to fly to Australia. While descending from their flight at Kingsford Smith Airport, Mrs Hlaing fell down the stairs landing heavily on the tarmac and sustained a deep laceration to her thigh. She had considerable blood loss and was given first aid at the scene. Mrs Hlaing was then transported to the nearest emergency department (ED).

The Rohingya people are an ethnic minority who mostly reside in Rakhine State on the west coast of Myanmar. The Rohingyan community, the majority of whom are Muslim, have been in Rakhine State for generations (United Nations Human Rights Office of the High Commissioner [OHCHR], 2017). Since 1962, the Myanmar government have progressively stripped the Rohingya of their civil and political rights (OHCHR, 2017). Despite living in Myanmar for generations, the Myanmar government denies the Rohingya citizenship rights, effectively rendering them stateless people in their own home (Amnesty International, 2017). Since 2012, they have been stripped of their identity cards and their right to vote and form political parties (OHCHR, 2017).

An 'asylum seeker' is a person who has fled their country and applies to the government of another country for protection as a refugee. A 'refugee' is a person who is outside their own country and is unable or unwilling to return due to a well-founded fear of being persecuted because of their race, religion, nationality or political opinion.

The United Nations consider the Rohingya to be the most persecuted minority in the world (OHCHR, 2017). There are credible reports of widespread and systematic violent attacks against the Rohingyan community by the Myanmar government. Witnesses have reported the murder of adults and children, rape of women and girls, shooting of fleeing civilians, and burning and destruction of houses (Human Rights Council 36th Session, 2017).

By the end of 2017, approximately 626,000 Rohingyan refugees had fled to Bangladesh (Human Rights Council 36th Session, 2017). Some Rohingyan refugees have also fled to other neighbouring countries, such as Thailand, where they are vulnerable to human trafficking and forced labour (The Equal Rights Trust, 2014). Thailand is often a transit country for Rohingya who use it as a route to reach Malaysia or Australia (OHCHR, 2017).

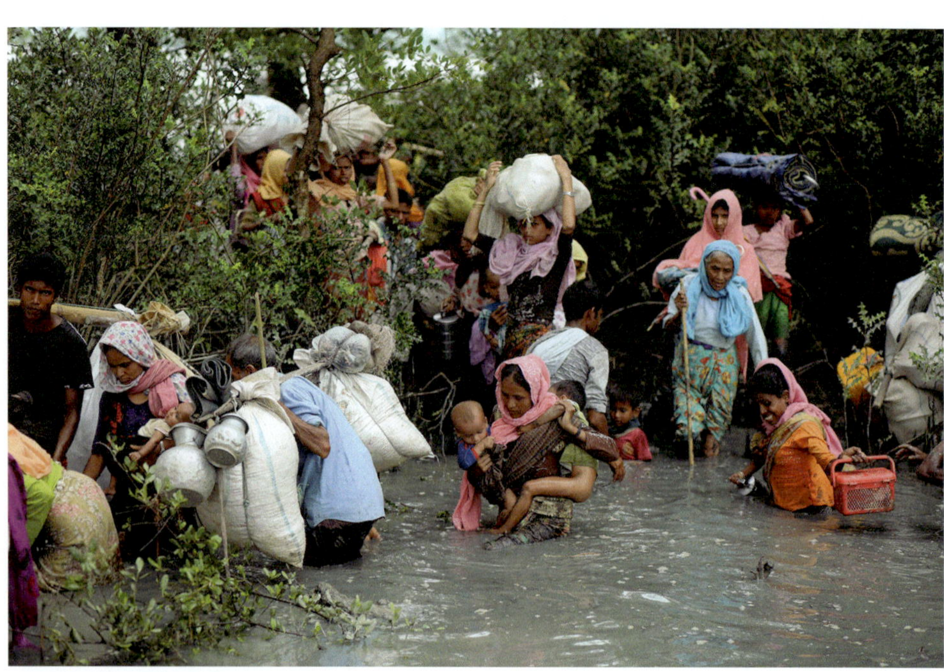

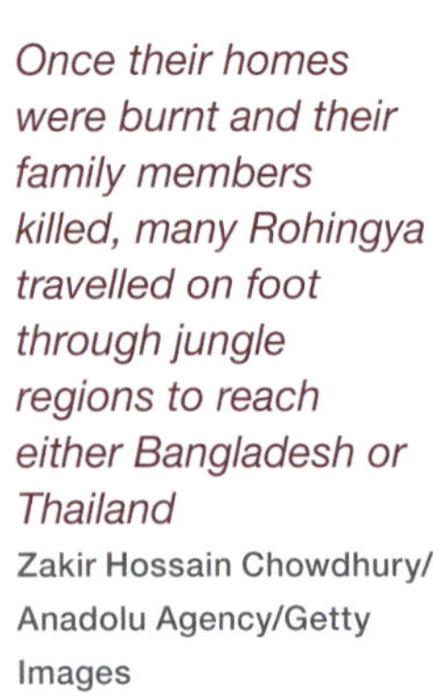

Once their homes were burnt and their family members killed, many Rohingya travelled on foot through jungle regions to reach either Bangladesh or Thailand
Zakir Hossain Chowdhury/Anadolu Agency/Getty Images

1. CONSIDER THE PATIENT SITUATION

You are a nurse working at the ED and will be responsible for Mrs Hlaing's care while she undergoes treatment for blood loss and suturing of her wound. You receive the following handover from the emergency personnel who attended the scene.

Handover report

We have Mrs Hayma Hlaing who is 42 years old. She has a deep and dirty penetrating laceration to her left thigh that she received when she fell down the stairs and onto the tarmac. We treated her at the scene and estimate at least 500 mL blood loss. The wound has been irrigated with sodium chloride and covered with a dressing and pressure bandage. Her BP was initially 100/50 but she developed a postural drop and her MAP fell to 60 so we inserted an 18 FG cannula and administered sodium chloride 0.9% 1000 mLs over 1 hour, her oxygen saturation was 89% so we commenced oxygen therapy via a Hudson mask and her oxygen saturation is now 95%. Her respiration rate is 26 breaths per minute, pulse 120 beats per minute and she's afebrile at 36.4 degrees celsius. She is accompanied by her husband who can speak limited English. He is insisting on staying with her saying that it's Sharia law. He couldn't tell us whether she has any allergies but, apparently, she hasn't seen a doctor for many years. We haven't given any analgesia. Their young daughter is also with them.

Sharia refers to Islam's legal system which is derived from the Quran, Islam's holy book.

National Safety and Quality Health Service (NSQH) Standards

Comprehensive care standard

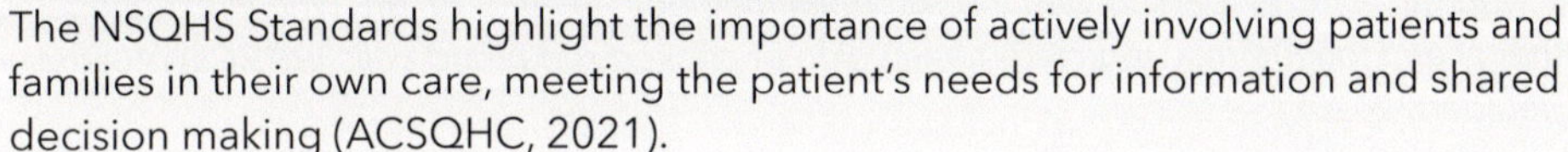

The NSQHS Standards highlight the importance of actively involving patients and families in their own care, meeting the patient's needs for information and shared decision making (ACSQHC, 2021).

Quick Quiz!

To ensure that you have a good understanding of the terms used in this handover, try this quick quiz.

Q1 Sodium chloride 0.9% is:

- a A sterile solution of water filtered to remove sodium chloride
- b A sterile solution that has the same tonicity as body fluids
- c A solution of 90 grams of sodium chloride in 1000 mL of water

Q2 FG means:

- a 'French gauge' and refers to the outside diameter of a cannula
- b 'Finish gauge' and refers to the number of lumens of a cannula
- c 'Finished grade' and refers to the quality of the cannula

Q3 What is the normal oxygen saturation parameter for a healthy person?

- a above 85%
- b above 90%
- c 95%–100%

Q4 MAP (mean arterial pressure) is a calculation that indicates:

- a Sufficient blood pressure to perfuse vital organs
- b Maximum blood volume
- c Sufficient blood pressure to perfuse the peripheries

MAP is calculated using the following formula:

$$\text{MAP} = \frac{(\text{Diastolic BP} \times 2) + \text{Systolic BP}}{3}$$

The doctor examines Mrs Hlaing and orders a full blood count, group and antibody screen and cross-match. However, because of her extensive bleeding, he does not wait for cross-matched packed red blood cells (PRBCs) to be available, instead ordering an immediate transfusion of emergency PRBCs. He notes that Mrs Hlaing appears dehydrated and exhausted, probably due to the hardships endured whilst trying to flee Myanmar to get to safety. The doctor cleans, sutures and dresses the wound. He observes several bruises of various sizes and ages and assumes that Mrs Hlaing suffered these from the fall from the plane onto the tarmac. The doctor then orders tests for tuberculosis (TB), human immunodeficiency virus (HIV), syphilis and malaria as part of the usual screening process.

Medical orders

- One unit of PRBCs over 3 hours followed by 1000 mLs 0.9% sodium chloride over 6 hours
- Morphine sulphate 5 mg via subcutaneous injection
- Prophylactic tetanus injection
- Prophylactic antibiotics: penicillin 500 mg IV; ceftriaxone 2 g IV

Something to think about . . .

While reasons for blood component transfusions vary, the aim is to supplement depleted components within the blood, in order to relieve clinical signs and symptoms and sometimes to prevent morbidity and mortality, but they are not without risks. Allogeneic transfusion can be associated with adverse patient outcomes, delay patient recovery and inadvertently increase morbidity and increase length of hospital stays (National Blood Authority, 2011–2016). The patient blood management guidelines (National Blood Authority) are evidence-based and do not promote unnecessary transfusions. For example, a person who is asymptomatic from anaemia (haemoglobin 85g/L) does not necessarily need a transfusion, whereas another person with the same haemoglobin level of 85 g/L who is experiencing increased lethargy and fatigue may require a transfusion of packed red blood cells (PRBCs) (Australian Red Cross Lifeblood, 2020).

Person-centred care

The focus of Mrs Hlaing's care so far has been the emergency management of her injury and bleeding, with the plan being to treat her injuries and return her to the detention centre where she will be processed for consideration as a refugee. However, you are concerned about Mrs Hlaing and her husband as they seem to be confused, distressed and frightened. You contact the interpreter service as you want to help the couple understand what is happening, establish a culturally safe environment and develop a therapeutic relationship.

Nursing and Midwifery Board of Australia (NMBA) *Registered Nurse Standards for Practice* The NMBA's *Registered Nurse Standards for Practice* (2016) state that RNs must work in partnership to determine factors that affect, or potentially affect, the health and wellbeing of people and to determine priorities for action and/or for referral.

The interpreter arrives and together you uncover the family's disturbing story. Mrs Hlaing was born in the Rohingyan Community in Myanmar where she watched her village burn to the ground, friends and family shot, and women and young girls raped. Mrs Hlaing had five children, all delivered at home by the village midwife. Two died soon after they were born and two were killed in ethnic cleansing programs. After their village was burnt down her husband gathered them together and they fled to Thailand. Healthcare in Mrs Hlaing's country was not readily available to them as they were displaced and the government had rescinded their national verification cards. Mrs Hlaing and her family are Muslim but were forbidden from practising their religion. As they were of Rohingya descent they were not permitted to rent, buy a home or work, they had lost their voting rights and could not marry without a permit—these can take years to be granted, if ever. Mrs Hlaing's husband tells you that she has not had any serious health issues.

Something to think about . . .

Communication with people from a refugee background may be affected by language and cultural differences as well as different social, economic and political experiences. Read Culturally sensitive communication in healthcare: A concept analysis *by Brooks, Manias & Bloomer (2019) to learn more about the concept of cultural communication with the use of interpreters.*

2. COLLECT CUES/INFORMATION

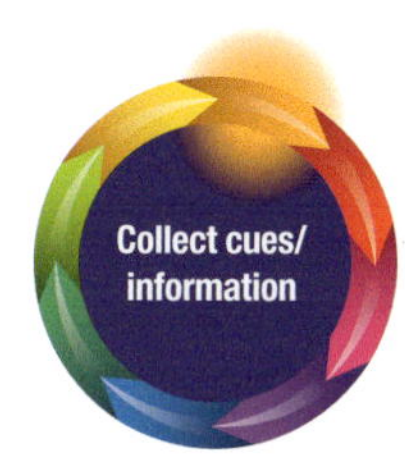

The unit of blood arrives from the facilities blood bank and you place it in the blood fridge in order to comply with cold chain storage requirements. About an hour later, you are able to start the transfusion; you remove the unit of blood from the blood fridge and complete the required cold chain documentation (Australia New Zealand Society of Blood Transfusion, 2018), placing it on the table behind the nurse's station. You then page the doctor to obtain consent to administer blood products. You also arrange for an unrelated translator so that the reason for the transfusion, along with possible side effects, can be explained to Mrs Hlaing and her husband. As they believe in Sharia law, you know that both Mrs Hlaing and her husband must be involved in any treatment decision; however, Mrs Hlaing is required to sign the consent form. You complete a set of baseline observations and prepare to commence the transfusion.

To ensure that Mrs Hlaing receives the right blood product, you undertake a number of checks at her bedside. The checks must be undertaken by two appropriate staff, one of whom must then connect and spike the bag.

Hint: This transfusion checklist will help you answer this question: https://transfusion.com.au/node/2196

Q These checks include the following (fill in the blanks):

a Blood pack label and ________________ /paperwork are all identical/compatible and correct.

b The blood pack and ________________ details are identical and correct.

c Patient name—ask them to state/spell their name and to clarify their ________________.

d ________________ and time of blood pack (ensure cross-match specimen current).

e Bag intact. No evidence of tampering or ________________.

f No clots or significant differences in ________________ between tube segments and blood in bag

g Ensure all documentation is completed and placed in the patient's medical record, with two nurses checking full printed names and ________________.

(a) Review current information

You review Mrs Hlaing's baseline observations:

Temperature	36ºC
Pulse rate	112
Respiratory rate	28
Blood pressure	90/50
Oxygen saturation level	95%

The blood administration rate will be unique for each pack as the volume differs. As this pack has been ordered over 3 hours and you note that the volume is 336 mLs, you calculate that 112 mLs/hr is the correct rate and enter this information into the pump. You observe Mrs Hlaing for the first 15 minutes of the transfusion and retake her observations, which are very similar to the baseline observations. You then leave to attend to another patient.

A few minutes later, Mrs Hlaing's husband runs to you and tells you to come quickly. When you return, you observe that Mrs Hlaing has started to shiver, and she is moaning and clutching her head with her hands. You stop the transfusion immediately and check Mrs Hlaing's vital signs.

(b) Gather new information

Revise your knowledge about blood transfusions by accessing the Clinical Transfusion e-learning package at: https://bloodsafelearning.org.au/course/clinical-transfusion-practice

Q1 From the list below, identify the *four* cues that you need to collect immediately.

- a Respiratory rate
- b Pain score
- c Level of consciousness
- d Skin colour
- e Temperature
- f Pulse rate
- g Blood pressure
- h Condition of the wound

Q2 What else would you check at this stage?

(c) Recall knowledge

Quick Quiz!

Caring for someone undergoing a blood transfusion and experiencing a possible reaction requires a sound knowledge base. Try this quiz to test your knowledge.

Q1 The process of red blood cell destruction is called:

- a Erythrocytosis
- b Erythropoiesis
- c Haemocytosis
- d Haemolysis

Q2 If someone's blood agglutinates with both anti-A and anti-B antisera, what is their blood type?

- a B
- b AB
- c O
- d A

Q3 If someone's blood type is O and they have the RhD factor on the membrane of their red cells, their blood group is O+ve. What two blood groups are suitable for a transfusion for this person?

- a O–ve
- b O+ve
- c A+ve
- d A–ve
- e B+ve
- f B–ve
- g AB+ve
- h AB–ve

Q4 Blood with what blood group would be appropriate for Mrs Hlaing's emergency transfusion?

- a Type A (the most common group for Middle-Eastern people)
- b Type B (least likely to be a mismatch)
- c Type AB (universal recipient)
- d Type O (universal donor)

Q5 Transfusion request forms in Australia should include a signed declaration verifying correct patient identification procedures have been followed. This declaration is designed to:

- a Confirm that the patient has consented to the blood transfusion
- b Ensure the right blood is collected from the right patient and labelled correctly
- c Document the collector's identity for the transfusion service provider's records
- d Record the collector's details in case the transfusion service provider needs the specimen label amended

Q6 How often, or for how long, should transfusion observations be attended?

- a During the transfusion of each unit according to hospital policy
- b 15 minutes after the transfusion commences
- c Before the start of each unit of blood commences
- d When the transfusion is complete
- e All of the options

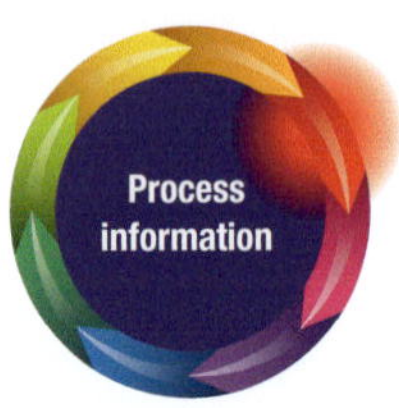

3. PROCESS INFORMATION

(a) Interpret and (b) Discriminate

You now review and interpret Mrs Hlaing's current observations.

Q1 Which two of the observations below are within normal parameters for Mrs Hlaing?

Temperature	38.2ºC
Pulse rate	118 beats/min
Respiratory rate	24 breaths/min
Blood pressure	100/60
Oxygen saturation level	95%

Q2 You identify that Mrs Hlaing has been given Type O–ve blood. Is this of concern? Why or why not?

Access the following resources if you need help with this question: https://transfusion.com.au/blood_basics/compatibility

(c) Relate and (d) Infer

Cluster the cues together to identify relationships between them and draw inferences based on what you know about Mrs Hlaing's history and signs and symptoms.

Further information on blood transfusion reactions can be reviewed using the following resource: https://transfusion.com.au/adverse_events_overview

Q Which one of the following statements is *true*?

a Mrs Hlaing could be hypertensive and tachycardic from a rapid IV rate.
b Mrs Hlaing could be hypoxic and tachypnoeic as a result of pulmonary oedema.
c Mrs Hlaing could be normotensive and bradycardic because she is anxious and frightened.
d Mrs Hlaing could be hypotensive and tachycardic from the initial trauma and low blood volume.
e Mrs Hlaing could be febrile and tachycardic due to a transfusion reaction.

(e) Predict

Q What could happen to Mrs Hlaing if no action is taken and this situation is not corrected? Select the *incorrect* statement.

When answering this question, think about the causes and consequences of transfusion reactions.

a Mrs Hlaing's condition will gradually improve over the next few days.
b Mrs Hlaing could develop acute kidney injury.
c Mrs Hlaing could develop circulatory overload.
d Mrs Hlaing could lose consciousness.
e Mrs Hlaing could die.

4. IDENTIFY THE PROBLEM/ISSUE

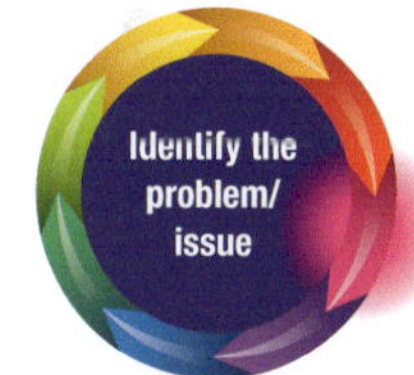

At this stage, you bring together (synthesise) all of the facts you've collected and inferences you've made to make a nursing diagnosis of Mrs Hlaing's main problems or issues.

Q Select from the following list two most likely nursing diagnoses for Mrs Hlaing.

a Transfusion-related acute lung injury (TRALI), evidenced by fever hypoxia and tachypnoea
b A febrile transfusion reaction related to possible bacterial contamination, evidenced by chills, tachycardia, fever and hypotension
c An anaphylactic reaction to an incompatible blood transfusion, evidenced by headache, chills, tachycardia, fever, urticaria and itching
d Hypervolaemia related to a fluid overload, evidenced by tachycardia, headache and hypertension
e A febrile non-haemolytic transfusion reaction related to possible antibody/antigen reaction, evidenced by headache, chills, tachycardia, fever and hypotension

5. ESTABLISH GOALS

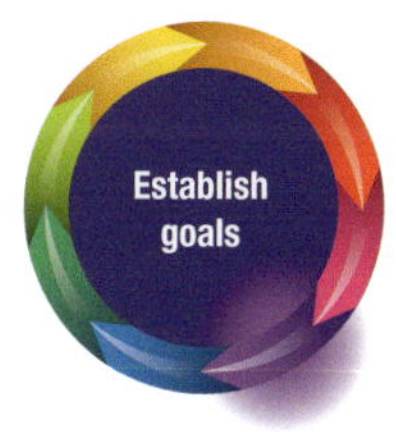

Q Before implementing any actions to improve Mrs Hlaing's condition, it is important to clearly specify what you want to happen and when. Which of the following are correct goals?

a For Mrs Hlaing to be afebrile and without shivering, headache, tachycardia or hypotension within 2 hours (and over the next week)
b For Mrs Hlaing to be afebrile and without headache, tachycardia or hypertension within 24 hours (and over the next month)

c For Mrs Hlaing to be febrile and without dark urine or urticaria within 4 hours (and over the next day)
d For Mrs Hlaing to be normotensive and without headache, tachycardia or urticaria within 48 hours (and over the next week)

6. TAKE ACTION

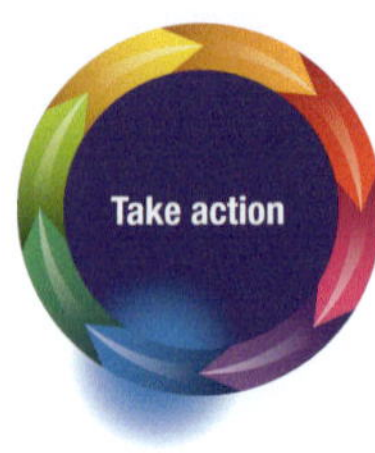

Q1 From the list below, choose the four *most immediate actions* you should take at this stage.
a Maintain IV access.
b Flush the existing IV line.
c Notify the doctor immediately.
d Re-perform steps 1 to 4 of the pre-transfusion check.
e Monitor Mrs Hlaing's pain score.
f Monitor Mrs Hlaing's vital signs and oxygen saturation level.
g Notify the transfusion service (in this case blood bank) provider.

A medical review is conducted and the doctor agrees with your nursing diagnosis. He believes Mrs Hlaing is most likely experiencing a febrile non-haemolytic transfusion reaction, probably due to an antibody/antigen interaction. However, he does not rule out bacterial contamination, especially when you tell him that the blood sat on the nurse's desk for over an hour before being administered.

The doctor orders paracetamol and asks you to restart Mrs Hlaing's transfusion if her symptoms resolve when the paracetamol takes effect. He wants you to monitor Mrs Hlaing's condition very closely for the remainder of the transfusion and if there is any reoccurrence of her symptoms, the transfusion is to be ceased completely. However, the doctor specifies that if another unit of blood is required, cross-matching with full antibody screening will be necessary. Once Mrs Hlaing's transfusion is completed, the doctor wants the intravenous sodium chloride 0.9% started, as he is still concerned about her dehydration and hypovolaemia.

Q2 In the following table, match the rationales for care to the corresponding nursing action.

Rationales

- To identify improvement or deterioration in Mrs Hliang's condition
- Dark-coloured urine may indicate haemolysis
- To ensure cannula is patent; pain along the IV line may indicate haemolysis
- Anxiety and restlessness may indicate worsening antigen/antibody reaction
- To ensure adequate oxygen delivery; deterioration may indicate laryngeal oedema, bronchospasm or TRALI
- To immediately identify an urticarial rash and any abnormal, unexplained bleeding

Nursing action	Rationale
Check cognitive status regularly	
Monitor haemodynamic status closely	
Examine skin regularly	
Maintain patent IV access and monitor IV site regularly	
Maintain oxygen therapy via nasal prongs and hourly oxygen saturation	
Check colour in each specimen of urine	

7. EVALUATE

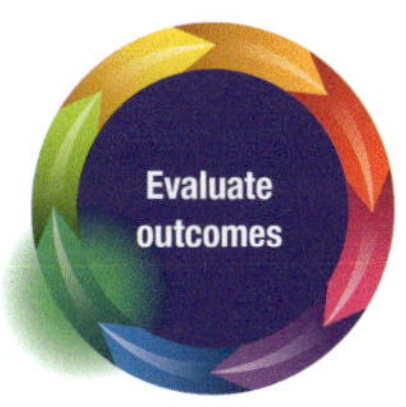

Q It is now two hours since Mrs Hlaing's blood transfusion was completed and her sodium chloride 0.9% IV commenced. Review the following signs and symptoms to determine whether Mrs Hlaing's condition has improved. Label them as *unchanged, improving* or *deteriorating*.

Cognitive status	Patient restless and anxious
Pulse rate	105
Blood pressure	100/55 lying; 90/50 sitting
Respirations	26
Oxygen saturation level	95%
Skin	No rash evident
Shivering	Ceased
Temperature	37.2°C

8. REFLECT

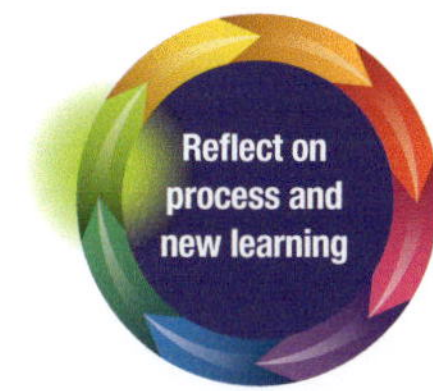

Reflect on your learning from this scenario and consider the following questions.

Q1 What are three of the most important things that you have learnt from this scenario?

Q2 Could anything have prevented Mrs Hlaing's transfusion reaction?

Q3 What actions will you take in clinical practice as a result of your learning from this scenario?

Q4 How do you think that your own cultural beliefs and values influence your ability to provide culturally competent care for your patients?

SCENARIO 9.2 Caring for a person undergoing a transfusion of platelets and fresh frozen plasma

CHANGING THE SCENE

In Scenario 9.1, Mrs Hlaing experienced a febrile non-haemolytic blood transfusion reaction. Despite the treatment provided, her haemoglobin remained low and she still experienced symptoms of anaemia, so a second unit of cross-matched PRBCs was transfused without complications. Following treatment in the emergency department (ED), Mrs Hlaing was transferred to a detention facility and waited for the processing of her refugee application. Mrs Hlaing and her husband plus their daughter were granted refugee status and six months later were settled in the Western Downs, about 350 kilometres from Brisbane, Queensland.

Over the ensuing 12 months, Mrs Hlaing's fatigue did not resolve and she continued to experience bruising unrelated to trauma. Her gums also bled repeatedly, despite paying strict attention to her oral hygiene. Eventually, Mrs Hlaing presented to the ED of the local hospital. A full blood count was ordered and it revealed that she had severe anaemia and thrombocytopaenia. She was diagnosed with acute myeloid leukaemia.

The epidemiology of leukaemia

In Australia, leukaemia is the seventh most commonly diagnosed cancer. It is estimated that 4,903 people will be diagnosed with leukaemia in 2021—1,898 females and 3,005 males. Survival rates from leukaemia have increased markedly over the past 20 years and the five-year survival rate is now 63 per cent (Cancer Australia, 2021).

The aetiology and pathogenesis of leukaemia

Leukaemia is a disease in which malignant white blood cells (WBCs) proliferate in the bone marrow and peripheral blood supply, replacing normal cells. The aetiology of leukaemia is unknown; however, there are several predisposing factors associated with the development of the disease. These include high doses of radiation, exposure to benzenes and some viruses. There are also some genetic conditions that have been identified as risk factors, such as Down syndrome, Fanconi's anaemia and Klinefelter's syndrome. A family history of leukaemia is also a risk factor as an abnormal gene can be passed down from one generation to the next (Leukaemia Foundation, 2021).

Person-centred care

Mrs Hlaing was admitted to the haematology/oncology unit, and her initial treatment included three units of packed red blood cells (PRBCs) and one unit of platelets. Her husband told the team about her previous experience in the ED when they first arrived in Australia.

Chemotherapy was prescribed for Mrs Hlaing. As she was to have many transfusions and intravenous therapies, Mrs Hlaing had a Hickman's line inserted (see Figure 9.1) in the radiology department. She was then discharged and attended the outpatient haematology/oncology clinic for an aggressive regimen of chemotherapeutic agents.

Patient Safety Competency Framework (PSCF)

Domain 1—Person-centred care

The PSCF specifies that nurses must have the ability to plan and provide care that is respectful of the person's individual needs, values and life experiences.

Source: *The Patient Safety Competency Framework for Nursing Students*, https://patientsafetyfornursingstudents.org

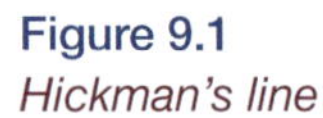

Figure 9.1
Hickman's line

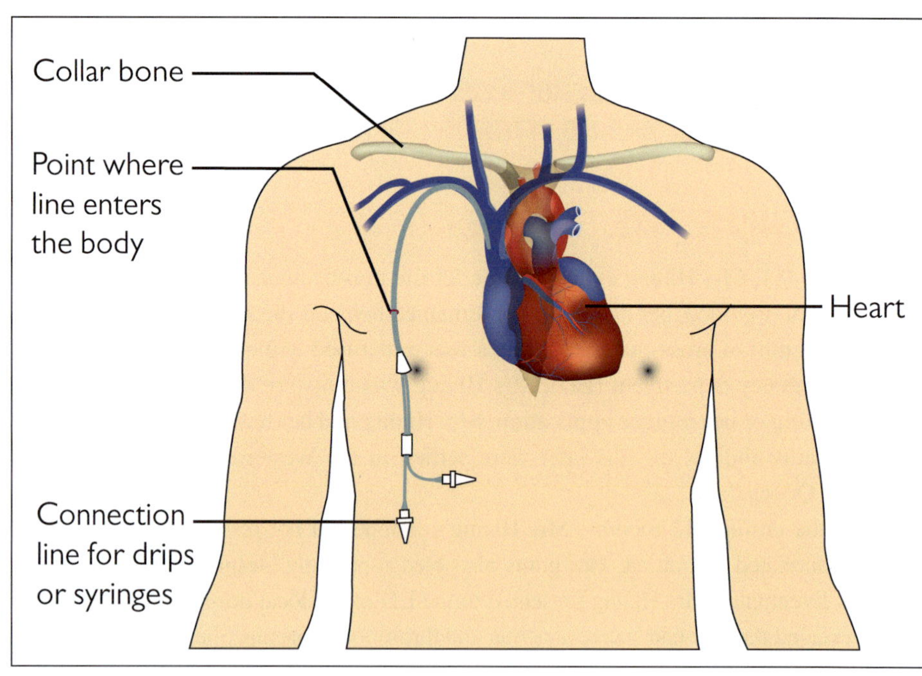

A Hickman's line is a type of central venous access device (CVAD). CVAD's may be utilised for chemotherapy, blood products, intravenous fluids, total parenteral nutrition and apheresis. These devices can stay in place for an extended period of time. A Hickman's line is inserted into the superior vena cava and the lumen's exit site is from the chest wall.

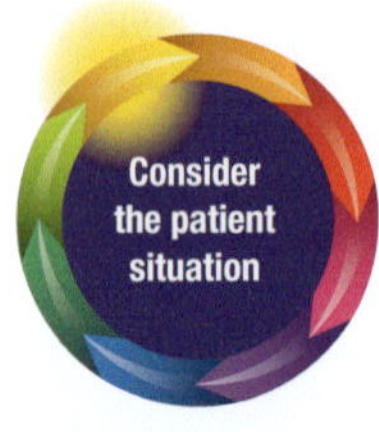

1. CONSIDER THE PATIENT SITUATION

On one of the days that Mrs Hlaing attends the haematology/oncology clinic, she tells the nurse on arrival that she 'feels strange and not very well'. She is assessed and immediately admitted to the haematology/oncology ward. When you arrive for your shift, you are given the following handover report:

What are pancytopaenia and neutropaenia?

Mrs Hlaing has acute myeloid leukaemia and is on her third cycle of chemo. Today she told the clinic staff she felt unwell. Her gums are bleeding slightly and she is pancytopaenic and neutropaenic, probably from her

chemo. She is febrile—38.3ºC; other vital signs are between the flags. She needs a septic work-up for the source of infection and had been prescribed with three units of packed cells. She is charted for 4.5 g of IV Tazocin/ piperacillin TDS and daily 1 g vancomycin IV.

The doctor visits Mrs Hlaing to discuss her pathology results, which show that she might have an underlying liver abnormality. He explains that this may account for some of her coagulopathies (bleeding tendencies). The doctor talks with Mrs Hlaing about her history and explains her current liver problems and leukaemia. Mrs Hlaing becomes very upset by the memories raised in this discussion and a counsellor from the local migrant and refugee resource centre is asked to come and support her.

Access the Edith Cowan University video resource titled: 'He's not from here' to examine the impact of cultural insensitivity towards people from a refugee background: https://www.ecu.edu.au/schools/medical-and-health-sciences/training-for-health-professionals-and-teachers/interprofessional-learning-resources/resources/hes-not-from-here

Something to think about ...

Most people from refugee backgrounds will have been exposed to traumatic events such as prolonged periods of deprivation, human rights abuses, the loss of loved ones or a perilous escape from their homelands. Read pages 24–28 and 45–75 of the Foundation House (2012) resource to understand more about trauma and torture experiences, and the role of health professions in promoting refugee health: http://refugeehealthnetwork.org.au/wp-content/uploads/PRH-online-edition_July2012.pdf

Mrs Hlaing completed her first 2 of 3 units of PRBC transfusion without any adverse reactions. She had a clinical assessment and a full blood count blood test after her second unit. Mrs Hlaing no longer felt lethargic and breathless and her haemoglobin had increased to 102 g/L. Therefore, the 3rd unit of PRBC was no longer required. Mrs Hlaing also had attended as part of her septic workup: an MSU, CXR, swab at exit site of Hickman's line, serum lactate and blood cultures (both peripheral and from the Hickman's line).

The patient blood management guidelines (National Blood Authority, 2011–2016), recommend that a clinical assessment is required after every unit transfused to assess if further blood transfusions are required. Once initial signs and symptoms of anaemia have been resolved, no further units are required despite a low laboratory haemoglobin level. Single unit transfusions help to reduce the number of unnecessary transfusions.

2. COLLECT CUES/INFORMATION

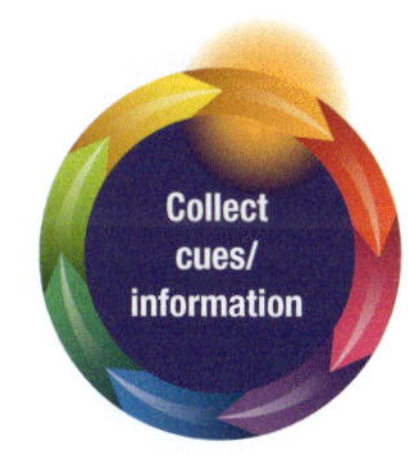

(a) Review current information

The following day you are caring for Mrs Hlaing again. Most of the results from her investigations are available so you begin to review them and think about Mrs Hlaing's septic work-up:

- CXR: No collapse or consolidation is detected. No pleural effusion seen. No rib fractures seen
- Lactate: Mildly elevated
- MSU: Anti-bacterial activity—not detected. Culture—no significant growth
- Blood culture: No growth to date. A further report will follow if growth occurs.

(b) Gather new information

What other clinical assessment information do you need to collect?

Q1 From the following list, identify the two cues that you believe are *most* relevant to your assessment of Mrs Hlaing at this time.

a Respiratory rate
b Sputum culture
c Pain
d Cognitive state
e Swab of the catheter site
f Mobility

Review the approved abbreviations on this site: http://nursing.flinders.edu.au/students/studyaids/clinicalcommunication/page_glossary.php?id=13

Q2 One of your colleagues says in passing, 'I bet the infection is because of where she lives. "They" always live in dirty, overcrowded places.' Which clinical reasoning error is this nurse's comment an example of?

a Racism
b Pattern matching
c Diagnostic momentum
d Fundamental attribution error

Something to think about ...

The notion of cultural competence being integral to safe and effective clinical practice, and a key attribute of professional competence, is undisputed (Federation of Ethnic Communities' Councils of Australia, 2019). Yet cultural empathy, a driving motivation for culturally competent practice, is not well understood. Cultural empathy refers to the ability to perceive and share experiences through the unique lens of values, beliefs and perspectives of people from cultural backgrounds different to one's own (Moudatsou, Stravropoulos, Philalithis & Koukouli, 2020). To what extent do you think your practice is informed by cultural empathy?

Patient Safety Competency Framework (PSCF)

Domain 3–Cultural competence

The PSCF specifies that nurses must demonstrate cultural empathy by seeking to understand each person's cultural and spiritual values, needs, practices and perspectives; and avoid generalisations and stereotypes when discussing people from different cultural groups.

Source: *The Patient Safety Competency Framework for Nursing Students*, https://patientsafetyfornursingstudents.org

(c) Recall knowledge

Quick Quiz!

To ensure that you have a good understanding of the key concepts related to sepsis, immunity and allergic reactions, test yourself with the following questions.

Q1 Which of the following is not a type of leukocyte?

a Macrophage
b Eosinophil
c Monocyte
d Keracyte

Q2 Malaise, fever, heat, swelling, pain and pus are all signs of infection. Currently, the only sign exhibited by Mrs Hlaing is fever. Which of the following statements is correct?

a Mrs Hlaing is neutropaenic, so her total white cell count is compromised.
b Mrs Hlaing is neutropaenic and she does not have enough neutrophils to produce the classic signs of infection.
c Mrs Hlaing is neutropaenic, so her lack of thrombocytes prevents redness and swelling.
d Mrs Hlaing is pancytopaenic, so her lack of erythrocytes prevents redness and swelling.

Q3 A normal leucocyte count is 4.9–11.0 × 10^9/L (values may vary slightly between laboratories).

a True
b False

Q4 A differential count is the percentage of each cell type in the blood. The differential for neutrophils is:

a 2–8%
b 0.5%
c 55%
d 20–40%

Q5 Which of the following constitutes a risk for a neutropaenic patient?

a Presence of chronic illness
b Altered immune response
c Skin breakdown
d Presence of invasive or indwelling medical device
e Non-refrigerated food
f All of these options

Q6 Symptoms of an anaphylactic reaction include:

- a Hypovolaemia and hypertension
- b Bradycardia and hypotension
- c Broncho-constriction and bronchospasm
- d Urticaria and flushed skin

Q7 The first phase of haemostasis is:

- a Separation of globin and haeme
- b Activation of prothrombinase
- c Platelet aggregation
- d Vascular spasm

The source of Mrs Hlaing's infection is found to be her Hickman's line and she is scheduled to return to radiology to have it replaced. In view of her coagulopathy and her impending surgery, she is ordered a platelet transfusion which she has without incident. This is to be followed by a transfusion of two units of extended life plasma (ELP).

Q8 What process should be followed when commencing a platelet transfusion?

- a The same process as red blood cells but without the need to do vital signs as a baseline
- b The same process as red blood cells
- c The same process as red blood cells but non-ABO identical platelets are not uncommon
- d The same process as red blood cells but without the need to check expiry date

Q9 Which of the following statements is the *most* correct?

- a One unit of ELP is the plasma taken from a unit of whole blood.
- b ELP is frozen within eight hours of collection.
- c ELP contains all coagulation factors in normal concentrations.
- d ELP may be transfused up to five days after thawing.
- e ELP may have two expiry dates to be checked (one for collection and one for thawing).
- f All of the options.

Visit the Australian Red Cross Lifeblood resource, *Blood Book: Australian Blood Administration Handbook* 2020, pp. 10–11 to revise your knowledge of platelet transfusions: https://transfusion.com.au/bloodbook

3. PROCESS INFORMATION

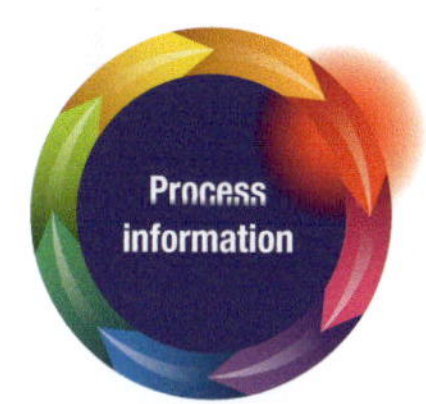

The ELP may be delivered to the organisation's blood bank frozen and must be thawed before delivery to the ward. The process takes approximately 30 minutes using a water bath. *Never* improvise by using other methods such as hot water or a microwave, as this could damage the product and make it unsafe.

You do another set of baseline observations and review Mrs Hlaing's pathology results before giving the ELP. Her results are as follows:

Temperature	38.0ºC
Pulse rate	98 beats/min
Respiratory rate	20 breaths/min
Blood pressure	110/60
Oxygen saturation level	95%
Haemoglobin	102 g/dL
Total white cell count	3.0×10^9/L
Blood group	O+ve

You then begin the checking procedure for the transfusion of the ELP. You notice that the ELP is from a number of different ABO groups.

Why can ELP come from different blood groups? Access the Australian Red Cross Lifeblood resource, *Blood Book* (2020, pp. 12–13) for more information about FFP and ELP transfusions: https://transfusion.com.au/bloodbook

(a) Interpret

Q Which of the following units are considered to be appropriate for Mrs Hlaing's ELP transfusion?

- a Unit labelled A
- b Unit labelled AB
- c Unit labelled B
- d Unit labelled O
- e All of the options

(b) Discriminate and (c) Relate

Q After the first 15 minutes, you do a second set of observations. Which two of the following are considered to be within normal parameters for Mrs Hlaing while she is receiving this blood transfusion?

a Temperature: 37.5ºC
b Pulse rate: 122 beats/min
c Respiratory rate: 28 breaths/min
d Blood pressure: 112/60
e Oxygen saturation level: 95%

Mrs Hlaing is restless and scratching her arms. She says she is very thirsty and is having trouble breathing. She reaches for a glass of water and you observe that she has weakness in her hands. She tells you that she has a terrible headache and a pain in her right leg.

(d) Infer

Q From what you have observed and from what you have learnt about blood transfusions, what are four signs or symptoms that may indicate a transfusion reaction to ELP?

(e) Predict

Q What might happen if Mrs Hlaing's ELP transfusion is not stopped and appropriate actions taken at this time? Choose the response that is *most* correct for this situation.

a Mrs Hlaing could go into shock and cardiac arrest.
b Mrs Hlaing's condition will gradually improve over the next few days.
c Mrs Hlaing could develop acute kidney injury.
d Mrs Hlaing could lose consciousness.
e Mrs Hlaing could die.
f Mrs Hlaing could become hypoxic by developing a compromised airway.

Warning signs of adverse reaction to blood component therapies

Nurses have the primary responsibility for monitoring blood transfusions and it is imperative that they recognise and respond immediately to deterioration in the patient's condition. Reactions are classified as follows:

1 Immunological acute (<24 hours)
2 Non-immunological acute (<24 hours)
3 Immunological delayed (>24 hours)
4 Non-immunological delayed (>24 hours).

In Scenario 9.1, Mrs Hlaing's transfusion reaction would have been classified as an immunological acute (<24 hours) response.

Q The following list of eight signs and symptoms may indicate a transfusion reaction in Mrs Hlaing. From the list, enter the appropriate signs and symptoms for each type of reaction into the table below.

Signs and symptoms

- Headache
- Anxiety
- Rigors
- Tremor
- Flushing
- Tachycardia
- Fever
- Restlessness

Allergenic reaction–antibodies to proteins including IgA	Febrile non-haemolytic reaction–possible contamination with pyrogens and/or bacteria	Both
Palpitations		
Puritis		
Urticaria		
Mild dyspnoea		

(f) Match

Q In what way is this transfusion reaction similar to, or different from, the transfusion reaction that occurred in Scenario 9.1?

4. IDENTIFY THE PROBLEM/ISSUE

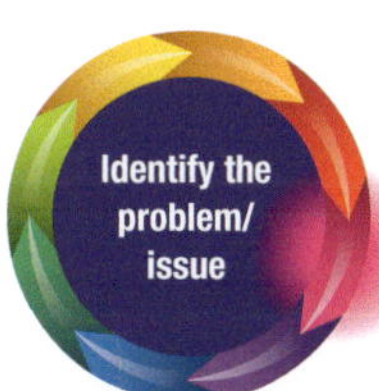

At this stage, you bring together (synthesise) all of the facts you've collected and inferences you've made to make nursing diagnoses of Mrs Hlaing's main problems or issues.

Q Select from the following, the *most* likely nursing diagnoses for Mrs Hlaing.

- a Transfusion-related acute lung injury (TRALI) related to fluid overload, evidenced by hypoxia and tachypnoea
- b A febrile transfusion reaction related to possible bacterial contamination, evidenced by chills, tachycardia, fever and hypotension
- c An allergic response related to a possible antibody/antigen reaction from the transfusion, evidenced by tachycardia, tachypnoea, low-grade temperature, headache and urticaria
- d Hypervolaemia related to a fluid overload, evidenced by tachycardia, headache and hypertension

Hint: Think about the causes and consequences of transfusion reactions. See www.transfusion.com.au/adverse_events/risks

5. ESTABLISH GOALS

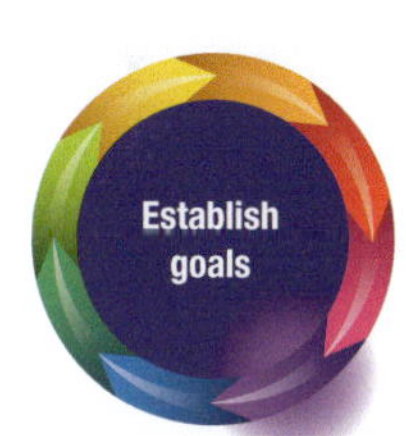

Q From the list below, choose the most important *immediate* goal for Mrs Hlaing's management at this time.

- a For Mrs Hlaing to be afebrile with respiratory distress, hypotension, headache or urticaria within the next 24 hours
- b For Mrs Hlaing to be afebrile with no respiratory distress, hypotension, chest tightness or headache, and with reducing urticaria, within the next 2 hours
- c For Mrs Hlaing to be afebrile with no shivering, respiratory distress, hypertension, headache or urticaria within the next 2–4 hours
- d For Mrs Hlaing to be afebrile with no shivering, respiratory distress, hypertension, headache or urticaria within the next 24 hours and for the following week

6. TAKE ACTION

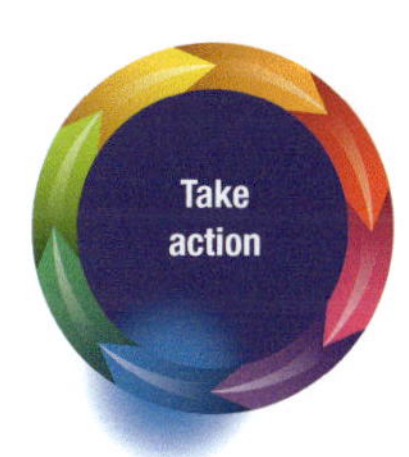

Q Which four of the following *would not* be nursing priorities at this time?

- a Consult a doctor for an order for an antihistamine.
- b Complete a transfusion reaction form and send it to the blood bank.
- c Give an adrenaline injection.
- d Give a diuretic.
- e Arrange for a repeat blood pathology.
- f Maintain IV access.
- g Flush the existing IV line.

h Request an immediate clinical review.
i Re-perform the pre-transfusion checklist.
j Monitor Mrs Hlaing's level of consciousness.
k Monitor Mrs Hlaing's vital signs and oxygen saturation level.

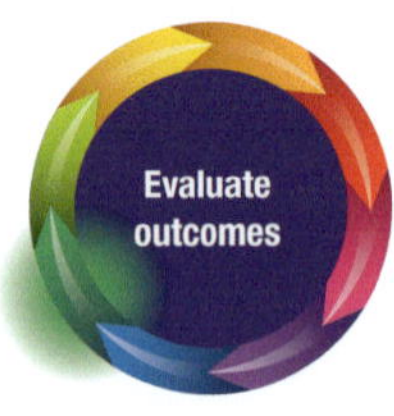

7. EVALUATE

Q Complete the following table, matching signs or symptoms to the desired observations indicating that Mrs Hlaing's condition has improved.

Sign or symptom

- Respiratory rate
- Pulse
- Skin
- Temperature
- Blood pressure

Sign or symptom	Desired observation
	No evidence of urticaria
	Normal rate with no signs of dyspnoea
	Normotensive with no postural drop
	No evidence of tachycardia
	Afebrile

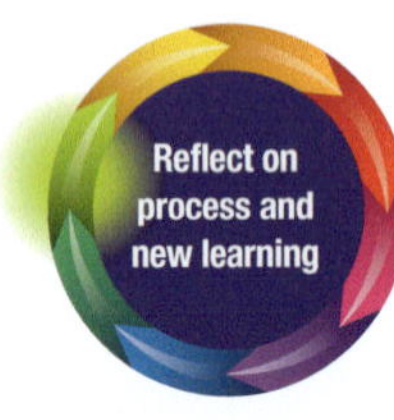

8. REFLECT

Reflect on your learning from this scenario and consider the following questions.

Q1 What are three of the most important things that you have learnt from this scenario?

Q2 What actions will you take in clinical practice as a result of your learning from this scenario?

Q3 If you had to teach another nurse about the key concepts related to the transfusion of red blood cells, platelets and extended life plasma, what key areas would you target?

Q4 How has your understanding of cultural competence and cultural empathy developed as a result of completing this scenario?

EPILOGUE

Mrs Hlaing recovered from her transfusion reaction and all future transfusions were managed with careful monitoring. She had her Hickman's catheter replaced and she completed her antineoplastic chemotherapeutic regimen. She then entered a period of remission. Unfortunately, six months later Mrs Hlaing's symptoms returned. A matched unrelated donor or MUD search was initiated and Mrs Hlaing was matched with a donor from an international stem cell bank. A successful allogeneic bone marrow transplant followed.

For more information about stem cell transplantation, access the EdCaN learning resources at http://edcan.org.au/edcan-learning-resources/supporting-resources/stem-cell-transplantation/principles-of-transplantation/role-in-cancer-control

Over the next two years, Mrs Hlaing's health improved and after the five-year waiting period all three family members became proud Australian citizens. Mrs Hlaing has learnt to speak English fluently and she now works as an interpreter and an assistant in nursing while she is studying to become a registered nurse. She attributes her commitment to nursing to the care she received during her many hospitalisations and to the empathetic and person-centred nurses she encountered.

FURTHER READING

Australian and New Zealand Society of Blood Transfusion & Australian College of Nursing. (2019). *Guidelines for the Administration of Blood Products*. ANZSBT Guidelines. Retrieved from: https://anzsbt.org.au/wp-content/uploads/2020/03/ANZSBT-Administration-Guidelines-Revised-3rd-edition-Publication-Version-FINAL-20191002.pdf

Australian Red Cross Lifeblood. (2020). *Blood Book: Australian Blood Administration Handbook*. Retrieved from: https://transfusion.com.au/bloodbook

Bielby, L., Peterson, D. & Spigiel, T. (2018). Transfusion education for nurses and transfusion practitioners in Australia. *ISBT Science Series*, *13*(3), 259–67. doi.org/10.1111/voxs.12409

BloodSafe eLearning Australia. (2018). *Clinical Transfusion Practice*. Retrieved from: https://bloodsafelearning.org.au/course/clinical-transfusion-practice

REFERENCES

Amnesty International. (2017). *Who are the Rohingya and What Is Happening in Myanmar?* Retrieved from: https://www.amnesty.org.au /who-are-the-rohingya-refugees/

Australian Commission on Safety and Quality in Health Care (ACSQHC). (2021). *National Safety and Quality Health Service Standards* (2nd edn). Sydney, Australia.

Australian & New Zealand Society of Blood Transfusion Ltd. (2018). *Guidelines for the Administration of Blood Products* (3rd edn). Retrieved from: https://anzsbt.org.au/wp-content/uploads/2018/06/ANZSBT_Guidelines_Administration_Blood_Products_3rdEd_Jan_2018.pdf

Australian Red Cross Lifeblood. (2020). *Blood Book: Australian Blood Administration Handbook*. Retrieved from: https://transfusion.com.au/system/files/resource_library/bloodbook_firstedition_june2020revised.pdf

Brooks, A. B., Manias, E. & Bloomer, M. J, (2019). Culturally sensitive communication in healthcare: A concept analysis. *Collegian*, *26*(3) 383–91. doi.org/10.1016/j.colegn.2018.09.007

Cancer Australia. (2021). *Leukaemia in Australia Statistics*. Retrieved from: https://www.canceraustralia.gov.au/cancer-types/leukaemia/statistics

EdCaN (2016a). *Supportive Care Needs During Treatment for NHL*. Retrieved from: https://www.edcan.org.au/edcan-learning-resources/case-based-learning-resources/lymphoma/active-treatment/supportive-care

EdCaN (2016b). *The Role of HSCT in Cancer Control*. Retrieved from: https://www.edcan.org.au/edcan-learning-resources/supporting-resources/stem-cell-transplantation/principles-of-transplantation/role-in-cancer-control

Federation of Ethnic Communities' Councils of Australia. (2019). *Cultural Competence in Australia: A Guide*. Retrieved from: http://fecca.org.au/wp-content/uploads/2019/05/Cultural-Competence-in-Australia-A-Guide.pdf

Foundation House. (2012). *Promoting Refugee Health: A Guide for Doctors, Nurses and Other Health Care Providers Caring for People from Refugee Backgrounds* (3rd edn). Brunswick, Vic.: Foundation House, Victorian Foundation for Survivors of Torture. Retrieved from: http://refugeehealthnetwork.org.au/wp-content/uploads/PRH-online-edition_July2012.pdf

Human Rights Council 36th session. (2017). *Darker and More Dangerous: High Commissioner Updates the Human Rights Council on Human Rights Issues in 40 Countries*. Retrieved from: https://www.ohchr.org/EN/NewsEvents/Pages/DisplayNews.aspx?NewsID=22041

Leukaemia Foundation. (2021). *Acute Myeloid Leukaemia (AML)*. Retrieved from: https://www.leukaemia.org.au/blood-cancer-information/types-of-blood-cancer/leukaemia/acute-myeloid-leukemia

Levett-Jones, T., Dwyer, T., Reid-Searl, K., Heaton, L., Flenady, T., Applegarth, J., Guinea, S. & Andersen, P. (2017). *The Patient Safety Competency Framework for Nursing Students*. Retrieved from: http://psframework.wpengine.com/wp-content/uploads/2018/01/PSCF_Brochure_UTS-version_FA2-Screen.pdf

Moudatsou, M., Stavropoulou, A., Philalithis, A. & Koukouli, S. (2020). The role of empathy in health and social care professionals. *Healthcare (Basel)*, *8*(1), 26. doi: 10.3390/healthcare8010026

National Blood Authority. (2011–2016). *Patient Blood Management Guidelines*. Retrieved from: https://www.blood.gov.au/pbm-guidelines

Nursing and Midwifery Board of Australia (NMBA). (2016). *Registered Nurse Standards for Practice*. Retrieved from: www.nursingmidwiferyboard.gov.au/Codes-Guidelines-Statements/Professional-standards.aspx

The Equal Rights Trust. (2014). *The Human Rights of Stateless Rohingya in Thailand*. London: The Equal Rights Trust.

United Nations Human Rights Office of the High Commissioner (OHCHR). (2017). *Human Rights Council Opens Special Session on the Situation of Human Rights of the Rohingya and Other Minorities in Rakhine State in Myanmar*. Retrieved from: http://www.ohchr.org/EN/NewsEvents/Pages/DisplayNews.aspxNewsID22491LangIDE

Chapter 10

Caring for a person with sepsis

NATALIE GOVIND and LESLEY FITZPATRICK

LEARNING OUTCOMES

Completion of the activities in this chapter will enable you to:

- explain why an understanding of sepsis is essential to competent practice (**recall** and **application**)
- identify the clinical manifestations of sepsis and septic shock that are used to guide the collection and interpretation of appropriate cues (**gather, review, interpret, discriminate, relate** and **infer**)
- identify risk factors for sepsis and septic shock (**match** and **predict**)
- review clinical information to identify the main nursing diagnoses for a patient with sepsis and/or septic shock (**synthesise**)
- describe the priorities of care for a patient with sepsis and septic shock (**goal setting** and **taking action**)
- identify clinical criteria for determining the effectiveness of nursing actions taken to manage sepsis and septic shock (**evaluate**)
- apply what you have learnt about sepsis to new situations (**reflection** and **translation**).

INTRODUCTION

The scenario introduced in this chapter focuses on the care of a person who experiences sepsis. You will be introduced to Damien Arnold and follow his healthcare journey from admission to discharge. Sepsis is a time-critical emergency and one of the leading causes of morbidity and mortality in hospitalised patients worldwide (Thompson, Venkatesh & Finfer, 2019). It affects more than 48 million people globally each year, accounts for almost 20% of all global deaths and is one of the most underestimated health risks (Rudd et al., 2020). Each year in Australia, more than 5000 people die from sepsis and this figure translates to a greater burden of death than either breast, prostate or colorectal cancer (Bauer et al., 2020). A reduction in the incidence of sepsis could be achieved through improved adherence to hygiene standards, detection and early recognition of signs and symptoms, and accurate and time-critical clinical management. Excellent clinical reasoning skills will help you to identify and manage people with sepsis, with the aim of preventing deterioration and adverse patient outcomes.

KEY CONCEPTS

sepsis
septic shock
lactate
deterioration
rapid response

SUGGESTED READINGS

P. LeMone, G. Bauldoff, P. Gubrud-Howe, M.-A. Carno, T. Levett-Jones, . . . D. Stanley (Eds). (2020). *LeMone and Burke's Medical–Surgical Nursing: Critical Thinking in Person-Centred Care* (4th edn). Melbourne: Pearson Australia. Chapter 10: Nursing care of people experiencing trauma and shock

J. Vaughan & A. Parry. (2016). Assessment and management of the septic patient: Part 1. *British Journal of Nursing, 25*(17), 958–64.

G. Casey. (2016). Could this be sepsis? *Kai Tiaki Nursing New Zealand, 22*(7), 20–24.

SCENARIO 10.1 Caring for a person with sepsis

SETTING THE SCENE

Damien Arnold, an 18-year-old male, was brought to the emergency department (ED) of a regional hospital by his mother, Margaret. She was very worried and told the triage nurse that, 'Damien is never sick! He hasn't even been coming out of his room to eat . . . it's just not like him.'

National Safety and Quality Health Service (NSQH) Standards

Recognising and responding to acute deterioration standard

The NSQHS Standards emphasise that parents know their children best and can be acutely aware when their child is unwell or 'just not right', sometimes before the physiological parameters become abnormal. Concern on the part of a parent should be given appropriate consideration and may require escalation (ACSQHC, 2021).

Margaret gave the nurse a letter from the after-hours general practice they had attended. It stated that 'Damien was playing football three days ago and sustained an abrasion on his left forearm, which is now cellulitic in appearance. He has been feeling unwell for the last two days with weakness, loss of appetite and thirst, but he assumed that it was due to alcohol consumption during post-game celebrations. Significant medical history is Wegener's granulomatosis (now in remission) resulting in a kidney transplant three years ago, which is currently managed with immunosuppressant medications.'

Damien was given an Australian Triage Score (ATS) of 2 and transferred to an acute bed.

Globally, someone dies from sepsis every 2.8 seconds. For more information about how sepsis impacts patients and families, go to *Faces of Sepsis* at: https://youtu.be/12Qbnn6XfH0

The epidemiology of sepsis

Due to the ageing population, the greater number of invasive procedures being performed and the increase in disease survival, the incidence of sepsis is increasing worldwide (Singer et al., 2016). In 2017, a Global Burden of Disease study estimated 49 million incidences of sepsis and 11 million deaths were recorded internationally (Rudd et al., 2020). In Australia, the sepsis incidence is 1,162 cases per 100,000 residents, with 22 per cent of patients requiring intensive care, a mortality rate of 12 per cent (10 times higher than non-septic patients) and stays in hospital seven times longer than for non-septic patients (Li et al., 2020).

For more information on septic shock, access: *The Third International Consensus Definitions for Sepsis and Septic Shock (Sepsis-3)* at: https://jamanetwork.com/journals/jama/fullarticle/2492881

Watch this brief animation to gain an understanding of the pathophysiology of septic shock: https://youtu.be/-bt-H5VQI5E

The aetiology and pathogenesis of sepsis and septic shock

In simple terms, sepsis is a life-threatening condition where the body's response to an infection causes injury to its own tissues and organs (Singer et al., 2016)—see Figure 10.1. In 2016, the definition of sepsis was revised by the Third International Consensus Definitions Task Force (Sepsis-3). Sepsis is now defined as 'a life-threatening organ dysfunction caused by a dysregulated host response to infection' (Singer et al., 2016, p. 804). Septic shock is defined as 'a subset of sepsis in which underlying circulatory and cellular/metabolic abnormalities are profound enough to substantially increase mortality' (Singer et al., 2016, p. 805).

Consider how a parent of a child who has had a transplant may feel if their child becomes suddenly unwell. How would you address their concerns?

Person-centred care

Damien was born in Wamberal, a coastal town on the New South Wales Central Coast, and lives with his parents Margaret and David. He enjoys being physically active, surfs, and plays basketball and football. When Damien was 14 years old, he was diagnosed with Wegener's granulomatosis, a rare type

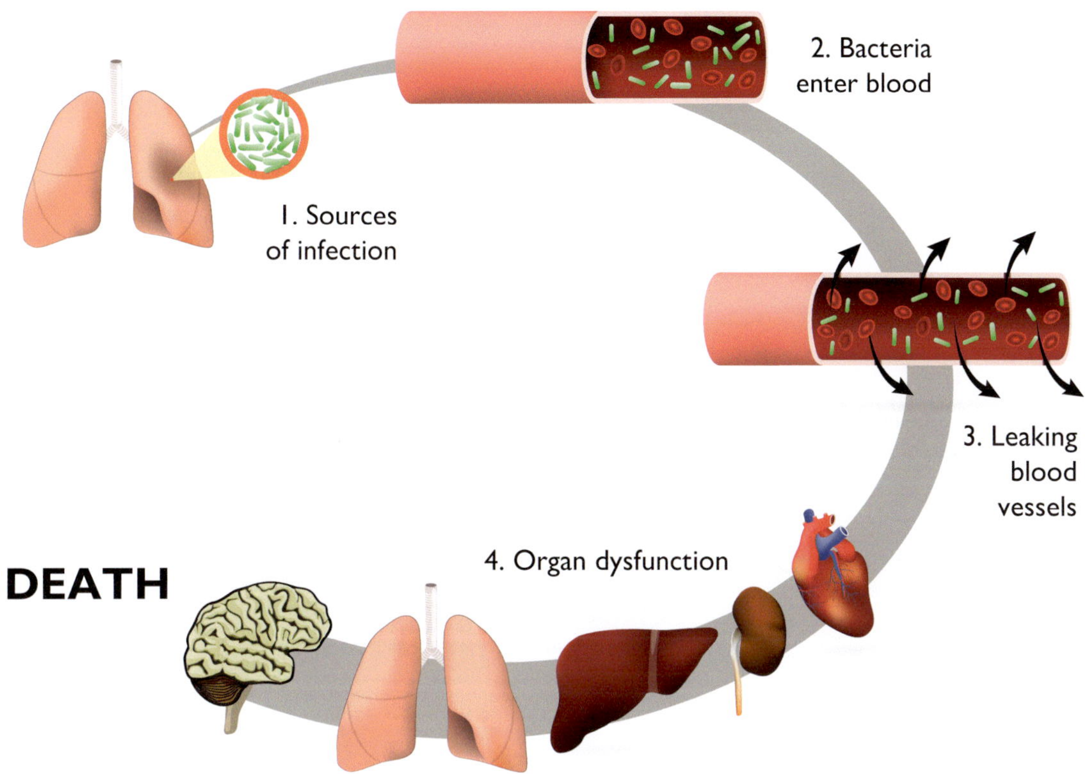

Figure 10.1
Cascade of events in simulation
Source: © Designua/ Shutterstock

of inflammation that targets the arteries, veins and capillaries of the kidneys and the respiratory system. By the time he was diagnosed, Damien had sustained significant and irreversible damage to his right kidney, and his left kidney function was also deteriorating, so he was given a kidney transplant from an anonymous donor. Since then, Damien has been in remission and takes immunosuppressant medications for maintenance therapy. Due to his illness, Damien was absent from school for long periods of time, so at the age of 17 he decided to leave school and take up an apprenticeship with his father's electrical business.

1. CONSIDER THE PATIENT SITUATION

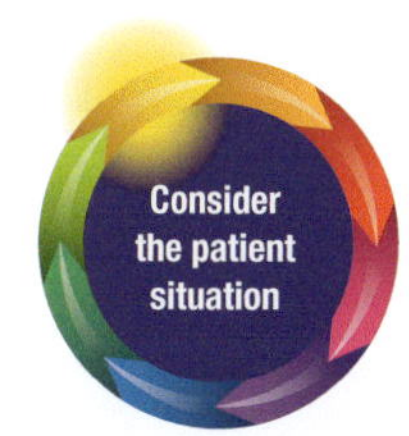

At 2100 hours, Damien is allocated to your care. He is pale and is lying in a supine position with his eyes closed. You receive the following handover report from the triage nurse.

This is Damien Arnold, an 18-year-old with suspected sepsis. He has a history of feeling unwell for the last two days with weakness, loss of appetite and thirst. There is a 3-day-old abrasion on his left forearm. Medical history includes Wegener's granulomatosis, which resulted in a kidney transplant three years ago; he is now in remission. His only medications are immunosuppressants.

Damien states that he has no pain in his arm or anywhere else in his body. He has an ATS 2 and I have commenced the adult sepsis pathway. The senior medical officer has been informed and is on his way to assess Damien. His mum, Margaret, has gone to call his father. I have asked the administration staff to send her straight through when she returns.

Admission observations

Airway	Patent
Respiratory rate	26 breaths/min
SpO_2	97% on room air
Heart rate	110 beats/min
Blood pressure	135/90 mmHg
AVPU	Voice
Temperature	38.6°C
Fluids in	Last intake at 2000 hrs, approximately 400 mL H_2O
Fluid out	Last voided small amount at 1730 hrs, dark urine appearance
BGL	6.5 mmol/L

Refer to the article 'Could this be sepsis?' (Casey, 2016) for information about the development and risks of sepsis.

Quick Quiz!

Q1 An ATS score of 2 indicates that the maximum waiting time for a person to receive medical assessment and treatment is:

a 120 minutes
b Immediately
c 10 minutes
d 20 minutes

Q2 The AVPU scale is a system by which a healthcare professional can measure and record a patient's responsiveness, indicating their level of consciousness. The acronym stands for:

a Alert, Vision, Pain, Unconscious
b Appearance, Verbal, Pain, Unresponsive
c Alert, Voice, Pain, Unresponsive
d Aware, Voice, Pain, Unconscious

Medical assessment of Damien

At 2110 hours, the senior medical officer arrives to examine Damien. A trauma call is received so, after she completes her assessment, she asks the junior medical officer to insert two peripheral intravenous catheters (PIVC) and collect two sets of blood cultures from two separate sites. Other bloods collected include VBG for lactate and glucose, FBC, EUC, CRP, LFTs and coags. The senior medical officer prescribes 2 g IV cephazolin 8-hourly and an IV fluid bolus of 20 mL/kg stat. She asks you to swab the wound to send to pathology and to continue monitoring Damien's observations. She states that she will return as soon as possible to review his condition and that Damien is to stay in overnight.

Q1 Why might the senior medical officer have decided to hospitalise Damien overnight?

You assist the junior medical officer to prepare for cannula insertion, but he appears hurried and you notice that he has forgotten gloves and alcohol-based swabs. You go and get the equipment, but by the time you return the first cannula has been inserted. You suggest that he perform hand hygiene, don gloves and use the alcohol-based swabs before he inserts the second peripheral cannula, but he shakes his head saying, 'It's all good, I washed my hands before and gloves make it too difficult to find the vein. Don't worry, I have never had any issues.'

Q2 How would you respond if you were to encounter a similar situation in your future practice?

National Safety and Quality Health Service (NSQH) Standards

Preventing and controlling infections standard

Preventing and controlling healthcare-associated infections is one of the NSQHS Standards. The purpose of this standard is to minimise risk and exposure to preventable infections, and if they do occur, to use evidence-based treatment approaches (ACSQHC, 2021).

Quick Quiz!

The medical orders included a number of abbreviations. Before progressing to the next stage of the clinical reasoning cycle, test your understanding of these terms.

Q Match each abbreviation to the correct definition.

Abbreviation

- Peripheral intravenous cannula/catheter (PIVC)
- Full blood count (FBC)
- Liver function tests (LFT)
- C-reactive protein (CRP)
- Stat
- Electrolytes, urea, creatinine (EUC)
- Coags
- Venous blood gas (VBG)

Abbreviation	Definition
	Protein made by the liver and secreted into the blood—often the first evidence of inflammation or an infection in the body
	From the Latin word *statim* meaning 'immediately'
	A test to determine a person's coagulation activity
	A device inserted into a small peripheral vein for therapeutic management such as administration of medications and fluids
	A screening panel that examines different components of the blood, checking for conditions such as anaemia, infection and many other disorders
	A test to look at the basic chemical balance of the blood, as well as kidney function
	A test for ALT, AST, alkaline phosphatase, PT, INR, albumin and bilirubin
	An alternative technique of estimating lactate and pH levels that does not require arterial blood sampling

Caring for an immunocompromised patient suspected of having sepsis is challenging. For further information, access the article by Donnelly et al. (2016).

2. COLLECT CUES/INFORMATION

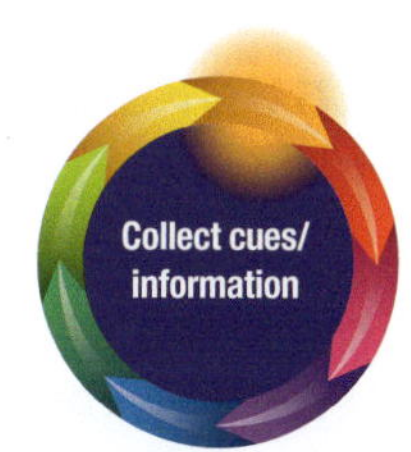

The Sepsis Alliance (2021) developed SEPSIS as an acronym to aid in recognition of the signs and symptoms of this condition:

S—Shivering, fever or feeling very cold

E—Extreme pain or general discomfort

P—Pallor or discolouration of skin

S—Sleepiness, difficult to rouse, confusion

I—'I feel like I might die' (sense of impending doom)

S—Shortness of breath (dyspnoea)

For more information, refer to the Clinical Excellence Commission's Adult Sepsis Pathway at: https://www.cec.health.nsw.gov.au/keep-patients-safe/deteriorating-patient-program/sepsis/sepsis-tools

For special populations, refer to the drop downs for maternal, paediatric and newborn pathways, or the Clinical Excellence Queensland paediatric sepsis project for clinical pathways and resources at: https://clinicalexcellence.qld.gov.au/priority-areas/safety-and-quality/sepsis/sepsis-resources/paediatric-sepsis-pathways

(a) Review current information

The next stage of the clinical reasoning cycle is to collect relevant cues and information. Start by reviewing Damien's current observations:

Airway	Patent
Respiratory rate	28 breaths/min
SpO_2	93% on room air
Heart rate	118 beats/min
Blood pressure	115/70 mmHg
Temperature	38.6°C
BGL	5.5 mmol/L
Lactate	2 mmol/L

Q The triage nurse stated that the adult sepsis pathway had been commenced. Using the information you now have, identify two relevant risk factors for Damien.

Nursing and Midwifery Board of Australia (NMBA) *Registered Nurse Standards for Practice* The NMBA *Registered Nurse Standards for Practice* (2016) state that RNs must comply with legislation, regulations, policies, guidelines and other standards or requirements relevant to the context of practice when making decisions.

(b) Gather new information

Q From the list below, identify the three additional cues that are *most* relevant to your assessment of Damien at this time.

a Weight (75 kg)
b Capillary return (<2 secs)
c Level of consciousness (voice)
d Pain 1/10
e Alcohol withdrawal score of 2
f Urine output (nil since presentation to ED)

(c) Recall knowledge

While cue collection involves reviewing current information and gathering new information, it also requires you to recall related knowledge.

Quick Quiz!

To build on your understanding of the key concepts related to sepsis, test yourself with the following questions.

Q1 Sepsis is a progressive condition that _________ capillary permeability due to a rise in _________ acid and _________ oxide. This triggers _________ and interrupts the body's ability to provide adequate _________, oxygen and nutrients to the _________ and cells.

Q2 What signs and symptoms are *most common* in patients presenting with sepsis? (Match the sign/symptom to the correct percentage.)

Sign/symptoms

- Tachypnoea
- Fever >38.5°C
- Acute oliguria
- Changes in mental status
- Tachycardia
- Hypothermia <36°C
- Metabolic acidosis

Sign/symptoms	Percentage
	99%
	45%
	54%
	97%
	70%
	13%
	38%

3. PROCESS INFORMATION

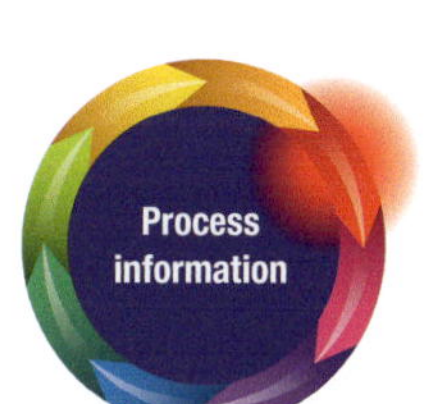

(a) Interpret

The next step of the clinical reasoning cycle is to interpret the data (cues) that you have collected by careful analysis and applying your knowledge of sepsis. By comparing normal versus abnormal, you will come to a more complete understanding of Damien's signs and symptoms.

Q1 Which two of the following are considered to be within normal parameters for Damien?

- a BGL: 5.5 mmol/L
- b Heart rate: 118 beats/min
- c Respiratory rate: 28 breaths/min
- d Blood pressure: 115/70 mmHg
- e Urine output: nil since presentation to ED

You review Damien's recent venous blood gas (VBG). His lactate is 2.0 mmol/L and his pH is 7.28, indicating metabolic acidosis.

Q2 What is the normal lactate level in both arterial and venous blood?

- a <1.0 mmol/L
- b >1.0 mmol/L

Q3 Damien's current observations indicate that he is tachypnoeic. Tachypnoea is the most common early detectable clinical sign of sepsis.

- a True
- b False

Q4 Tachypnoea occurs when the respiratory system is compensating for metabolic acidosis. Damien's brain is sending a message to stimulate an increase in respiratory rate in order to increase the carbon dioxide levels within his body.

- a True
- b False

Q5 Damien's current observations indicate that he is tachycardic. Unless a person has a cardiac conduction defect or is taking beta-blockers, tachycardia is an early detectable sign of sepsis. Tachycardia is a vital compensatory mechanism that aims to maintain _______________ in response to _______________ volume deficits, decreased cardiac contractility and _______________.

(b) Discriminate

You have gathered cues and information. Now you need to narrow them down to the most important.

Q From the list below, select five cues that you believe are *most relevant* to Damien's condition *at this time*.

a Blood pressure
b Respiratory rate
c Temperature
d Heart rate
e Condition of wound
f Oxygen saturation
g Level of consciousness
h Appetite
i Urine output
j Pain
k BGL
l Lactate level

(c) Relate

It is important to cluster the cues together and to identify relationships between them (based on the information you have collected so far).

Q Which of the following statements are *true* and which are *false*?

a Damien is normotensive due to the beta-blocker medications he is prescribed.
b Damien is febrile because his inflammatory response has been activated as a result of the invasion of pathogens.
c Damien has an increased heart rate as a compensatory mechanism to increased cardiac output.
d Damien has decreased oxygen saturations as a result of hypertension and tachypnoea.
e Damien has a wound and is immunocompromised, which are two factors that increase his risk of developing sepsis.

Something to think about ...

Following renal transplant, a regimen of immunosuppressive medications are prescribed to prevent organ rejection. However, these medications reduce the function of the naturally occurring immune system within the body, making patients more susceptible to infection. Treatment of infections is complicated by the fact that drug interactions frequently occur between antibiotics and the immunosuppressive regimen (Bhagat et al., 2021).

(d) Infer

It is time to think about all the cues you have collected about Damien's condition, and to make inferences based on your analysis and interpretation of those cues.

Q From what you know about Damien's history, and signs and symptoms (as well as your knowledge about sepsis), identify which *three* of the following inferences are correct.

a Damien is normotensive and bradycardic.
b Damien is oliguric and tachycardic.
c Damien is hypertensive and tachycardic.
d Damien is febrile and normotensive.
e Damien is hypoxic and febrile.

(e) Predict

At this stage, you begin to consider the consequences of your actions, or inaction, by predicting potential outcomes for your patient.

Q If you do not take the appropriate actions at this time and Damien's condition is not managed correctly, what could happen? (Select the *two incorrect* responses.)

a Damien could develop disseminated intravascular coagulation (DIC).
b Damien's condition will gradually improve over the next few days.
c Damien could develop acute kidney injury.
d Damien could develop acute respiratory distress syndrome.
e Damien could die.
f Damien could become hypertensive and hypoglycaemic.
g Damien could develop septic shock.

4. IDENTIFY THE PROBLEM/ISSUE

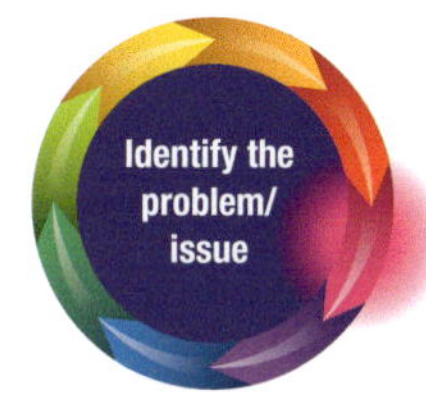

Q Select from the following list, the *four* correct nursing diagnoses for Damien.

a Ineffective tissue perfusion related to an inflammatory response to infectious pathogens, as evidenced by decreased oxygen saturation level, tachypnoea, tachycardia, oliguria and increased lactate level
b Fluid volume overload related to damaged capillary walls and vasodilation, as evidenced by hypotension, oliguria and bradycardia
c Risk of decreased cardiac output related to decreased preload
d Impaired skin integrity related to poor hygiene, as evidenced by abrasion on left forearm, increased temperature and tachycardia
e Acute pain related to cellulitic wound on left forearm, as evidenced by hyperthermia, tachypnoea, hyperglycaemia and hypertension
f Hypovolaemia related to damaged capillary walls and vasodilation, as evidenced by hypotension, oliguria and tachycardia
g Risk of septic shock related to inflammatory response to infectious pathogens, ineffective tissue perfusion and hypovolaemia

Patient Safety Competency Framework (PSCF)

Domain 5–Clinical reasoning

Remember, time is critical when caring for a person with sepsis, as early recognition and treatment improves patient outcomes. The PSCF states that nursing students demonstrate the ability to accurately assess, interpret and respond to individual patient data in a systematic and timely way.

Source: *The Patient Safety Competency Framework for Nursing Students*, https://patientsafetyfornursingstudents.org

5. ESTABLISH GOALS

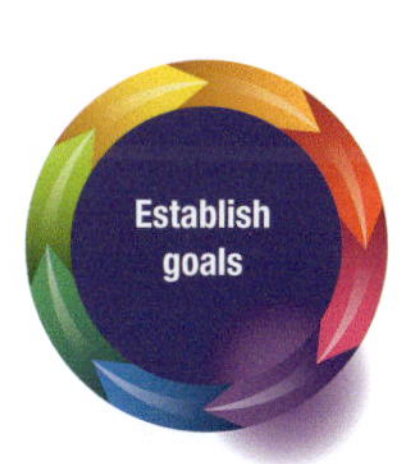

Q Before implementing any actions to improve Damien's condition, it is important to specify what you want to happen and when. From the list below, choose the *most important* short-term goal for Damien's management at this time.

a Damien's wound will be cleaned and a sterile dressing applied within the next 15 minutes.
b Damien will be discharged home from the ED within the next 3 hours.
c Damien will have no evidence of further deterioration within the next 60 minutes.
d Damien will be normotensive with urine output greater than 80–100 mL/hr within the next 24 hours.

6. TAKE ACTION

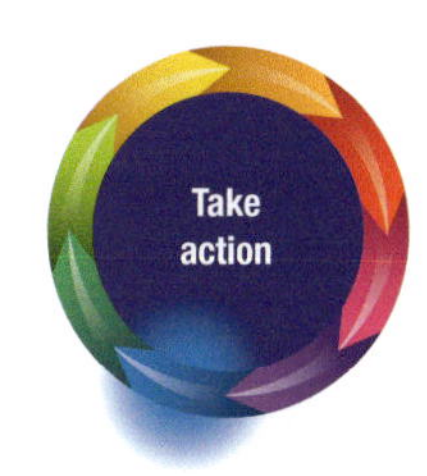

This stage of the clinical reasoning cycle requires knowledge, clinical skills, effective communication skills and sophisticated clinical reasoning ability. The nurse has to decide which actions take priority, who should be notified and who is best placed to undertake each nursing action.

Q From the list of immediate actions below, choose the three actions you would *not* take at this time.

a Administer oxygen therapy to maintain saturations ≥95%.

b Monitor Damien's pain score.
c Continuously monitor and document Damien's vital signs and oxygen saturation level.
d Monitor and document the condition of Damien's wound.
e Administer IV antibiotics as ordered within 60 minutes.
f Administer a normal saline fluid bolus as ordered (20 mL/kg stat).
g Collect a venous blood sample for lactate and glucose levels.
h Position Damien in a semi-Fowler's to high-Fowler's position as tolerated.
i Assess Damien's level of consciousness using AVPU every 30 minutes.
j Reposition Damien to minimise pressure area development.
k Strictly monitor and document Damien's fluid input/output and maintain hourly urine measures.

Something to think about …

Antimicrobial resistance is an ever-increasing threat to safe patient care. For further information about the use of antibiotics and microbial resistance, access:

Joshua S. Davis, Cheryl A. Jones, Allen C. Cheng & Benjamin P. Howden (2019). Australia's response to the global threat of antimicrobial resistance. Medical Journal of Australia, 211*(3), 106–108e1. doi: 10.5694/mja2.50264*

and

Antimicrobial Stewardship *at:*

https://www.cec.health.nsw.gov.au/keep-patients-safe/medication-safety/antimicrobial-stewardship

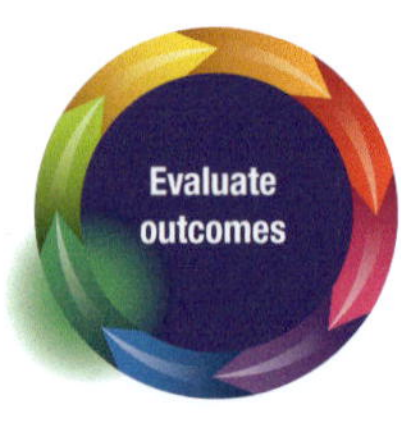

7. EVALUATE

It is now 2300, two hours since Damien presented to the ED. He has been given a 1500 mL fluid bolus (20 mL/75 kg) stat; broad-spectrum IV antibiotics have been administered as ordered; and he has oxygen therapy at 3 L/min via nasal prongs. Damien's signs and symptoms provide you with data to make a determination of whether or not the nursing and medical interventions have been effective, and whether his condition is improving.

Q1 Rate each of the following signs and symptoms as *unchanged, improving* or *deteriorating*.
a Oxygen saturations: 97%
b Heart rate: 90 beats/min
c AVPU: voice
d Respirations: 23 breaths/min
e Temperature: 38.0°C
f Lactate: 1.5 mmol/L
g Urine output: 20 mL/hr
h Blood pressure: 110/75
i Colour: pale
j BGL: 7.5 mmol/L

Q2 You now need to synthesise these parameters to decide whether Damien's condition has improved overall. Which of the following statements is the *most correct*?
a Damien's condition has improved significantly.
b Damien's condition has not improved and you need to call a rapid response.
c Damien's condition has improved but still requires careful monitoring and reassessment. You will need to contact the doctor again if further improvement is not seen in the next hour.
d Damien's condition has not improved but you will monitor his condition carefully for the next 24 hours.

8. REFLECT

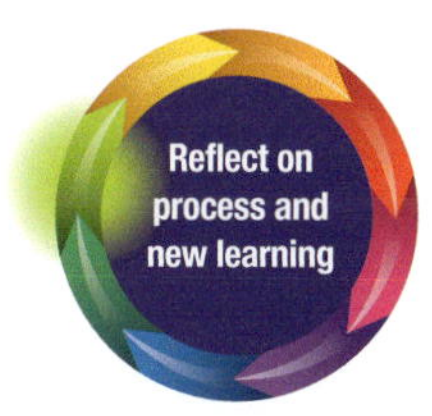

The final stage of the clinical reasoning cycle is 'reflection'. Reflect on your learning from this scenario and consider the following questions.

Q1 What are three of the most important things you have learnt from this scenario?

Q2 What actions will you take in clinical practice as a result of your learning from this scenario?

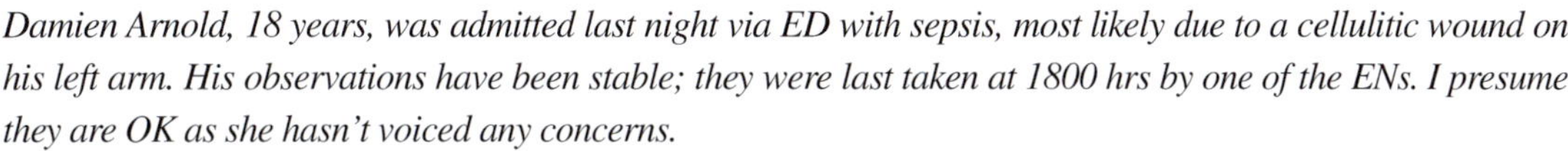

CHANGING THE SCENE

1. CONSIDER THE PATIENT SITUATION

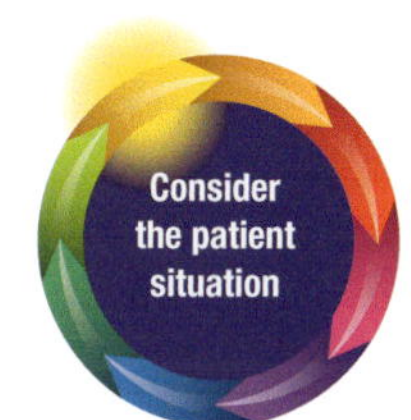

At 2330 hours, Damien's condition is stable and he is transferred to the short-stay ward for observation. He has IV fluids running at 100 mL/hr and is to have IV antibiotics as prescribed.

The following day you return for another night shift. It is quiet in the ED so you are sent to the short-stay ward which is busy and short staffed. By chance, you are allocated to the care of Damien and you look forward to seeing how he is progressing. The afternoon staff provide the following handover report:

Damien Arnold, 18 years, was admitted last night via ED with sepsis, most likely due to a cellulitic wound on his left arm. His observations have been stable; they were last taken at 1800 hrs by one of the ENs. I presume they are OK as she hasn't voiced any concerns.

Nursing and Midwifery Board of Australia (NMBA) Registered Nurse Standards for Practice The NMBA Standards (2016) specify that RNs can delegate nursing care activities only when the appropriate level of supervision can be provided. When an RN delegates care to an enrolled nurse (EN), they must provide guidance, assistance, support and clinically focused supervision.

Damien's medications have been administered as charted, although his 1600 hrs IV antibiotic wasn't given until 1800 hrs because we've been so busy. He has an IV at 100 mL/hr via PIVC in the right cubical fossa; it's patent but a bit red. His mum keeps saying 'it should come out', but Damien is not complaining. The other PIVC is in the left hand and currently capped.

Overdue doses (i.e. medications that are prescribed but not administered on time) are the second largest cause of reported medication incidents. Importantly, failure to administer antibiotics at the prescribed time can lead to serious patient harm (Härkänen et al., 2019).

Damien is taking sips of water but has not eaten today; he says he is not hungry. He is passing small amounts of urine. He was getting up to the bathroom this morning but has been sleeping for most of the afternoon/evening. We've just let him sleep as we have been flat out. We are still waiting for results from his blood cultures and wound swab; I've asked the medical team to follow this up. Also, as per the sepsis pathway, another VBG was collected for lactate; I haven't had a chance to see if the results are back yet. Damien's mother has been here all day. She keeps saying to anyone who will listen that he is not getting better … she requires lots of reassurance. I think because Damien had a kidney transplant three years ago, Margaret is overprotective.

Q1 Based on the handover report, what are your initial concerns about Damien's current situation?

Q2 The nurse's comment about Margaret being 'overprotective' is an example of which clinical reasoning error?

- a Ascertainment bias
- b Premature closure
- c Overconfidence bias
- d Fundamental attribution error

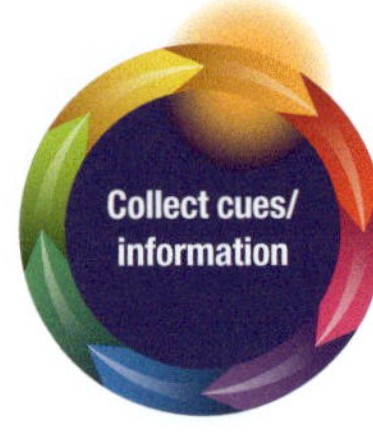

2. COLLECT CUES/INFORMATION

(a) Review current information

You review Damien's charts and identify that the following observations were documented at 1800 hours:

Respiratory rate	26
Oxygen saturation level	94% 3 L O_2 via NP
Heart rate	105 beats/min
Blood pressure	105/70 mmHg
AVPU	Voice
Temperature	38°C
Fluids IN	100 mL/hr (total IN from midnight: 1900 mL)
Fluids OUT	380 mL (since midnight)
BGL	6.2 mmol/L

(b) Gather new information

When you enter Damien's room at 1920 hours, Margaret says, 'Oh, you're the nurse from ED; I am so glad to see you. He's not getting better; he can't keep his eyes open, his breathing sounds funny and no one will listen to me! Please help him.'

You note that Damien is lying on his left side with his eyes closed. You observe that his nasal prongs have slipped down to his chin and there is increased work of breathing. You touch his arm and it feels cool. When you ask, 'How are you feeling, Damien?' he doesn't open his eyes, but quietly moans. You then conduct a head-to-toe assessment.

Q From the following list, select the four cues that are *least relevant* at this stage.

a Respiratory rate: 32 and observed increase work of breathing
b Oxygen saturations: 90% 3 L O_2 via NP
c Heart rate: 115 beats/min
d Blood pressure: 90/55 mmHg
e Glasgow Coma Scale: 11
f Pupillary response: PEARL (Pupils Equal and Reactive to Light)
g Mobility status: 1 X assistance
h BGL: 7.8 mmol/L
i Temperature: 38.0°C
j Lactate: 4 mmol/L
k Condition of wound to forearm: dressing dry and intact, no ooze
l PIVC in right cubical fossa: redness and tracking along vein noted

(c) Recall knowledge

Quick Quiz!

Q1 Fill in the missing words in this paragraph.

Shock is a life-threatening condition related to the failure of the ________________ system, characterised by ________________ leading to poor oxygenation and nutrition delivery to the tissues. Due to the body's compensatory mechanisms, the effects of shock are initially ________________. However, the person's condition will rapidly deteriorate without appropriate and timely management and the shock will become ________________ resulting in multi-organ dysfunction syndrome (MODS) and ________________.

Q2 Septic shock is a form of:

a Cardiogenic shock—reduction in cardiac output due to a primary cardiac disorder
b Obstructive shock—interference with the mechanical mechanisms of the heart
c Distributive shock—maldistribution of intravascular volume
d Hypovolaemic shock—decreased intravascular volume

Q3 Lactate is an indicator of tissue hyperperfusion.

a True
b False

Q4 What are the normal levels of serum lactate?

a <1.0 mmol/L
b 1.0–2.0 mmol/L
c 2.0–4.0 mmol/L
d 4.0–6.0 mmol/L

Something to think about ...

Lactate is a normal product of anaerobic cell metabolism. It is released into the blood and metabolised by the liver when there is insufficient oxygen for cellular activity. Elevated lactate is typically present in patients with severe sepsis or septic shock. Lactate levels taken 6 hours after initial identification have better prognostic value in predicting 30-day mortality in comparison to initial lactate levels, with one study demonstrating a 40% mortality rate with a median lactate level of 4.6 mmol/L (2.7 mmol/L to 7.1 mmol/L) (Lee et al., 2021). Therefore, a lactate level above 4.0 mmol/L should activate an immediate rapid response call.

3. PROCESS INFORMATION

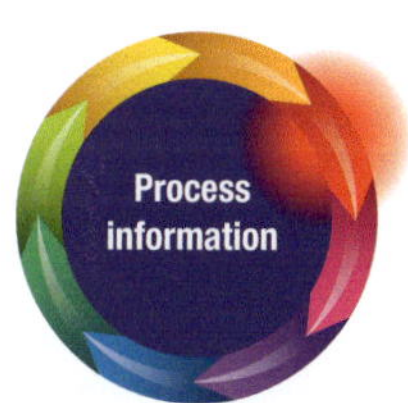

To learn more about lactate and sepsis, access the Lactate information sheet at: https://www.cec.health.nsw.gov.au/keep-patients-safe/deteriorating-patient-program/sepsis/education

(a) Interpret, (b) Discriminate, (c) Relate and (d) Infer

Q Which seven of the following signs and symptoms is Damien displaying that are suggestive of septic shock?

a Tachypnoea
b High pain score
c Hypertension
d Decreased level of consciousness
e Hyperglycaemia
f Pupillary response: PEARL
g Hypotension
h ECG rhythm: sinus tachycardia
i Temperature: 38°C
j Lactate: 4 mmol/L
k Hypoglycaemia
l Hypoxia
m Oliguria

(e) Predict

Q What could happen to Damien if appropriate action is not taken at this time? (Select all that apply.)

a Damien could have a cardiac arrest.
b Damien could develop multi-organ dysfunction syndrome (MODS).
c Damien's condition will gradually improve over the next few days.
d Damien could develop pulmonary oedema.
e Damien could die.
f Damien could develop disseminated intravascular coagulation (DIC).

(f) Match

Q Have you ever seen someone with the same signs and symptoms as Damien? If so, what was done to manage the situation?

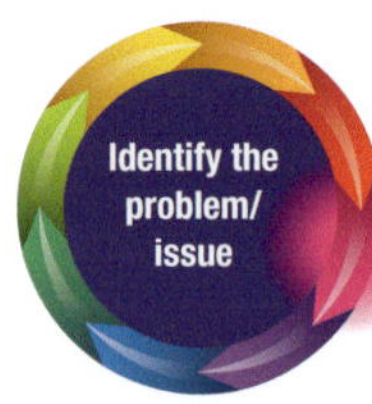

4. IDENTIFY THE PROBLEM/ISSUE

Q1 From the information that you currently have, identify the *three correct* nursing diagnoses for Damien.

a Hypoxia related to increased airway secretions, as evidenced by coughing, tachypneoa and decreased saturations

b Ineffective tissue perfusion related to decreased cardiac output and massive vasodilation, as evidenced by hypotension, tachycardia, decreased level of consciousness and cool peripheries

c Fluid volume deficit related to maldistribution of intravascular volume to the interstitial spaces, as evidenced by tachypneoa, tachycardia, hypotension and oliguria

d Ineffective breathing pattern related to shallow respirations and increased work of breathing, as evidenced by decreased oxygen saturations, increased respirations and tachycardia

e Impaired gas exchange related to interference with oxygen delivery from endotoxin-induced damage to the cells and capillaries, as evidenced by tachypnoea, increased work of breathing and hypoxia

Q2 Factors contributing to a failure to recognise and respond to a deteriorating patient are multifaceted. With reference to James Reason's 'Swiss Cheese Model' (see Figure 10.2), list the factors that may have contributed to Damien's deterioration.

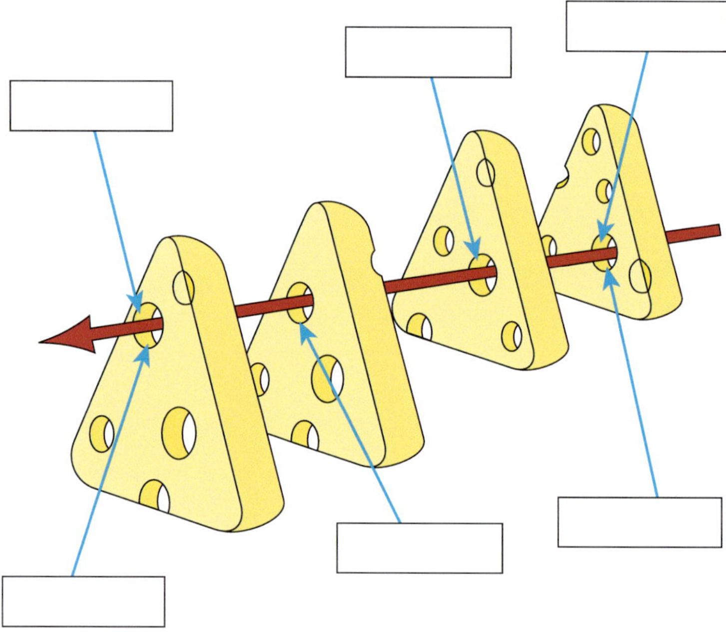

Figure 10.2 *Reason's Swiss Cheese Model*
Source: Based on J. Reason (2000). Human error: Models and management. *British Medical Journal, 320*, 768–70.

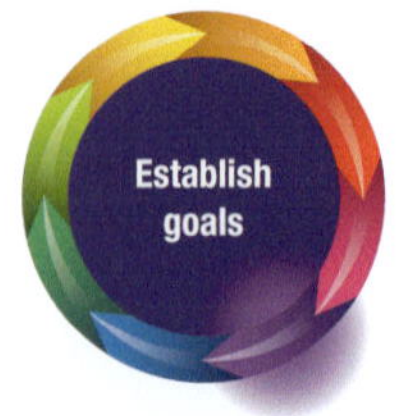

5. ESTABLISH GOALS

Before implementing any actions to improve Damien's condition, it is important to clearly specify what you want to happen and when.

Q From the list below, choose the four *most important* goals for Damien's management at this time.

a Damien will be self-caring and ambulant within the next 24 hours.

b Damien will be haemodynamically stable with an adequate circulating blood volume within 4–6 hours.

c Oral food and fluid intake will be established within 60 minutes.

d The potential source of infection will be identified and/or removed within 15 minutes.

e Damien will maintain his airway and will achieve adequate oxygenation saturations (>95%) within 30 minutes.

f Damien's urine output will be at least 37.5 mL/hr (0.5 mL/kg/hr) within 4 hours.

g Damien will not display evidence of pressure area development within 30 minutes.

If you do not understand the analogy of the Swiss Cheese Model, read the relevant information in the chapter on *Caring for a person experiencing an adverse drug reaction.*

6. TAKE ACTION

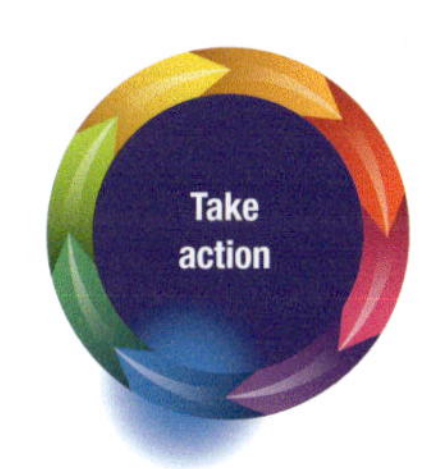

Q1 From the list below, choose the six *most immediate* actions you should take at this stage.

a Call a rapid response.
b Administer a diuretic.
c Continue to monitor haemodynamic status and vital signs closely.
d Administer oxygen therapy to maintain saturations >95%.
e Remove the PIVC from right cubical fossa and collect tip to send to pathology.
f Check weight each day.
g Decrease IV rate TKVO pending medical orders.
h Maintain patent IV access.
i Administer oxygen 2 L/min via nasal prongs.
j Assess and maintain patent airway.

Q2 Using ISBAR (Identity, Situation, Background, Assessment, Request/Recommendation), document how you would communicate with the rapid response team leader.

7. EVALUATE

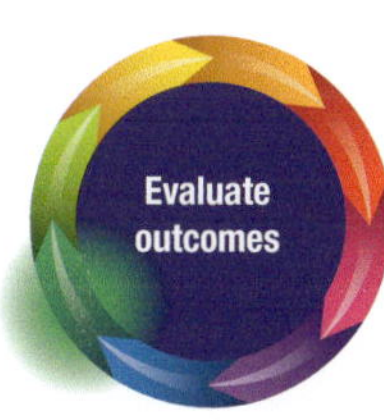

Q From the list below, identify the signs and symptoms that would indicate Damien's condition has improved following the rapid response call and initiation of appropriate actions.

a decreased respiratory rate or increased respiratory rate
b decreased oxygen saturation level or increased oxygen saturation level
c reduced heart rate or increased heart rate
d increased blood pressure or decreased blood pressure
e decreased lactate level or increase lactate level
f decreased urine output or increased urine output

8. REFLECT

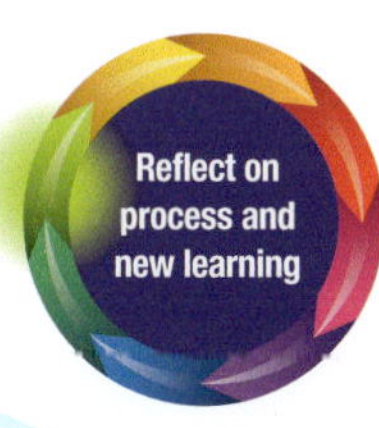

Contemplate what you have learnt from this scenario and how this learning will inform your practice. Respond to the following questions with reference to Scenario 10.2.

Q1 How could Damien's deterioration have been prevented?

Q2 What have you learnt from the scenario that you can apply to your future practice?

Access UHD NHS's *Sepsis—a patient story* to gain a deeper understanding of the risk's associated with complacency when caring for a person with sepsis: https://youtu.be/Ch-XuVY_T9M.

EPILOGUE

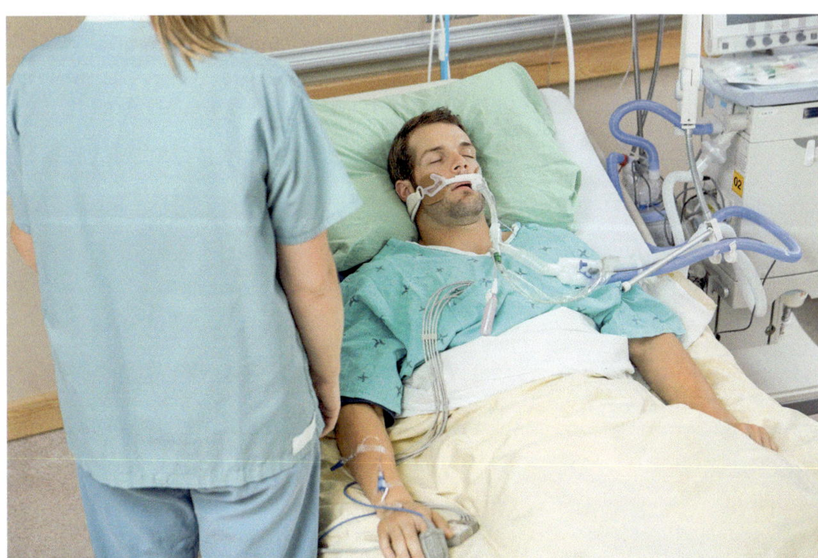

Damien being treated for septic shock in the ICU

Damien was assessed by the rapid response team and transferred to the intensive care unit (ICU) for ongoing clinical management. A central line and arterial line were inserted and Damien was intubated and ventilated. Despite fluid resuscitation, his blood pressure remained low and a noradrenaline (vasopressor) infusion was commenced to maintain his blood pressure to the target of MAP >65 mmHg. Damien continued to deteriorate and he was diagnosed with acute kidney injury. On days 6–10, he required continuous renal replacement therapy (CRRT) (dialysis). He also required an insulin infusion as his BGLs were unstable due to his critical illness. Throughout this time, Damien remained sedated with morphine and midazolam infusions. On day 12, Damien displayed signs of respiratory and haemodynamic stabilisation and by day 14 he was extubated and the noradrenaline ceased. Damien remained in ICU for another three days and was then transferred to the high dependency unit (HDU).

Damien spent 35 days in hospital before being discharged. He still suffers from disabling fatigue, poor concentration, insomnia and nightmares. Fortunately, his kidneys did not suffer any further damage and, despite the insult on his body systems, his Wegener's granulomatosis remained in remission. Damien hopes to return to work, at least part-time, within two to three months. Margaret believes that it was the ED nurse who saved her son's life, as no one else would listen to her concerns.

FURTHER READING

Clinical Excellence Commission (CEC). (2011). *Sepsis Kills Program.* Retrieved from: www.cec.health.nsw.gov.au/patient-safety-programs/adult-patient-safety/sepsis-kills

Surviving Sepsis Campaign. (2016). Retrieved from: www.survivingsepsis.org

World Sepsis Day. Retrieved from: www.world-sepsis-day.org

REFERENCES

Australian Commission on Safety and Quality in Health Care (ACSQHC). (2021). *National Safety and Quality Health Service Standards* (2nd edn). Sydney, Australia.

Bauer, M., Gerlach, H., Vogelmann, T., Preissing, F., Stiefel, J. & Adam, D. (2020). Mortality in sepsis and septic shock in Europe, North America and Australia between 2009 and 2019—results from a systematic review and meta-analysis. *Critical Care*, *24*(1). doi.org/10.1186/s13054-020-02950-2

Bhagat, V., Pandit, R. A., Ambapurkar, S., Sengar, M. & Kulkarni, A. P. (2021). Drug interactions between antimicrobial and immunosuppressive agents in solid organ transplant recipients. *Indian Journal of Critical Care Medicine*, *25*(1), 67–76.

Casey, G. (2016). Could this be sepsis? *Kai Tiaki Nursing New Zealand*, *22*(7), 20–24.

Donnelly, J. P., Locke, J. E., MacLennan, P. A., McGwin, G., Jr., Mannon, R. B., Safford, M. M., ... Wang, H. E. (2016). Inpatient mortality among solid organ transplant recipients hospitalized for sepsis and severe sepsis. *Clinical Infectious Diseases*, *63*(2), 186–94.

Härkänen, M., Vehviläinen-Julkunen, K., Murrells, T., Rafferty, A. M. & Franklin, B. D. (2019). Medication administration errors and mortality: Incidents reported in England and Wales between 2007 – 2016. *Research in Social and Administrative Pharmacy*, *15*(7), 858–63. doi.org/10.1016/j.sapharm.2018.11.010

Lee, S. G., Song, J., Park, D. W., Moon, S., Cho, H. J., Kim, J. Y., Park, J. & Cha, J. H. (2021). Prognostic value of lactate levels and lactate clearance in sepsis and septic shock with initial hyperlactatemia: A retrospective cohort study according to the Sepsis-3 definitions. *Medicine*, *100*(7).

Levett-Jones, T., Dwyer, T., Reid-Searl, K., Heaton, L., Flenady, T., Applegarth, J., Guinea, S. & Andersen, P. (2017). *The Patient Safety Competency Framework for Nursing Students.* Retrieved from: http://psframework.wpengine.com/wp-content/uploads/2018/01/PSCF_Brochure_UTS-version_FA2-Screen.pdf

Li, L., Sunderland, N., Rathnayake, K. & Westbrook, J. I. (2020). *Epidemiology of Sepsis in Australian Public Hospitals.* Sydney: ACSQHC.

Nursing and Midwifery Board of Australia (NMBA). (2016). *Registered Nurse Standards for Practice*. Retrieved from: www.nursingmidwiferyboard.gov.au/Codes-Guidelines-Statements/Professional-standards.aspx

Rudd, K. E., Johnson, S. C., Agesa, K. M., Shackelford, K. A., Tsoi, D., Kievlan, D. R., ... Naghavi, M. (2020). Global, regional, and national sepsis incidence and mortality, 1990–2017: Analysis for the Global Burden of Disease Study. *The Lancet*, *395*(10219), 200–11. doi.org/10.1016/s0140-6736(19)32989-7

Sepsis Alliance. (2021). Retrieved from: www.sepsis.org

Singer, M., Deutschman, C. S., Seymour, C. W., Shankar-Hari, M., Annane, D., Bauer, M., ... Angus, D. C. (2016). The Third International Consensus Definitions for Sepsis and Septic Shock (Sepsis-3). *JAMA*, *315*(8), 801–10.

Thompson, K., Venkatesh, B. & Finfer, S. (2019). Sepsis and septic shock: Current approaches to management. *Internal Medicine Journal*, *49*(2), 160–70. doi.org/10.1111/imj.14199

Chapter 11

Caring for a person with substance dependence and complex post-traumatic distress syndrome

MARK GOODHEW and TRACY ROBINSON

LEARNING OUTCOMES

Completion of the activities in this chapter will enable you to:

- define the terms 'substance use dependence', 'harm reduction', 'complex PTSD (post-traumatic stress disorder)' and 'trauma-informed care' (**gather information, interpret** and **discriminate**)
- explain why an understanding of substance use dependence, harm reduction, complex PTSD and trauma-informed care is essential to competent nursing practice (**recall** and **application**)
- outline the clinical manifestations of a substance use dependence, harm reduction, complex PTSD and trauma-informed care, that will guide your collection of appropriate cues (**gather information, interpret** and **discriminate**)
- identify risk factors for substance use dependence (**matching** and **predicting**)
- review clinical information to identify the main nursing diagnoses for a person experiencing substance dependence and complex PTSD (**synthesise**)
- describe the priorities of care for the management of a person experiencing substance dependence and complex PTSD (**goal setting** and **taking action**)
- consider how stigma may interfere with person-centred care (**reflection** and **translation**)
- reflect on personal reactions to people who use alcohol or other drugs and identify appropriate self-management strategies (**reflection** and **translation**).

INTRODUCTION

The scenarios introduced in this chapter focus on the care of a person with substance use dependence and complex post-traumatic stress disorder (PTSD). This chapter will use the term 'substance use dependence' instead of commonly used terms such as 'substance use disorder' and 'addiction'. We made this decision because language is powerful, and these negative terms can further stigmatise already highly marginalised groups, such as people who inject drugs (Network of Alcohol and other Drugs [NADA], 2019).

The Australian community has a long history of struggling with drugs and alcohol. Alcohol use has been widespread throughout Australia's colonial past and continues to be a fundamental part of many social activities. However, harmful consumption levels are a significant health issue, and alcohol has consistently remained the most common drug of concern among people accessing specialist treatment services. In the nineteenth century, the medical use of opioids was common and continued until the mid1950s when heroin was prohibited (Alcohol and Drug Foundation, 2019).

For the past 100 years, governments worldwide have effectively waged war on drugs, and people who experience substance dependence have often been viewed as undeserving of care. Instead of being viewed as individuals who require compassionate medical and psychological care, substance users are predominantly portrayed as criminals and mainly managed via the criminal justice system (Hari, 2016).

This stigmatising view has extended into healthcare settings where nurses too often view people with substance dependence as manipulative and violent criminal drug seekers who are unworthy of care (Copeland, 2020; Horner et al., 2019; Neville & Roan, 2014).

Seeing and responding to substance dependence as a legal rather than a health 'problem' means other contributing factors are overlooked. For example, there is strong evidence that interpersonal childhood trauma is linked to an increased vulnerability to substance use dependence (Lotzin et al., 2019; Moustafa et al., 2018). In addition, the pervasive influence of racism is evident with Australian Indigenous people often feeling judged by mainstream health services and being denied treatment for substance dependence (Queensland Mental Health Commission, 2020). Further, use of prescription opioids for chronic medical conditions has substantially increased. These factors highlight how trauma, racism and chronic pain are all factors that may underlie substance dependence, and that legal approaches, alone, have failed to stem the growing prevalence of substance use dependence.

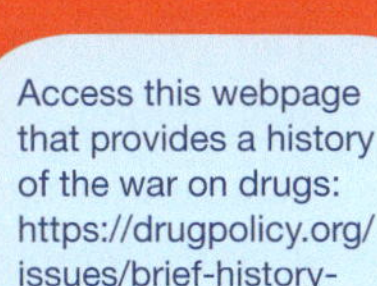

KEY CONCEPTS

substance use dependence
harm reduction
complex post-traumatic stress disorder
trauma-informed care

SUGGESTED READINGS

P. LeMone, G. Bauldoff, P. Gubrud-Howe, M.-A. Carno, T. Levett-Jones, . . . D. Stanley (Eds). (2020). *LeMone and Burke's Medical–Surgical Nursing: Critical Thinking in Person-Centred Care* (4th edn). Melbourne: Pearson Australia.

Chapter 5: Nursing Care of People with Problems of Substance Misuse

Chapter 50: Mental Healthcare in the Australian Context

Drug and Alcohol Withdrawal Clinical Practice Guidelines–NSW (NSW Health, 2008). https://www1.health.nsw.gov.au/pds/ActivePDSDocuments/GL2008_011.pdf

SCENARIO 11.1 Caring for a young man with substance use dependence

SETTING THE SCENE

Mr Shawn Bolton is a 25-year-old male who self-presented to the emergency department (ED) with a temperature of 39°C and an infected abscess on his left arm from injecting heroin. Shawn has been admitted to your ward for observation, and has been prescribed IV antibiotics to treat the abscess and prevent infective endocarditis—a severe cardiac infection that is associated with injecting drug use.

Shawn was released from prison six weeks ago for a drug-related offence. Unfortunately, he was released without accommodation, support or money and, as a result, he has been sleeping rough. Due to Shawn's drug use and criminal history, a number of the nurses on the ward are reluctant to care for Shawn. One of the nurses said he hopes Shawn will discharge himself so his bed can be given to a more 'deserving' patient.

Aetiology of substance use dependence

The *Diagnostic and Statistical Manual of Mental Disorders-V* (DSM-V) (American Psychiatric Association, 2013) states that an essential feature of a substance use dependence is a cluster of cognitive, behavioural and physiological symptoms resulting in the individual continuing to use the substance despite significant substance-related problems. The aetiology of substance use is complex and factors including trauma, genetic background, and medical and mental illness have all been associated with increased substance use (Bujarski, Lim & Ray, 2018).

Recently, the understanding of the effects of trauma on the brain, sympathetic nervous system and endocrine system has dramatically increased, and brain imaging has shown that traumatic stress can produce lasting changes in brain areas, including the amygdala, hippocampus and prefrontal cortex (Henigsberg et al., 2019). Stress hormones, such as cortisol and norepinephrine, are also likely to induce negative thoughts, aggressive (or passive-aggressive) behaviours and a survival mentality driven by the amygdala (Raber et al., 2019).

Traumatised people often have difficulties managing emotional impulses. What nurses often perceive to be challenging behaviours could actually be fight, flight and freeze responses that are common when people are traumatised. Recognising the complex aetiology of substance use allows us to reframe the concept of 'challenging behaviours' as 'survival skills'.

Epidemiology of mental health and substance use dependence

In Australia, mental illnesses are one of the leading causes of disease burden. In 2017–18, one in five (20.1%) or 4.8 million Australians had a mental or behavioural condition (Australian Bureau of Statistics, 2018). Further, one in six (16.1%) people aged 18 and over consume more than two standard drinks per day (exceeding the lifetime risk guidelines) (Australian Bureau of Statistics, 2018). The *Australian Burden of Disease Study* (Australian Institute of Health and Wellbeing [AIHW], 2019) demonstrated that substance use disorders account for 45 per cent of the disease burden in Australians aged under 50. Overall, mental and substance use disorders accounted for 12 per cent of the disease burden. However, it is essential to note that the burden of disease is not equally shared across the lifespan or across population cohorts, with some age groups and populations more vulnerable to mental health and substance dependence.

Alcohol and other drugs (AOD) use is a significant public health issue. Over 2 per cent of the world's population are diagnosed with AOD dependence (Ritchie, 2019). Every year, 11.8 million people die prematurely from smoking, alcohol and substance use (Ritchie, 2019). Over the past few decades, there has been a dramatic rise in opioid-related deaths, with 109,520 deaths recorded in 2017 (Ritchie, 2019). This rise is primarily attributed to the doubling of opioid prescriptions between 2001 and 2013 in the United States, Canada, Australia and some Western European countries (Berterame et al., 2016).

Access this link to the opioid diaries that provide devastating stories from people who are affected by the opioid crisis in the USA: https://time.com/james-nachtwey-opioid-addiction-america

There are many ethical challenges concerning Shawn's care. Using your clinical reasoning skills can help you recognise, better understand and respond to dilemmas such as those portrayed here, resulting in empathic, accurate, timely and person-centred care.

Stigma

Because drug use has been stigmatised, many nurses will find it challenging to develop a therapeutic alliance with Shawn, which may compromise his care. Goffman (1986) conceptualised stigma as an attribute that is deeply discrediting and makes the person carrying it 'different from others and of a less desirable kind' (p. 3). Stigma diminishes self-esteem and robs people of social opportunities because of stereotyping, prejudice and discrimination (Corrigan, 2004).

Many people with substance dependence have experienced this kind of stigma and shame and, unfortunately, this is often reinforced when they encounter the health system. Trying to access and navigate healthcare systems can be traumatising, particularly if people are 'judged' as unworthy of receiving help or are seen as somehow to blame for their situation. Patient experience is now recognised as a central pillar of a quality healthcare system, and equally as important as clinical care (The Health Foundation, 2021). Hence, Shawn's experience in hospital is not simply an important consideration when assessing him but could also significantly influence his clinical outcomes.

1. CONSIDER THE PATIENT SITUATION

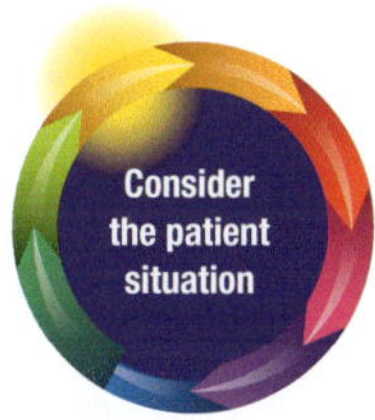

National Safety and Quality Health Service (NSQH) Standard

Communicating for safety standard

The NSQHS Standards emphasise the importance of effective communication in healthcare settings, including the importance of structured, effective clinical handovers to communicate critical patient information (ACSQHC, 2021).

This factsheet will provide you with more information about OxyContin: https://adf.org.au/drug-facts/oxycodone

It is now 0700 hours. You are allocated to care for Shawn on the morning shift, and you are provided with the following handover report:

Shawn Bolton is in room 4. He was transferred from ED last night with infected abscess on his left arm from injecting heroin use. He is prescribed intravenous antibiotics. Shawn has not slept overnight, has been highly agitated, complaining of severe stomach cramps, and has been demanding that he be prescribed OxyContin and be given a cigarette.

Shawn's behaviour and symptoms indicate that he may be withdrawing from heroin. Refer to pages 34–40 of the drug and alcohol withdrawal guidelines to find out about the management of opioid withdrawals: https://www1.health.nsw.gov.au/pds/ActivePDSDocuments/GL2008_011.pdf

Medical orders

- Paracetamol 500 mg—1 g every 4–6 hours, no more than eight tablets in 24 hours
- Ampicillin 2 g IVI every four hours
- Full set of observations every four hours

The nurse reports that Shawn swore when told he was only charted paracetamol for his pain and that the hospital has a strict no-smoking policy. Shawn was told his behaviour was inappropriate and the nurse walked out and has left him alone 'to calm down'. Staff have been told to limit contact with him because he is drug seeking and has a criminal record. Security has been notified and will monitor his behaviour.

Something to think about . . .

NSW Health has a clear policy for preventing and managing violence in the NSW Health Workplace (NSW Health, 2015). This policy defines violence as 'any incident in which an individual is abused, threatened or assaulted' (NSW Health, 2015, p. 2) and includes verbal, physical or psychological abuse, threats or other intimidating behaviours. However, it is important to distinguish between behaviour resulting from a number of medical conditions (such as delirium) and potentially violent behaviours (NSW Health, 2015).

Zero tolerance policies were introduced in NSW Heath sector in 2005 (Morphet et al., 2014) and, although well meaning, they suggest that any violence, threats or intimidation should be viewed as entirely negative and should not be accepted from anyone under any circumstances. Zero tolerance policies also suggest there is no discretion on the part of the nurse, which may invite an inflexible adherence to the rules and adversarial attitudes towards patients. This differs from legislation, such as the NSW Mental Health Act *and the* Anti-Discrimination Act 1977, *that enshrines a person's right to be treated with respect and in the least restrictive environment.*

Nursing and Midwifery Board of Australia (NMBA) *Registered Nurse Standards for Practice* The NMBA's *Registered Nurse Standards for Practice* (2016) state that care must be based on purposefully engaging a person in effective therapeutic and professional relationships, communicating effectively and being respectful of a person's dignity, culture, values, beliefs and rights.

Q1 In the nurse's handover report, there are significant gaps in information.

- a True
- b False

Q2 What personal assumptions or biases might influence the care provided to Shawn from hospital staff?

- a He is a criminal.
- b He is a drug addict.
- c He is undeserving of care.
- d All of the options.

Q3 Any aggressive acts by a patient, including physical violence, threats, abuse and intimidation, should always be viewed as entirely negative and should never be accepted from anyone.

- a True
- b False

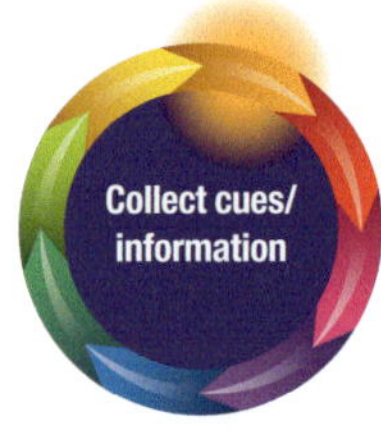

2. COLLECT CUES/INFORMATION

In this stage of the clinical reasoning cycle, it is essential that you collect both subjective and objective cues to gain a deeper understanding of Shawn's situation and healthcare issues (Levett-Jones et al., 2010). Subjective data is what the person tells you about their symptoms, feelings, perceptions and concerns (such as asking people to rate their pain on a scale from 1 to 10). As you can see, this is open to interpretation on the part of the nurse and even misinterpretation. In contrast, objective data is observable and measurable and is obtained through physical examination, vital signs and tests.

(a) Review current information

Although you are not sure what is happening with Shawn, based on the handover provided, you are concerned about heroin withdrawal and that he may be at risk of endocarditis. From the handover and a brief conversation with Shawn, you review his subjective cues, including fatigue, aching joints, restlessness, irritability, anxiety, sweating, shortness of breath, swelling feet and cravings for drugs.

(b) Gather new information

You realise that to keep Shawn comfortable and provide safe nursing care, you need to gather more information about his drug and alcohol use. You decide to assess his withdrawal symptoms and take his vital signs (listed below).

Clinical Opiate Withdrawal Scale (COWS)	28
Temperature	38.7 C
Pulse rate	112
Respiratory rate	22
Blood pressure	150/90

Q From the following list, select the four *best* responses to help you engage Shawn and collect more information about his drug and alcohol use.

- a 'Have some respect, and don't swear at me.'
- b 'I see that you are uncomfortable and worried because you are withdrawing. So can I ask you some questions about your drug use?'

c 'I would like to help you, as I can see that you are upset.'
d 'I am concerned about you. Are you happy to have a chat about your drug use?'
e 'Shawn, I want to better understand your experience and current health concerns. Is it okay if we talk more about your use of alcohol and other drugs?'
f 'If you continue behaving like that, I will call security.'

Comprehensive drug and alcohol assessment

A comprehensive drug and alcohol assessment aims to obtain a relevant history and better understand a person's readiness to change. This information is then used to formulate a management plan based on the individual's needs. In the past, confrontational approaches to dealing with substance use have been used, but assessment should be a therapeutic process and an opportunity to understand the person's situation and goals. Therefore, nurses should preface any assessment by explaining why they are taking a history and re-establishing appropriate confidentiality.

To determine Shawn's current and past use of drugs and alcohol, the following questions should guide your thinking:

- What are the patterns of use and route of administration?
- Has the person experienced any physical and psychosocial consequences?
- What is their motivation for taking substances? What effect does it have?
- What is the frequency/duration/amount used?
- Have there been previous attempts at reduction or cessation of substance use and does your patient want to stop or cut down?
- What harm reduction interventions (e.g. using clean injecting equipment, injecting in a supervised injecting facility) has Shawn used to reduce the harms associated with drug use?

Nurses must be well-informed about harm reduction interventions as there is strong evidence that they reduce disability and death associated with opioid use. Further, it is unethical for nurses not to adopt harm reduction interventions into their practice as this philosophy is closely aligned with the International Council of Nurses (2012) Code of Ethics (Iammarino & Pauly, 2020).

You complete a comprehensive drug assessment, and ascertain the following subjective cues:

- Last alcohol drink: 4 days ago (drinks once a week)
- Last heroin use: 24 hours ago (uses 3–4 times a day)
- Last cannabis use: 21 days ago (smokes once a month)
- Tobacco intake: 30 per day—last cigarette one day ago
- Commenced all of the above in early adolescence.

(c) Recall knowledge

At this point, you carefully consider Shawn's past medical history, his presenting complaints, current treatment plan and current vital signs, and start to analyse your findings. You may decide to gather more information by accessing the *Drug and Alcohol Withdrawal Clinical Practice Guidelines—NSW* (NSW Health, 2008). From your research and previous knowledge, you know that restlessness, perspiration, insomnia, joint pain and intense cravings are key symptoms of withdrawal from opioids and your findings indicate that this could be an issue for Shawn. You also ascertain that withdrawal may have an onset of 8–24 hours and a duration of 4–10 days, and anticipate that Shawn's behaviour could become unpredictable.

To complicate matters further, your comprehensive drug and alcohol assessment indicates that Shawn is also at high risk of withdrawing from tobacco. Tobacco is an addictive substance and abrupt cessation produces a withdrawal syndrome. Many of the nicotine withdrawal symptoms are similar to those of other drug withdrawal syndromes: anxiety, awakening during sleep, depression, difficulty concentrating, impatience, irritability/anger and restlessness (Quit Victoria, 2021).

Before proceeding to the next stage of the clinical reasoning cycle, you consider any gaps in the information you received from the handover and history, and think about the potential impact these may have on Shawn's care.

Q1 In the handover, the nurse communicated all the important and relevant clinical information.

a True

b False

Q2 From the list below, identify how the tone and content of the nursing handover provided to you and the other nurses might influence the care provided to Shawn? (Select two correct answers.)

a Staff are more likely to be empathic towards Shawn.

b Staff are more likely to like Shawn.

c Staff are more likely to provide excellent care to Shawn.

d Staff are more likely to stigmatise Shawn.

e Staff are more likely to fear Shawn.

Quick Quiz!

To ensure that you have a good understanding of the key concepts related to substance use, test yourself with the following questions.

Q1 Which medication would be prescribed to lessen Shawn's discomfort when he is withdrawing from heroin?

a OxyContin

b Panadol

c Buprenorphine

d Morphine

Q2 Match the medication that will help lessen Shawn's opioid withdrawal symptoms.

Medication

- Diazepam
- Hyoscine
- Metoclopramide
- Clonidine

Medication	Withdrawal symptom
	Nausea
	Sweating or agitation
	Abdominal cramps
	Agitation or restless legs

Q3 Healthcare professionals too often perceive people who use drugs as:

a People who are traumatised and therefore deserving of care

b People who have a legitimate medical condition and are therefore deserving of care

c People who are criminals and manipulative, and therefore undeserving of care

d People who don't help themselves and are therefore undeserving of care

Q4 Fill in the missing words from the choices given:

a In Australia one in ______________ people will be diagnosed with a mental health problem in their life time. (five, ten, twenty)

b Substance use disorders account for ______________ per cent of the disease burden in Australians aged under 50. (25, 45, 65)

c Over the past few decades there has been a dramatic increase in ______________ related deaths. (opioid, alcohol, cannabis)

d Many people who are diagnosed with substance dependence have experienced ______________ ______________ early in life. (malnutrition, medical issues, traumatic events)

Q5 Combining smoking-cessation medications with a referral to a specialised support service would provide Shawn with the best chances of quitting.

a True

b False

Q6 Mark each of the following signs or symptoms of opioid withdrawal as *true* or *false*.

- Restricted pupils
- Perspiration
- Constipation
- Intense hunger and overeating
- Cramps
- Intense craving for opioids
- Vomiting
- Chest pain
- Yawning
- Piloerection

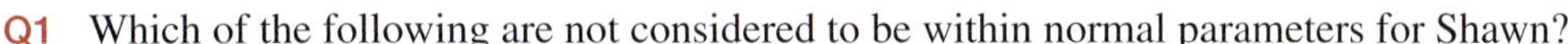

3. PROCESS INFORMATION

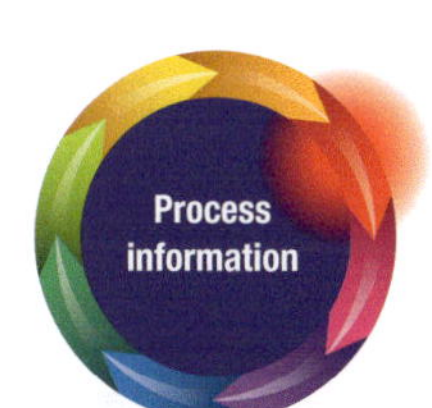

(a) Interpret

The next step of the clinical reasoning cycle is to interpret the data (cues) that you have collected by carefully analysing and comparing normal versus abnormal. This step is critical in the clinical reasoning cycle as it enables you to identify relationships between cues and make inferences about the subjective and objective data that you have collected.

Q1 Which of the following are not considered to be within normal parameters for Shawn?

a Temperature: 38.7 C

b Pulse rate: 112

c Respiratory rate: 22

d Blood pressure: 150/90

e COWs score: 28

f All options

Q2 The Clinical Opioid Withdrawal Scale (COWS) is an 11-item scale which is used to monitor and rate symptoms of opioid withdrawal. A score of 28 would indicate:

a Mild withdrawal

b Moderate withdrawal

c Moderately severe withdrawal

d Severe withdrawal

(b) Discriminate

From the cues and information you now have, you need to narrow down the information to what is most important.

Q1 From the list below, identify the three cues that would most concern you when assessing Shawn at this time.

a High respiratory rate

b High temperature

c High pulse rate

d Craving for drugs

e Increasing levels of agitation

f Sweating

g Aching joints

Q2 Are there any gaps in the information that has been collected so far?

(c) Relate

You now have a list of important cues that you need to cluster to find patterns or interrelationships between them, and to better understand Shawn's situation.

Q The following are *true* statements or *false*?

- a Shawn's blood pressure and pulse are too high for a person of his age.
- b Shawn's agitation and behaviour are likely to be related to opioid and nicotine withdrawals.
- c A high temperature, sweating, high pulse rate, shortness of breath and swelling feet may indicate that Shawn has infective endocarditis.
- d Shawn's irritability, insomnia and craving for nicotine and heroin suggest that he may be withdrawing from these substances.

(d) Infer

It is now time to consider all the cues you have collected about Shawn and make inferences based on your analysis and interpretation of the cues.

Q From what you know about Shawn, identify which three of the following inferences are correct.

- a Shawn is withdrawing from opioids.
- b Shawn is a risk for aggression and/or violence due to his withdrawal symptoms.
- c He is withdrawing from nicotine.
- d He is reacting badly to hospitalisation because of how staff are stigmatising him.
- e He is reacting badly to hospitalisation because he is a drug addict and recently discharged from jail.

(e) Match

Think back to your last clinical placement or past experience. Have you seen anyone presenting in a similar way? How were they managed? What were the key concerns of the healthcare professionals involved?

(f) Predict

Now is the time to consider the consequences of your actions or inaction by predicting potential outcomes for Shawn.

Shawn is thinking of discharging himself against medical advice because of how the nursing staff are treating him. If you do nothing, what might be the consequences?

Q The following outcomes have a *high, possible* or *low* likelihood.

- a Shawn's dependence on opioid and nicotine will remain untreated.
- b Shawn's drug use will increase because of his social circumstances.
- c Shawn is at risk of becoming seriously unwell if he discharges himself, as he could develop endocarditis.
- d Shawn's psychosocial issues will not be resolved.

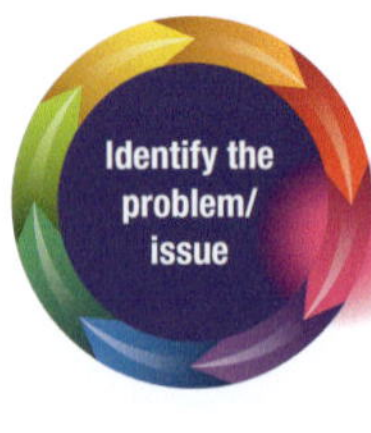

4. IDENTIFY THE PROBLEM/ISSUE

At this stage of the clinical reasoning cycle, you bring together (synthesise) all of the information and inferences you have made in order to make a definitive nursing diagnosis of Shawn's main problems.

Q Select from the following list, the incorrect nursing diagnosis for Shawn.

- a Opioid withdrawal related to the recent cessation of intravenous heroin use, evidenced by a high COWS score
- b Nicotine withdrawal related to limited access to cigarettes whilst hospitalised, evidenced by agitation, insomnia and headache
- c Homelessness related to being recently discharged from prison, evidenced by sleeping rough
- d Antisocial behaviour related to verbal aggression to staff and total disregard for the hospital's zero tolerance policy

5. ESTABLISH GOALS

Before implementing any actions to improve Shawn's condition, it is important to clearly specify what you want to happen and when. By building trust and a therapeutic relationship with Shawn, you will better understand his situation and the factors likely to influence clinical outcomes. Communicating with Shawn will help you collect and verify subjective data that can inform your treatment goals.

Q From the list below, choose the three *most important* short-term goals for Shawn's management at this time.

- a To be discharged as soon as possible to avoid further difficulties with his behaviour
- b To encourage him not to self-discharge so that he can receive treatment for his heroin dependence
- c To have counselling for his substance abuse issues
- d To minimise the effects of heroin and nicotine withdrawal
- e To access psychosocial support for Shawn so he will have suitable accommodation on discharge
- f To inform Shawn that his behaviour could be seen as a violation of the hospital's zero tolerance policy

6. TAKE ACTION

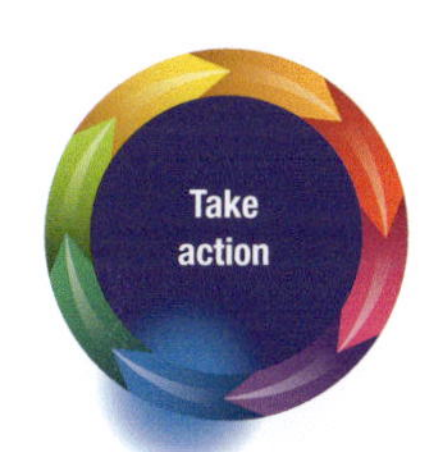

Q Which of the following actions would be most helpful in caring for Shawn at this time? (Select the *three* correct answers.)

- a Continue to monitor and document Shawn's withdrawal from opiates and nicotine.
- b Remind Shawn that the hospital has a zero tolerance policy for physical and verbal aggression.
- c Agree on a clear management plan with Shawn and the treatment team.
- d Respond to the person not the label.
- e Reassure Shawn that his abscess will abate with antibiotics.
- f Try to spend more time with Shawn so that you can help him solve some of his problems.
- g Set appropriate limits and boundaries about appropriate and inappropriate behaviours.

7. EVALUATE

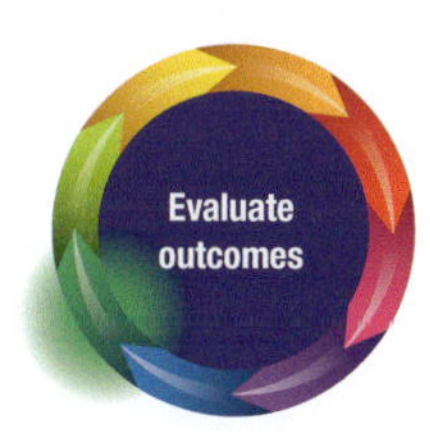

You talk to Shawn about how his heroin withdrawal will be monitored and you suggest that he tries a nicotine replacement patch to help with nicotine withdrawal. You also discuss with Shawn ways that you can communicate and work together so that he feels more settled.

Q If these communication strategies are successful, you should notice which *five* of the following:

- a Shawn's COWS score decreases.
- b Shawn discharges himself.
- c Shawn's cravings for heroin and nicotine decrease.
- d Shawn is not asking to be discharged.
- e Shawn is starting to trust you more.
- f Shawn apologises to the nurses and keeps quiet.
- g Shawn is feeling less agitated and anxious.
- h There is an improvement in Shawn's vital signs.

8. REFLECT

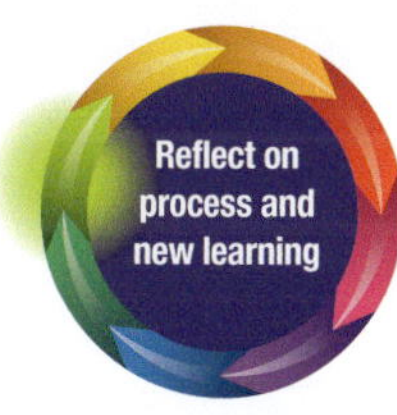

Q1 From the following, identify three factors that negatively influenced the nurse's attitudes towards Shawn and his subsequent management.

- a Not attempting to create a therapeutic relationship with Shawn
- b Focusing on Shawn's intravenous drug use and criminal history
- c Empathising with Shawn's situation
- d Taking the zero tolerance policy
- e Judgement, referring to clinical handover and notes

Q2 How could Shawn's admission and initial hospitalisation have been managed more effectively?

Q3 What have you learned from this scenario that you can apply to your future practice?

Q4 While reflecting on this scenario, consider how you would be feeling when caring for Shawn and how you might react to him. Nursing can be stressful and we often lack the resources or experience to deal effectively with all the situations we encounter. Please ask yourself the following questions if you are caring for someone like Shawn.

- a What are my feelings about caring for someone with an addiction to illicit substances? Could my feelings affect my reasoning?
- b What are my moral beliefs about people who use substances, and could my beliefs affect my reasoning?
- c What are my own patterns of using alcohol and other substances? Have I ever felt annoyed if someone made comments about my drinking and/or smoking?
- d What are my beliefs about people who continue using tobacco? Do I see smoking as a personal choice or health-related issue?

SCENARIO 11.2 The story unfolds: More than just substance abuse

CHANGING THE SCENE

1. CONSIDER THE PATIENT SITUATION

Consider the patient situation

It is nearing the end of your shift and you feel concerned that Shawn's 'real' issues may not have been properly addressed. You also feel a little guilty, as you think your attitude towards Shawn may have been influenced by the comments of other nurses and by your previous experiences with 'challenging' patients. You decide to talk to Shawn and, because you were the nurse who 'sorted out' the buprenorphine and the nicotine patches for him, he seems to trust you.

Shawn tells you he was removed from his parents when he was 18 months old as they were young and couldn't cope with a baby. As a result, Shawn was placed into foster care. He lived in 10 different homes until the age of 15 when he was put in juvenile detention for drug dealing. Shawn said that he started drinking alcohol and smoking weed at the age of 12 to cope with feeling neglected and unloved, and to block out memories of being physically, emotionally and sexually abused in the foster homes. Shawn's abuse has made him distrustful of most people, making it difficult to form close relationships. The abuse has also impacted his self-esteem and made him feel worthless. He tells you that it is sometimes hard for him to control or make sense of his emotions.

Substance use and dependence frequently co-occurs with post-traumatic stress disorder (PTSD). People may use alcohol and other drugs to help them cope but this can lead to further difficulties. Shawn said he would like to give up drugs but they block out his negative feelings and distressing memories. Shawn also said that abuse is a recurring theme in his life. He was abused throughout his childhood, beaten in jail, kicked in the head while sleeping rough, and is made to feel like a 'junkie' by healthcare professionals each time he enters a medical service.

Access the Uniting Sydney Medically Supervised Injecting Centre's (MSIC) website; read the aims of the MSIC, what happens and its impressive record of success: https://www.uniting.org/community-impact/uniting-medically-supervised-injecting-centre--msic

Shawn mentioned that he recently started injecting in a supervised injecting facility where he can inject legally and more safely under the supervision of healthcare professionals. He likes the service as the staff are nonjudgmental, and it provides him with a safe place to inject, clean injecting equipment and nurses who can save his life if he overdoses. Shawn also saw a mental health nurse at the facility, and she said he has complex PTSD and that she could refer him to someone for therapy.

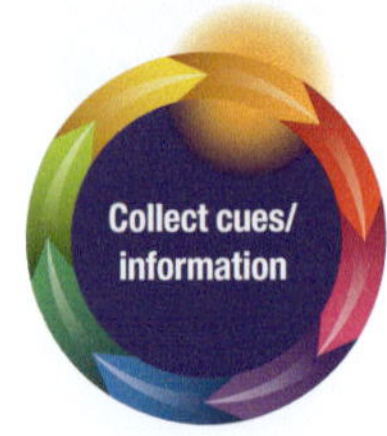

2. COLLECT CUES/INFORMATION

(a) Review current information

You decide you need more specific information in order to plan Shawn's care. You review his admission documentation again, including his drug and alcohol history. Although Shawn is exhibiting some symptoms of opioid withdrawal, you start to wonder whether this is the primary problem or if Shawn's substance use is his attempt to deal with another problem. You realise the trauma he experienced as a child might be a factor in his substance use and that he might be 'self-medicating' as a way of coping with his distress.

(b) Gather new information

You decide to gather further information about Shawn's situation by accessing the *Australian Guidelines for the Prevention and Treatment of Acute Stress Disorder, Post-traumatic Stress Disorder and Complex PTSD* (Phoenix Australia, 2021).

For more information on the prevention and treatment of acute stress disorders PTSD and CPTSD, see Chapter 7 of the guidelines at: https://www.phoenixaustralia.org/australian-guidelines-for-ptsd/

Q1 Which of the following would not be consistent with a diagnosis of PTSD?

- a Avoidance of situations that bring back memories of trauma
- b Feeling on edge and looking out for danger
- c Nightmares
- d Constant worrying over minor things

Q2 Which of the following commonly contribute to complex PTSD?

- a Events in early childhood
- b A single traumatic event
- c Vicariously seeing a person experience trauma
- d Dissociation from traumatic memories

Patient Safety Competency Framework (PSCF)

Domain 2–Therapeutic communication

The PSCF specifies that nurses need to be skilled in verbal and nonverbal communication skills so they can show empathy and respect, and encourage people to express their feelings and needs. Therapeutic communication occurs within professional boundaries and is an essential skill for all nurses.

Source: *The Patient Safety Competency Framework for Nursing Students*, https://patientsafetyfornursingstudents.org

Because you feel a little confused, you decide to see if you can talk more with Shawn and attempt to better understand his situation. You ask him if you can clarify some things he raised in your earlier discussion and he agrees.

RN: *Hi, Shawn, thank you for sharing your story with me. I can now see you have had some really tough times in your life, and the fact that you survived all these challenges clearly shows your strength and resilience. I am wondering if we can discuss how best we can support you at this point?*

Shawn: *I will be just fine when I get out of here and I don't think you can do much after that.*

RN: *Well, can I just check that I have understood? So, you had a lot of grief and loss as a child in terms of being put in foster care. You also had some very traumatic experiences, which we don't need to go into at the moment. Using drugs is one way you have found to cope with your memories and painful feelings. You also said you would like to stop using but you are scared the memories will return. Lately, you have been accessing the safe injecting room where the staff are very supportive and one of the nurses there mentioned to you that you could have complex PTSD. Have I understood correctly, Shawn?*

When people present with complex and chronic issues, it is important to ensure you have understood all the issues from the person's point of view. Paraphrasing and reflecting are communication techniques you can use when gathering new information. This is a way of 'checking in' with the person to ensure you have understood them properly.

Shawn: *Yep, that's it in a nutshell. I don't really know much about PTSD. All I know is that the injecting room is the one place where the staff don't treat me like a junkie.*

RN: *It must be good to have finally found a place where you feel safe.*

Shawn: *Yeah, it is, and that's how I met the mental health nurse who told me I could have PTSD.*

RN: *Shawn, I wonder if that is something you would like to know more about?*

Shawn: *At the moment, I just want this headache and sweating to stop.*

RN: *That's understandable. With the antibiotics and the buprenorphine, you should be feeling better soon. Thanks for being so open with me. I now have a better understanding of why you are using heroin. If you ever need to talk, I am happy to listen.*

Shawn: *Well, I want to stop using but I don't even know where to start—I'm just trying to get through each day, you know? And it's awful in here—the nurses ignore me and I have to fight just to get some pain relief.*

RN: *Shawn, would it help if I got some information together for you. I know you're not up to reading it now, but what if I find out about treatment options for heroin dependence and homeless health services, and how we can make sure you are safe when you leave hospital?*

Shawn: *Yeah, that would be good but I can't think about all that now.*

How commonly is substance use dependence co-morbid with trauma?

Early life stress and exposure to adverse childhood experiences are common, and have been found to be a significant contributing factor for substance use dependence, PTSD, borderline personality disorder (BPD) and various medical illnesses including cardiovascular disease (Kirsch et al., 2020). For people with substance use dependence, early life stress is associated with increased risk of relapse and poor treatment response (Kirsch et al., 2020).

Given that complex PTSD (CPTSD) is a more severe and long-term form of PTSD (Cloitre, 2020), it is important to understand that Shawn's coping mechanisms and behaviour may, in times past, have protected him from the many adverse events he experienced. The risk of him developing disorders such as depression, substance use, PTSD and BPD was increased as a result of his prolonged trauma at particular physical and psychological developmental stages (Phoenix Australia, 2021).

For more information on BPD, access: https://www.bpdfoundation.org.au

and for information about available services, access: https://www.uow.edu.au/project-air/find-a-service

A person with complex PTSD experiences problems with emotion regulation, self-identity and relationships (Cloitre, 2020). A better understanding of these 'symptoms' allows us to unravel the complexities of how trauma and substance use commonly co-occur and give rise to the 'survival skills' and behaviours that healthcare professionals often conceptualise as 'challenging' (such as anger, explosive outbursts and withdrawal).

Something to think about...

View a personal video account (FlightMediocrity, 2020) of what it is like to live with addiction and trauma:
https://www.youtube.com/watch?v=ys6TCO_olOc

(c) Recall knowledge

Q. What could you say to Shawn about his opioid use and complex PTSD? Select the two *most appropriate* statements from those listed below.

a Complex PTSD is a lifelong condition and is commonly associated with substance use dependence.
b Complex PTSD is common and affects a significant proportion of the population.
c Complex PTSD is associated with increased smoking rates across genders.
d Shawn needs to stop using heroin if he wants to address his history of trauma.
e Shawn could stop using drugs if he really wanted to.
f Shawn's self-sabotaging behaviour is a result of his traumatic childhood.

3. PROCESS INFORMATION

Process information

(a) Interpret

The next step of the clinical reasoning cycle is to interpret the data (cues) that you have collected while applying your knowledge about Shawn. It would be easy to feel overwhelmed in the face of Shawn's complex presentation given that he has a range of emotional and relational issues, with his substance use being only one consequence of his past traumatic experiences. Because you have a therapeutic relationship with Shawn, your interpretation of cues collected so far is that, when he is discharged, it is important to ensure that if he decides to continue injecting heroin that he does so safely with clean injecting equipment and in company to avoid any further risk of blood borne viruses or overdose.

It can be helpful to use a case formulation format to assist you to see what information you have about Shawn and what information may be missing. Case formulation can help you develop the foundation for a mutually agreed treatment plan and involves consideration of the following:

- predisposing factors (those that increase a client's vulnerability to drug use)
- precipitating factors (triggers for using a substance)
- maintaining factors (such as homelessness or drug-using friends, etc.)
- relationship between mental health problems and drug use
- protective factors.

For more information on case formulation see: https://tpcjournal.nbcc.org/case-formulation-and-intervention-application-of-the-five-ps-framework-in-substance-use-counseling

and

doi.org/10.1192/apt.bp.115.014670

Q Complete the following table by matching the term to the correct descriptions.

Term

- Psychological
- Physical
- Social
- Biological

Term	Predisposing factors	Precipitating factors	Perpetuating factors	Prognostic indicators (including protective)
	Societal stigma against substance dependence	Prolonged exposure to traumatic events in childhood and adolescence	Government's war on drugs policy	Stays in hospital to have physical health needs addressed
	Family history of substance dependence	Long term use of opioids	Unable to access treatment for substance dependence	Nurses engaging Shawn in a therapeutic relationship
	Has developed tolerance to opioids and nicotine	Opioid and nicotine withdrawal symptoms	Low self-esteem	Hospital staff recognising that Shawn's issues need to be seen through a trauma-informed lens
	Trauma	Homelessness and incarceration	Physical tolerance to substances	Intelligent

(b) Discriminate

It is important to now focus on the most relevant information that you have. You realise that Shawn's symptoms are broadly consistent with both complex PTSD and BPD. Although it is out of your scope of practice to diagnose a mental health condition, it is evident that a common feature of both is a history of prolonged trauma. You have also heard staff speak disparagingly about people with BPD so you are reluctant to 'label' Shawn in this way. Establishing a medical diagnosis for Shawn is not a priority at this stage. What is more important is that Shawn trusts the staff who are caring for him.

Access the following website for information about the principles of trauma-informed care: https://www.health.nsw.gov.au/mentalhealth/psychosocial/principles/Pages/trauma-informed.aspx

This trust can be achieved through the provision of trauma-informed care. If Shawn feels safe and trusts staff, he will be less likely to discharge himself.

Given the complexity of Shawn's presentation, you are unsure whether it is appropriate to simply refer him to a drug and alcohol service when he is discharged, and you wonder whether they will have the capacity to help Shawn address his complex PTSD. Because he has told you he needs the drugs to cope with intrusive memories, you realise that Shawn may not cease using opioids in the short term. You discern that, in addition to drug treatment options, you need to provide him with safe injecting information. With Shawn's permission, you decide to inform the mental health nurse at the supervised injecting centre of his admission, if Shawn decides to return there. You also decide to contact the consult liaison psychiatry (CLP) team that assesses and manages psychological problems and psychiatric disorders in general hospitals, because you think they may be able to help organise some psychological interventions for Shawn's trauma. Another consideration is to refer Shawn to the local drug and alcohol service for ongoing support with harm-reduction strategies.

For more information on homelessness services access the following:

https://www.svhs.org.au/our-services/list-of-services/homeless-health-service

https://www.aihw.gov.au/reports/australias-health/health-of-people-experiencing-homelessness

https://www.redcross.org.au/get-help/community-services/homelessness-services

Because Shawn does not have a fixed address and you are aware that homelessness is a risk factor for his substance dependence, you decide to contact various homelessness services to try and organise some crisis accommodation and ongoing healthcare for him.

(c) Relate

Q Based on what you have discovered about Shawn so far, are the following statements *true* or *false*?

- a Shawn's prolonged experience of childhood abuse and neglect by primary caregivers is an antecedent for both complex PTSD and substance use dependence.
- b Shawn's symptoms of complex PTSD may account for his problems with opioids.
- c Responses from staff have an important impact on Shawn's future help-seeking behaviours.
- d Shawn's complex presentation means he is at risk of harm to self or others.
- e Shawn has no motivation to stop using drugs.

(d) Infer

Q From what you know about Shawn's history, identify which of the following inferences is the *most* correct.

- a Shawn is verbally aggressive to staff because he has been in prison and has no respect for authority.
- b As Shawn has complex PTSD, you could conduct a comprehensive trauma assessment with him, but only if he is ready.
- c Shawn needs to stop using drugs before his complex PTSD can be effectively treated.
- d Shawn's problems with opioids should be treated at the same time as his complex PTSD.
- e Shawn's problems with the law precipitated his current problems.
- f Shawn's detachment from staff and his anger mean that he is not likely to engage with services.
- g Ensuring that Shawn feels emotionally and physically safe is paramount to him engaging in treatment and care and not discharging himself.

(e) Predict

Now is the time to consider the consequences of your actions or inaction by predicting potential outcomes for your patient.

Q If you do not take the appropriate actions, what could happen if Shawn is discharged at this point? (Select the *three* most correct responses.)

- a Shawn is unlikely to seek treatment for either his opioid use or his complex PTSD.
- b Shawn's drug use is likely to get worse.
- c Shawn is likely to end up in the criminal justice system.
- d Shawn will have an elevated risk of harm to others.

4. IDENTIFY THE PROBLEM/ISSUE

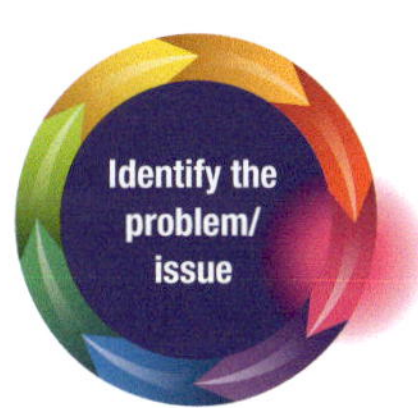

At this stage, you bring together (synthesise) all of the facts you've collected and inferences you've made to make a definitive nursing diagnosis of Shawn's main problems.

Q Select from the following list the *most correct* nursing diagnoses for Shawn.

a Aggressive behaviour related to nicotine withdrawal, evidenced by agitation and moodiness
b Ineffective impulse control related to opioid withdrawal, evidenced by verbal outbursts and anger
c Chronic low self-esteem related to childhood trauma, evidenced by refusal to engage with staff
d Ineffective coping related to childhood trauma, evidenced by substance dependence and decreased ability to manage stress
e Risk for other directed violence related to opioid withdrawal, evidenced by angry outbursts and verbal abuse

5. ESTABLISH GOALS

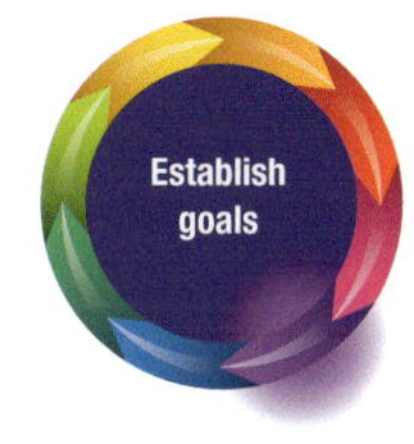

Before implementing any actions to improve Shawn's condition, it is important to clearly specify what you want to happen and when.

Q From the list below, choose the three most important *short-term* goals for Shawn when he leaves the hospital.

a Referral for psychological treatment in order to understand and address his CPTSD
b To take prescribed medication to treat CPTSD
c To be abstinent of opioids
d To increase Shawn's knowledge about harm reduction strategies (such as using clean injecting equipment)
e To contact local homelessness services and agencies to organise short-term accommodation for Shawn
f To contact staff at the safe injecting room and inform them of Shawn's hospitalisation

For more information about the concept of harm reduction, access: https://www.hri.global/what-is-harm-reduction

6. TAKE ACTION

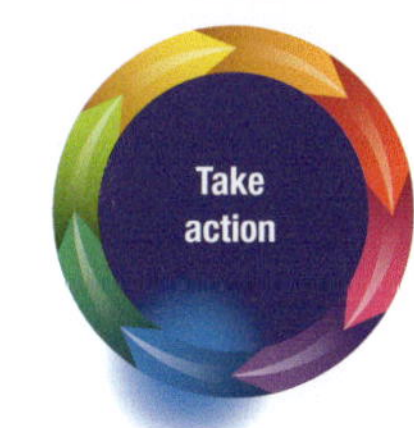

Q You decide to talk with Shawn about treatment options for his complex PTSD, substance dependence and harm reduction interventions. Which of the following interventions would be recommended for Shawn in the first instance? (Select *two* correct responses.)

a Refer Shawn to a drug and alcohol consultant.
b Refer Shawn to a specialist in trauma informed care.
c Provide information about meditation breathing and relaxation techniques.
d Promote Shawn's sense of safety and help him connect/reconnect with support services.
e Discuss the importance of using clean injecting equipment and using a supervised injecting facility to prevent blood borne infections, abscesses, endocarditis, and death or disability due to overdose.

7. EVALUATE

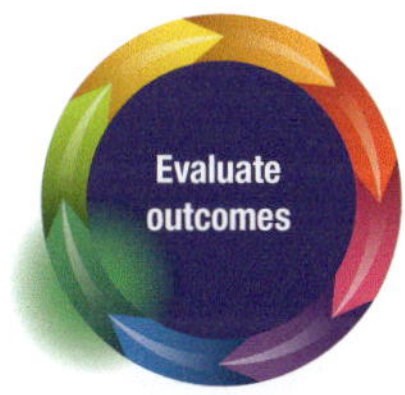

In complex clinical situations such as the one portrayed in this scenario, it can be difficult to evaluate the effectiveness of your intervention(s) in the short term. This is compounded when there is a short length of stay and you have very little time to build up a therapeutic relationship.

Q How would you determine whether you have made a positive difference to Shawn's nursing care?

8. REFLECT

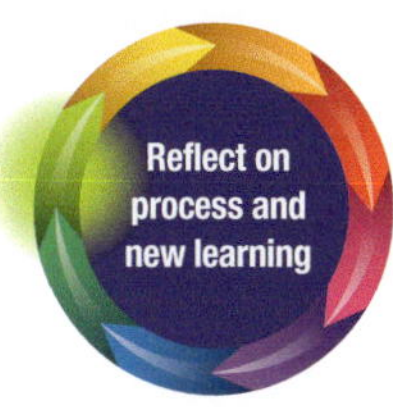

Reflect on your learning from this scenario and consider the following questions.

Q1 What are three of the most important things that you have learnt from this scenario?

Q2 What actions will you take in clinical practice as a result of your learning from this scenario?

Q3 How does therapeutic communication lead to improved outcomes for a marginalised person such as Shawn?

Q4 If you come across an 'unpopular patient', what might you change in your approach to their care?

Q5 Next time you hear a handover where the term 'challenging' or 'difficult patient' is used, how could you respond?

Q6 When you are 'challenged' by a patient's behaviour, how do you ensure that you continue to maintain a therapeutic alliance?

Q7 Iammarino and Pauly (2020) state that the principles of harm reduction are closely aligned with those of nursing ethics. What are your thoughts about this statement?

Something to think about...

You might want to ask yourself the following questions if you are looking after someone like Shawn.

1. *Are Shawn's problems too difficult to address with my current knowledge and skills?*
2. *Am I concerned that I might be acting out of my scope of practice?*
3. *Am I trying too hard to rescue him?*

Time Out!

If, while working through this scenario, you have identified that you may be at risk of having PTSD or a substance use disorder, it is important to talk with your doctor and discuss your concerns. It might also be time to evaluate what stresses you are under. Common signs of stress include chronic fatigue, difficulties sleeping, change in appetite, frustration, self-criticism and negativity, inability to 'switch off' from work, over-emotional reactions to stressors and minor physical illnesses (Edward et al., 2011). What are you doing to look after yourself? The following can be useful:

- Have fun outside work.
- Debrief with colleagues/mentor/educator.
- Have regular exercise, get adequate sleep and eat a balanced diet.
- See your mistakes as opportunities to learn.
- Do something enjoyable every day.
- Consider meditation, relaxation, mindfulness or yoga.

FURTHER READING

Krediet, E., Bostoen, T., Breeksema, J., van Schagen, J., Passie, T. & Vermetten, E. (2020). Reviewing the potential of psychedelics for the treatment of PTSD, *International Journal of Neuropsychopharmacology*, *23*(6), 385–400. doi.org/10.1093/ijnp/pyaa018

Maercker, A. (2021). Development of the new CPTSD diagnosis for ICD-11. *Borderline Personality Disorder and Emotion Dysregulation*, *8*, 7. doi.org/10.1186/s40479-021-00148-8

Te Pou. (2018). *Trauma Informed Care Resources for Leaders and Managers*. https://www.tepou.co.nz/uploads/files/resources/Trauma-informed-care-resources-for-Leaders-and-managers-1.pdf

REFERENCES

Alcohol and Drug Foundation. (2019). *Drugs and Stigma: A Short History.* Retrieved from: https://adf.org.au/insights/drug-stigma-history/

American Psychiatric Association. (2013). *Diagnostic and Statistical Manual of Mental Disorders* (5th edn). Arlington, VA: American Psychiatric Association.

Australian Bureau of Statistics. (2018). *National Health Survey: First Results, 2017–18.* Canberra: ABS; 2018. Catalogue No. 4364.0.55.001.

Australian Commission on Safety and Quality in Health Care (ACSQHC). (2021). *National Safety and Quality Health Service Standards* (2nd edn). Sydney, Australia.

Australian Institute of Health and Welfare. (2019). Australian Burden of Disease Study: Impact and Causes of Illness and Death in Australia 2015*. Australian Burden of Disease series no. 19.* Cat. no. BOD 22. Canberra: AIHW.

Berterame, S., Erthal, J., Thomas, J., Fellner, S., Vosse, B., Clare, P., … Mattick, R. P. (2016). Use of and barriers to access to opioid analgesics: A worldwide, regional, and national study. *The Lancet*, *387*(10028), 1644–56. doi.org/10.1016/s0140-6736(16)00161-6

Bujarski, S., Lim, A. & Ray, L. (2018). Prevalence, causes, and treatment of substance use disorders: A PRIMER. *The Judges' Journal*, *57*(1), 10–15.

Cloitre, M. (2020). ICD-11 complex post-traumatic stress disorder: Simplifying diagnosis in trauma populations. *British Journal of Psychiatry*, *216*(3), 129–31. doi.org/10.1192/bjp.2020.43

Copeland, D. (2020). Drug-seeking: A literature review (and an exemplar of stigmatization in nursing). *Nursing Inquiry*, *27*(1), e12329. doi.org/10.1111/nin.12329

Corrigan, P. (2004). How stigma interferes with mental health care. *American Psychologist*, *59*(7), 614–25.

Edward, K., Munro, I., Robins, A. & Welch, A. J. (2011). *Mental Health Nursing: Dimensions of Praxis.* South Melbourne: Oxford University Press.

Goffman, I. (1986). *Stigma. Notes on the Management of Spoiled Identity.* New York, NY: Simon & Schuster.

FightMediocrity. (2020). *The Best Explanation of Addiction I've Ever Heard—Dr. Gabor Maté.* Retrieved from: *YouTube.* https://youtu.be/ys6TCO_olOc

Hari, J. (2016). *Chasing The Scream: the First and Last Days of the War On Drugs*. Bloomsbury.

Henigsberg, N., Kalember, P., Petrovic, Z. K. & Secic, A. (2019). Neuroimaging research in posttraumatic stress disorder—Focus on amygdala, hippocampus and prefrontal cortex. *Progress in Neuro-Psychopharmacology and Biological Psychiatry*, *90*, 37–42. doi.org/10.1016/j.pnpbp.2018.11.003

Horner, G., Daddona, J., Burke, D. J., Cullinane, J., Skeer, M. & Wurcel, A. G. (2019). 'You're kind of at war with yourself as a nurse': Perspectives of inpatient nurses on treating people who present with a comorbid opioid use disorder. *PLoS One*, *14*(10), e0224335. doi.org/10.1371/journal.pone.0224335

Iammarino, C. & Pauly, B. (2020). Harm reduction as an approach to ethical nursing care of people who use illicit substances: An integrative literature review of micro and meso influences. *Drugs: Education, Prevention and Policy*, 1–14. doi.org/10.1080/09687637.2020.1840515

International Council of Nurses. (2012). *The ICN Code of Ethics for Nurses*. Retrieved from: https://www.icn.ch/sites/default/files/inline-files/2012_ICN_Codeofethicsfornurses_%20eng.pdf

Kirsch, D., Nemeroff, C. M. & Lippard, E. T. C. (2020). Early life stress and substance use disorders: Underlying neurobiology and pathways to adverse outcomes. *Adversity and Resilience Science*, *1*(1), 29–47. doi.org/10.1007/s42844-020-00005-7

Levett-Jones, T., Hoffman, K., Dempsey, J., Jeong, S. Y., Noble, D., Norton, C. A., Roche, J. & Hickey, N. (2010). The 'five rights' of clinical reasoning: An educational model to enhance nursing students' ability to identify and manage clinically 'at risk' patients. *Nurse Education Today*, *30*(6), 515–20. doi.org/10.1016/j.nedt.2009.10.020

Levett-Jones, T. Dwyer, T., Reid-Searl, K., Heaton, L., Flenady, T., Applegarth, J., Guinea, S. & Andersen, P. (2017). *The Patient Safety Competency Framework (PSCF) for Nursing Students*. Sydney, NSW.

Lotzin, A., Grundmann, J., Hiller, P., Pawils, S. & Schafer, I. (2019). Profiles of Childhood Trauma in Women With Substance Use Disorders and Comorbid Posttraumatic Stress Disorders. *Front Psychiatry*, *10*, 674. doi.org/10.3389/fpsyt.2019.00674

Morphet, J., Griffiths, D., Plummer, V., Innes, K., Fairhall, R. & Beattie, J. (2014). At the crossroads of violence and aggression in the emergency department: Perspectives of Australian emergency nurses. *Australian Health Review*, *38*(2), 194–201. doi.org/10.1071/AH13189

Moustafa, A. A., Parkes, D., Fitzgerald, L., Underhill, D., Garami, J., Levy-Gigi, E., Stramecki, F., Valikhani, A., Frydecka, D. & Misiak, B. (2018). The relationship between childhood trauma, early-life stress, and alcohol and drug use, abuse, and addiction: An integrative review. *Current Psychology*, *40*(2), 579–84. doi.org/10.1007/s12144-018-9973-9

NADA. (2019). *Language Matters*. Retrieved from: https://nada.org.au/wp-content/uploads/2021/01/language_matters_-_online_-_final.pdf

Neville, K. & Roan, N. (2014). Challenges in nursing practice: Nurses' perceptions in caring for hospitalized medical-surgical patients with substance abuse/dependence. *The Journal of Nursing Administration*, *44*(6), 339–46. doi.org/10.1097/NNA.0000000000000079

NSW Health. (2008). *Drug and Alcohol Withdrawal Clinical Practice Guidelines—NSW.* Retrieved from: https://www1.health.nsw.gov.au/pds/ActivePDSDocuments/GL2008_011.pdf

NSW Health. (2015). *Preventing and Managing Violence in the NSW Health Workplace: A Zero Tolerance Approach.* Retrieved from: https://www1.health.nsw.gov.au/pds/ActivePDSDocuments/PD2015_001.pdf

Nursing and Midwifery Board of Australia (NMBA). (2016). *Registered Nurse Standards for Practice*. https://www.nursingmidwiferyboard.gov.au/codes-guidelines-statements/professional-standards/registered-nurse-standards-for-practice.aspx

Phoenix Australia. (2021). *Australian Guidelines for the Prevention and Treatment of Acute Stress Disorder, Posttraumatic Stress Disorder and Complex PTSD*. https://www.phoenixaustralia.org/australian-guidelines-for-ptsd/

Queensland Mental Health Commission. (2020). *Don't Judge and Listen: Experiences of Stigma and Discrimination*

Related to Problematic Alcohol and Other Drug Use. Retrieved from: https://www.qmhc.qld.gov.au/sites/default/files/qmhc_dont_judge_and_listen_report.pdf

Quit Victoria. (2021). *What Is Nicotine Withdrawal?* Retrieved from: https://www.quit.org.au/articles/what-is-nicotine-withdrawal/

Raber, J., Arzy, S., Bertolus, J. B., Depue, B., Haas, H. E., Hofmann, S. G.,… Boutros, S. W. (2019). Current understanding of fear learning and memory in humans and animal models and the value of a linguistic approach for analyzing fear learning and memory in humans. *Neuroscience & Biobehavioral Reviews*, *105*, 136–77. doi.org/10.1016/j.neubiorev.2019.03.015

Ritchie, H. & Roser, M. (2019). Drug Use. OurWorldInData.org. https://ourworldindata.org/drug-use

The Health Foundation. (2021). *Quality Improvement Made Simple: What Everyone Should Know About Healthcare Quality Improvement*. Retrieved from: https://www.health.org.uk/sites/default/files/QualityImprovementMadeSimple.pdf

Chapter 12

Caring for a person with Parkinson's disease

RACHEL ROSSITER and VINCENT CARROLL

LEARNING OUTCOMES

Completion of the activities in this chapter will enable you to:

- explain why an understanding of the impact of Parkinson's disease on mental health is essential to competent practice (**recall** and **application**)
- identify the clinical manifestations and psychological impact of the neurodegenerative condition, Parkinson's disease, that will guide the collection and interpretation of cues (**gather, review, interpret, discriminate, relate** and **infer**)
- identify risk factors for people with Parkinson's disease (**match** and **predict**)
- review clinical information to identify the main nursing diagnoses for people with Parkinson's disease (**synthesise**)
- describe the priorities of care for a person with Parkinson's disease and associated surgical interventions (**goal setting** and **taking action**)
- identify criteria for determining the effectiveness of nursing actions taken to manage the clinical manifestations of Parkinson's disease (**evaluate**)
- apply what you have learnt about Parkinson's disease to new situations and with different people (**reflection** and **translation**).

INTRODUCTION

People diagnosed with Parkinson's disease (PD), a neurodegenerative disease, live with a variable combination of symptoms, both motor and non-motor, that increasingly impact upon their quality of life, daily functioning and social interactions. The fluctuating nature of this disease and the many different combinations of symptoms experienced requires individualised care and treatment planning. Increasing numbers of Australians are faced with living with PD. For the affected person and their carers, the challenges multiply as the condition progresses. Too often, healthcare professionals have a limited understanding of the complexity of PD, the complex interplay between the physical and psychosocial issues encountered, and the progressive nature of this condition. The two scenarios introduced in this chapter will give you the opportunity to explore some of these challenges. While this chapter follows the story of Mr Rory Maher and his PD, what you learn will be applicable to the care of people with similar neurodegenerative diseases across a range of clinical contexts.

For someone living with PD, learning to adapt to a body that no longer functions as it did prior to the onset of symptoms is a daily challenge. The contrast between a pre-Parkinson's ability to be 'dashing here and there all the time' and the increasing slowness and difficulty in functioning can be frustrating and distressing (Eatough & Shaw, 2019). As the disease progresses, fluctuating symptoms during the day combined with time-limited benefits from medications begin to significantly impair the person's ability to function (Gibson, 2016; Gibson & Kierans, 2017). This is accompanied by increasing psychological distress triggered by the impact of the disease, the physical reduction in the person's ability to function and increasing neurological deterioration. The person requires increasing levels of psychosocial support from carers (Lawson et al., 2018).

Depression and anxiety are both common non-motor symptoms of PD which affect a person's psychological wellbeing that may have presented up to 15 years prior to diagnosis (Nicoletti et al., 2017). Up to 50 per cent of people with PD will experience anxiety and depression while, later in the disease, hallucinations, psychosis, dementia and delirium may occur (Pontone & Weiss, 2018). For the younger person living with a condition such as PD, the difficulties are magnified. Many people experience both isolation and fear of the unknown upon receiving a diagnosis of a condition that is not widely understood and is often seen as a disease of old age. The fear returns again and again as the person encounters yet another healthcare professional who has a very limited understanding of their condition.

KEY CONCEPTS

time-critical medications
neurodegenerative condition
motor and non-motor symptoms
complexity
primary health care
caregiver burden
psychological wellbeing

SUGGESTED READINGS

P. LeMone, G. Bauldoff, P. Gubrud-Howe, M.-A. Carno, T. Levett-Jones, . . . D. Stanley (Eds). (2020). *LeMone and Burke's Medical-Surgical Nursing: Critical Thinking for Person-Centred Care* (4th edn). Melbourne: Pearson Australia.

Chapter 43: Nursing care of people with neurological disorders: The person with Parkinson's disease, pp. 1620–27

Chapter 40: A person-centred approach to assessing the nervous system, pp. 1484–1509

The importance of nurses providing advocacy and ensuring personalised and coordinated care that is tailored to the person's individual needs cannot be underestimated (Tenison et al., 2020; van Halteren, et al., 2020). However, increasing your knowledge of this disease in combination with excellent clinical reasoning skills will enable you to systematically address each component of the care required for people with PD and their carers. You will then be able to support a person by providing individualised care and facilitating access to integrated care.

SCENARIO 12.1 Caring for a person with Parkinson's disease

SETTING THE SCENE

Person-centred care

Mr Rory Maher is a 51-year-old man with a 14-year history of Parkinson's disease. He lives with his wife, Marie. They have a close and supportive relationship and have two children (now aged 22 and 25). Rory has worked as a banana farmer and a horticulturist for many years. One of his great joys in life has been as a musician, playing guitar and lead vocals in a band. In 2017, he stopped playing gigs due to the progressive deterioration in his health but Rory continues to play and sing socially. He and his family are active members of a local Christian church, enjoying the social interactions and support of the church community. Rory has a family history of PD with two paternal uncles being diagnosed with this disease.

For some years before Rory became aware of any difficulties with motor symptoms related to PD, he noticed that he seemed to be having trouble with temperature regulation when he went surfing. He quickly became cold and began shivering after a short time in the water. In 2004, three years before he was diagnosed with Parkinson's, Rory noticed some stiffening in his left hand when playing the guitar, that he was dragging his left foot when walking, and moving required extra effort. Rory also noticed a deterioration in his writing. His wife and children also noticed these changes. Although initially they did not have a great impact on his quality of life, Rory was concerned about these symptoms. They gradually worsened until Rory noticed a tremor that increased over time. At 39 years of age, he was formally diagnosed with PD.

Rory's condition continued to slowly deteriorate, affecting his ability to work as a horticulturist. At age 42, three years after his diagnosis, Rory retired. His motor symptoms had continued to increase, while the motor fluctuations occurring as a side effect from the medications being used to treat these symptoms were such that he could no longer function effectively.

Rory's motor and non-motor symptoms continued to deteriorate after his retirement and he experienced increasingly complicated and intrusive motor fluctuations.

The prevalence of neurodegenerative disorders

Neurodegenerative diseases affect neurons in different parts of the brain and nervous system (JPND Research, 2019) and, globally, millions of people are impacted (National Institute of Environmental Health Sciences, 2019). In some conditions, neurons responsible for motor functioning are impacted initially while in other conditions, a decline in cognitive functioning is the first indicator of a neurodegenerative condition. The following provides information about the four most commonly known neurodegenerative disorders.

1. Dementia is the most prevalent of the neurodegenerative disorders and for Australians is the second most likely cause of death (Dementia Australia, 2021). Caring for a person with dementia is explored in detail later in this text—see the chapter on *Caring for an older person with altered cognition.*
2. Increasing numbers of people are being diagnosed with Parkinson's disease, which is now recognised as the second most prevalent neurodegenerative disorder (Deloitte Access Economics, 2015).

3. Motor neurone diseases (MND) are a group of rapidly life-limiting and rare neurodegenerative disorders that affect motor neurons in the spinal cord and brain. MNDs 'have low prevalence and incidence, but cause severe disability with a high fatality rate' (Logroscino et al., 2018).
4. In contrast, Huntington's disease is classified as a 'genetic neurodegenerative condition' with prevalence varying markedly in different parts of the world and in differing populations (Rawlins et al., 2016). A person who develops Huntington's disease is born with abnormal genes that cause the symptoms of the condition in young to middle adulthood.

For more information about Huntington's disease, access: https://huntingtonsvic.org.au

Something to think about . . .

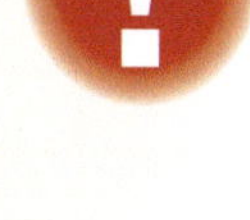

***Neurodegenerative diseases** 'occur when nerve cells in the brain or peripheral nervous system lose function over time and ultimately die. Although treatments may help relieve some of the physical or mental symptoms associated with neurodegenerative diseases, there is currently no way to slow disease progression and no known cures' (National Institute of Environmental Health Sciences, 2019, p. 1).*

***Complexity:** sometimes referred to as multi-morbidity, i.e. a person with more than one chronic condition. It is important to consider not only the complexity of the disease process/es, such as those in Parkinson's disease, but also concurrent physical and psychological conditions. Factors including chronic pain, suffering, poverty, social isolation and poor quality living conditions further contribute to the difficulties experienced by a person with complex health needs (Webster et al., 2019).*

***Caregiver burden:** 'the level of multifaceted strain perceived by the caregiver from caring for a family member and/or loved one over time' (Liu, Heffernan & Tan, 2020, p. 438).*

***Primary health care** 'is generally the first contact a person has with Australia's health system. It relates to the treatment of patients who are not admitted to hospital . . . [that] can be provided in the home or in community-based settings such as general practices, other private medical practices, community health centres, local government, and nongovernment service settings, such as Aboriginal Community Controlled Health Services' (Australian Government Department of Health, 2018).*

***Time-critical medications** for people with Parkinson's disease are individualised to the person. Minor delays in dosing of greater than 15 minutes may make a difference to symptom control, while prolonged withdrawal can cause a rare but fatal neuroleptic-like syndrome and dopamine agonist withdrawal syndrome characterised by fever, muscle rigidity, cognitive changes, autonomic instability and an altered level of consciousness (NSW Health, 2020).*

The prevalence of Parkinson's disease

Parkinson's disease (PD) is the second most common neurodegenerative condition in Australia and worldwide, after dementia. PD affects one per cent of the population of people 60 years and older (Deloitte Access Economics, 2015, 2011; Tel & Yalçin Çakmakli, 2017). A recent epidemiological study in Australia indicated that 1 in 117 people aged over 50 are living with PD—a total of 212,000 people (Ayton et al., 2019).

The prevalence of PD has been shown to be higher than a number of diseases considered national health priority areas, including breast cancer, kidney and bladder cancer, lymphoma and leukaemia, and uterine, cervical and ovarian cancers (Deloitte Access Economics, 2015). PD is reported to be higher in rural and regional areas than in metropolitan areas, with the health-related quality of life for people living with Parkinson's lower than for those living in urban areas (Soh et al., 2012).

Although the prevalence of PD increases with age, it is not limited to those over 65. Ten per cent of those diagnosed are under the age of 40 and a further 20 per cent are under the age of 50 (Parkinson's NSW, 2019). Many people living with PD lose the capacity to work and to live independently, becoming increasingly dependent on support and care from family and caregivers. PD affects a person's psychological wellbeing (Nicoletti et al., 2017) and places a high level of burden on the person with the disease, as well as their family, caregiver and society (Liu, Heffernan & Tan, 2020). The median time from onset of the disease to death is 12.2 years but many people live for more than 20 years. The duration is impacted by factors such as age of onset and presence of cognitive decline (Bäckström et al., 2018; Dommershuijsen et al., 2020). In Australia, an estimated 89 per cent living with Parkinson's disease live most of these years at home with family and carers, until the level of care needed is beyond what can be delivered at home. The remaining years of life are spent in residential aged care facilities (Bramble, Carroll & Rossiter, 2018).

Access these sites to learn more about Parkinson's disease and movement disorders: https://www.anna.asn.au/educational-publications

The aetiology and pathogenesis of Parkinson's disease

Challenge yourself further and watch this video: *The Basics of Parkinson's* https://youtu.be/FcvXEVBAG-U

You may need to brush up on your anatomy and physiology here. Parkinson's disease is described as a complex neurodegenerative disorder impacting on the neurotransmitter, dopamine. Check your knowledge of the role of dopamine here: https://www.atrainceu.com/content/2-pathophysiology-parkinson

'Non-motor symptoms' are often overlooked. This term refers to symptoms that are not associated with movement, such as pain, anxiety, depression, orthostatic hypotension, disordered sleep, fatigue, bladder and bowel problems, sexual difficulties and swallowing problems. (See the PD NMS questionnaire to build your knowledge of non-motor symptoms in Parkinson's disease: https://www.movementdisorders.org/MDS/MDS-Rating-Scales/Non-Motor-Symptoms-Questionnaire.htm)

As you read about PD, you will notice that there are a number of motor and non-motor symptoms that affect individuals very differently. PD is a progressive neurological disorder caused by the loss of dopaminergic neurons in the substantia nigra, causing motor, non-motor and cognitive impairments. Early symptoms such as loss of smell, constipation, sleep disorders, depression and anxiety (Schapira, Chaudhuri & Jenner, 2017) occur before motor symptoms appear. When a person begins to experience a combination of the following motor symptoms of tremor, bradykinesia, rigidity and postural instability, it then becomes possible for the diagnosis of PD to be made (Magrinelli et al., 2016). Although a definitive cause of PD is not known, increasing age and a combination of environmental factors and genetic susceptibility are thought to influence the development of the disease (Kouli, Torsney & Kuan, 2018).

As the disease progresses, increasing motor and non-motor complications are common. Motor complications with marked fluctuations in motor symptoms and dyskinesia worsen (Chaudhuri, Rizos & Sethi, 2013). Dyskinesia refers to involuntary dystonic or choreiform movements that occur with long-term levodopa treatment in people with PD (Chaudhuri, Rizos & Sethi, 2013; Edwards et al., 2016). Over time, the impact of dyskinesias and motor fluctuations can become troublesome, substantially affecting a person's level of mobility and ability to function, and hence their quality of life (Chaudhuri, Rizos & Sethi, 2013; Katzenschlager et al., 2018). Non-motor complications increase with worsening cognitive dysfunction—increasing anxiety, fatigue and depression, constipation and dysphagia (swallowing difficulties). These symptoms can be more disabling than the motor symptoms (Borgemeester, Drent & van Laar, 2016; Chaudhuri, Rizos & Sethi, 2013) and contribute to increasing social isolation and loss of identity. Social isolation increases as speech and swallowing problems, difficulties eating, and engaging in social activities increase (Sjödahl Hammarlund et al., 2018). A combination of motor and non-motor difficulties results in speech disorders in almost 90 per cent of people with PD (Dashtipour et al., 2018).

The only effective treatment at present is symptomatic therapy, with the gold standard treatment for motor symptoms being levodopa (a dopaminergic drug). The side effects of this class of drugs are complex in the long term with motor fluctuations and behavioural side effects, which lead to difficulties when planning changes or modifications to medication regimes (Tel & Yalçin Çakmakli, 2017).

As PD advances, the period when the beneficial effects of levodopa are experienced becomes shorter and shorter. This results in the medication wearing off before the next medication is due, with some doses variable in their effectiveness while some are not effective at all. The person experiences unpredictable fluctuations between 'ON' and 'OFF' (Chaudhuri, Rizos & Sethi, 2013).

Advances in disease management now provide some options to reduce the impact of persistent motor fluctuations and complications. In Australia, there are currently some advanced (assisted device) therapies available.

1. Deep brain stimulation (DBS)
2. Continuous dopaminergic drug delivery using either:
   a. intestinal infusion of levodopa-carbidopa gel, or
   b. subcutaneous infusion of apomorphine (a dopamine agonist) (Katzenschlager et al., 2018).

There is now high-level evidence demonstrating reduced severity of motor symptoms and improvements in a person's quality of life when an assisted device therapy is commenced. A higher level of assessment is required by the person's specialist to assess their suitability for these therapies (Chaudhuri, Rizos & Sethi, 2013; Katzenschlager et al., 2018; Merola et al., 2016). While people living in some of the capital cities in Australia have had access to the therapies for a number of years, people in regional areas may not have access to, or be aware of, advanced therapies that are now available.

Quick Quiz!

Before progressing to the first stage of the clinical reasoning cycle, test your understanding of the terminologies relevant to this chapter by selecting the correct response for each of the identified terms below.

Q1 Primary health care means:
- a Care provided in an emergency
- b End-of-life care
- c Care that includes general practice services, prevention and health screening, treatment and management
- d Early intervention for conditions such as cerebral palsy or autism spectrum disorder

Q2 Parkinson's disease:
- a Is a neurodegenerative disease
- b Occurs only in males
- c Is rapidly fatal
- d Is a rare condition in the Australian population

Q3 The principal *motor signs* of Parkinson's disease are:
- a Mood swings with irritability and aggression
- b Bilateral hand and jaw tremor
- c Tremor, rigidity, slowness and difficulty with initiation of movement, and impaired posture and balance
- d Sudden confusion, numbness and weakness

Q4 Prodromal symptoms of PD include:
- a Loss of smell, sleep disorders, constipation, mood disorders and rapid-eye-movement sleep behaviour disorder
- b Cognitive decline
- c Loss of hearing and ability to speak
- d Withdrawal from social activities and neglect of personal hygiene

Q5 Time-critical medications in PD must be administered:
- a Within 60 minutes of when the medication is due
- b Within 15 minutes of when the medication is due
- c When the person's motor symptoms are at their worst
- d When the person remembers to take them

1. CONSIDER THE PATIENT SITUATION

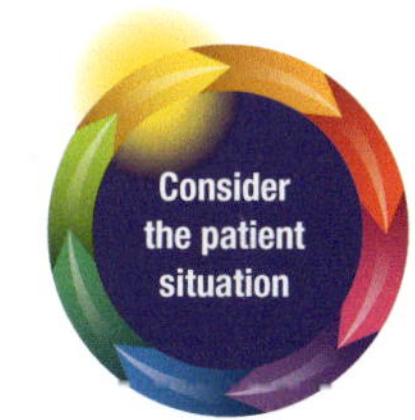

General practitioner appointment

You have recently commenced work as a primary healthcare nurse in a busy, regional, six-doctor general practice. The practice has a team of nurses who are actively involved in ensuring the people attending have access to comprehensive healthcare. One of your roles is to coordinate the care of people with complex long-term health problems, including assessing their health needs and their ability to manage their condition(s), preparing care plans and arranging new referrals as needed. You also collect and collate information from the different healthcare professionals to 'facilitate access to services and continuity of care' (Australian Nursing and Midwifery Federation Standards, 2014, p. 15). This is essential for a person with PD, which affects multiple body systems, requiring referrals to several different medical specialists and allied health services needing careful coordination. Importantly, a vital aspect of effective primary healthcare nursing is to foster the person's capacity to live as well as possible with long-term conditions such as PD (Australian Primary Health Care Nurses Association, 2012).

Patient Safety Competency Framework (PSCF)

Domain 4—Teamwork and collaborative practice

The PSCF specifies that nurses must have the ability to collaborate and communicate effectively with members of the healthcare team in ways that facilitate mutual respect and shared decision-making.

Source: *Patient Safety Competency Framework for Nursing Students*, https://patientsafetyfornursingstudents.org

Although this scenario is based in a primary healthcare setting, the information will also be relevant to acute care. Access the Australian Primary Health Care Nurses Association (APNA) to build your understanding of primary healthcare nursing: https://www.apna.asn.au

Rory's symptoms have now severely impacted upon his quality of life and independence, such that he needs increasing assistance from his family. His motor fluctuations, variable responses to medication and the side effect of dyskinesia further disrupt his functioning. Today, he is attending the general practice for follow-up with his general practitioner (GP) and for repeat prescriptions. At the conclusion of his appointment, you are asked to meet with Rory to develop a chronic disease management plan.

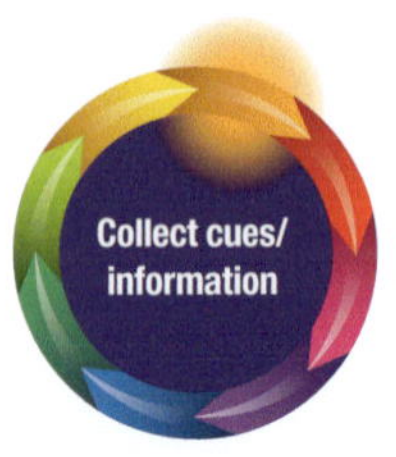

2. COLLECT CUES/INFORMATION

(a) Review current information

Review and think about Rory's presentation (see Figure 12.1). Although he is only 51 years of age, as he walks towards you, you observe his shuffling gait with his left foot dragging behind him. He is stooped over and it is evident that his mobility is impaired. Rory's face seems not to display any emotion and his speech is soft and somewhat difficult to understand. Once Rory has been seated for a few moments and is relaxed, you notice that he has a pronounced tremor in his left hand. Rory's wife has accompanied him and you observe the support she is providing, including prompting Rory with responses at times.

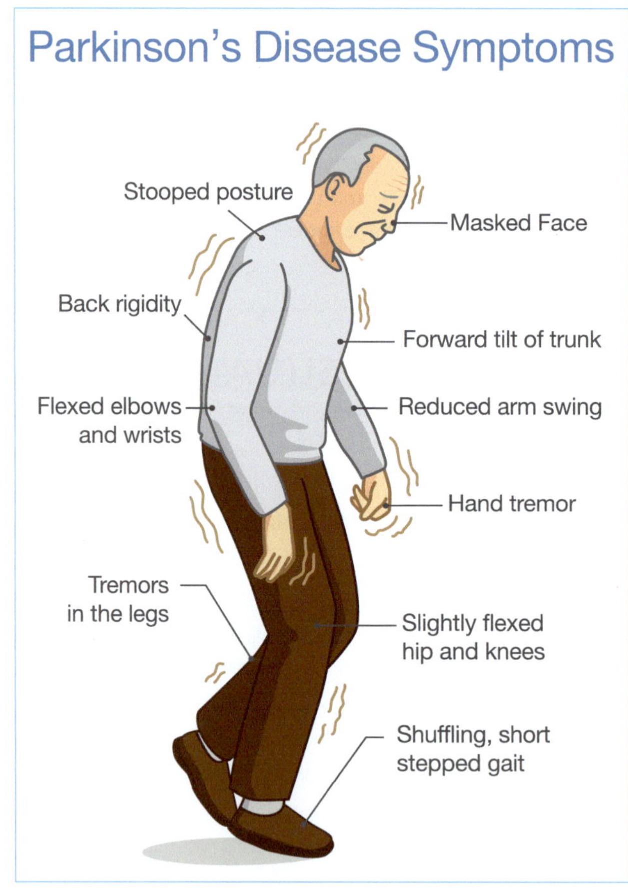

Figure 12.1 *The clinical manifestations of Parkinson's disease.*
Source: olar22/Shutterstock

The Isolated Patients Travel and Accommodation Assistance Scheme (IPTAAS) NSW government scheme provides financial assistance towards travel and accommodation costs when a person needs to travel long distances for treatment that is not available locally. See: http://www.iptaas.health.nsw.gov.au

Rory's clinical notes are somewhat limited. He has a recorded diagnosis of Parkinson's disease and is reviewed every six months by a neurologist in Sydney. These specialist reviews require Rory and Marie to travel five hours by car and stay overnight in Sydney. They use the Isolated Patient and Travel Accommodation Assistance Scheme (IPTAAS) for financial assistance to attend the appointments.

Rory is currently prescribed levodopa (Madopar) and trihexyphenidyl (Artane). You note that he had previously been prescribed pramipexole (Sifrol) but stopped this several years ago describing it as 'messing with my mind'.

There are no nursing notes as this is the first time that the GP has initiated a chronic disease management plan and requested your assistance.

(b) Gather new information

Rory's vital signs are as follows:

Temperature	36.2°C
Pulse	76
Respiratory rate	18
Blood pressure	L = 135/80, S = 130/75
Weight	63.0 kg
Height	175 cm
BMI	20.5

Hint: Think back to the information you have reviewed about Parkinson's disease.

Q As a primary healthcare nurse in this situation, what additional cues do you need to collect? From the list below, identify the *five* cues that you believe are most relevant to your assessment of Rory at this time.

a Mobility
b Non-motor symptoms
c Postural (orthostatic) hypotension
d Medication adherence
e Freezing of gait
f Past diagnosis of mental illness
g Motor fluctuations (on-off periods)
h Knowledge about his condition
i Speech difficulties
j Low body weight

An accurate collection of clinical assessment cues is integral to the role of a primary healthcare nurse. Here are some questions that would help to identify Rory's needs and concerns at this time:

- It seems to be difficult for you to walk easily, how long has this been an issue for you?
- Can you tell me about the impact that these difficulties have on your everyday activities?
- When were you first prescribed levodopa?
- Does it work as well as it did when you were first prescribed this medication?
- Are you sleeping well at night?
- What disturbs your sleep?
- How long have you been experiencing urinary urgency?
- How many times a night do you have to get up to pass urine?
- Has this urgency increased over the past few weeks?
- What impact is this having on how well you sleep?
- How long is it since you had a review with the neurologist?
- Would it be helpful for you to have more information about living with PD?

(c) Recall knowledge

You may have identified some gaps in your understanding about the care of a person with a neurodegenerative condition such as Parkinson's disease. If you are going to be able to provide evidence-informed and person-centred care, it is essential to recognise whether the person is newly diagnosed, has had PD for several years, has complex needs, or now requires palliative care. The following clinical scale (Table 12.1) can assist when developing a care plan appropriate to the needs of the individual.

Table 12.1 *A clinical scale for staging Parkinson's disease*

Stage	Name	Definition
1	Diagnosis	• From first recognition of symptoms/signs/problem • Diagnosis not established or accepted
2	Maintenance	• Established diagnosis of Parkinson's • Reconciled to diagnosis • No drugs or medication 4 or less doses/day • Stable medication for >3/12 • Absence of postural instability
3	Complex	• Drugs–5 or more doses/day • Any infusion therapy (apomorphine or duodopa) • Dyskinesia • Neurosurgery considered/DBS in situ • Psychiatric manifestations >mild symptoms of depression/anxiety/hallucinations/psychosis • Autonomic problems–hypotension either drug or nondrug induced • Unstable co-morbidities • Frequent changes to medication (<3/12) • Significant dysphagia or aspiration
4	Palliative	• Inability to tolerate adequate dopaminergic therapy • Unsuitable for surgery • Advanced co-morbidity (life-threatening or disabling)

Source: Parkinson's UK. (2019). UK Parkinson's Audit Patient Management: Elderly Care & Neurology—Standards and Guidance. Patient Audit Table, Parkinson's Phase (pp. 15–16). London, United Kingdom.

Explore these websites to help you answer the questions that follow. Australasian Neuroscience Nurses' Association, Movement Disorders chapter: https://www.anna.asn.au/educational-publications Parkinson's NSW: https://www.parkinsonsnsw.org.au 2019 UK Parkinson's Audit Patient Management: Elderly Care & Neurology: https://www.parkinsons.org.uk/professionals/uk-parkinsons-audit-transforming-care

Patient Safety Competency Framework (PSCF)

Domain 6–Evidence-based practice

The PSCF specifies that nurses must have the skills required to provide care that takes into account best available evidence, clinical expertise and a person's individual needs, values and preferences.

Source: *Patient Safety Competency Framework for Nursing Students*, https://patientsafetyfornursingstudents.org

Q1 Which of the following descriptions of the different phases of Parkinson's disease enable you to develop an effective care plan?

- a Diagnosis, maintenance, complex and palliative
- b Early, mid-stage and late
- c Mild, moderate, severe, very severe
- d Shock, reaction, processing and re-orientation

Q2 Dyskinesia is:

- a Involuntary, erratic, uncontrollable writhing movements of face, arms, legs or trunk
- b Slowness of movement
- c Rigidity and stiffness
- d Limited or absent movements

Q3 Non-motor symptoms in Parkinson's disease include:

- a Constipation
- b Sleep disturbances
- c Mood disturbances including anxiety, depression
- d All of the options

Q4 Potential factors contributing to a person developing Parkinson's disease are:

a Genetic
b Environmental factors
c Increasing age
d All of the options

3. PROCESS INFORMATION

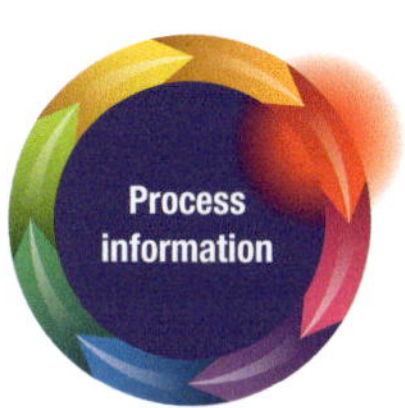

(a) Interpret

While it may be easier to identify the motor symptoms of PD, being aware of the non-motor symptoms that may be impacting on the person's quality of life, psychological wellbeing and functioning can be more challenging. Be aware that the person may have had limited education about their condition, with treatment focused primarily on the motor symptoms. This is a situation where you also need to be aware of any tendency to make the clinical reasoning error known as 'overconfidence bias'. PD is complex and multifaceted with everyone's presentation and combination of motor and non-motor symptoms unique to them. Common misconceptions, such as that PD is a condition that only affects motor functioning, will result in overlooking disabling non-motor symptoms which need assessment and appropriate interventions. PD impacts on multiple aspects of a person's wellbeing and can have a significant effect on others living with them. It is likely that the person will have more than one issue requiring attention. Unfortunately, as healthcare professionals, we are often working in a system that continues to focus on a single disease or issue. Remember, many people identify PD as impacting on their emotional health and limiting their ability to continue their social roles. This results in a marked reduction in the person's quality of life (Arky et al., 2020; Nicoletti et al., 2017).

Overconfidence bias: A universal tendency to believe we know more than we do. Overconfidence bias reflects a tendency to act on incomplete information, intuition, or hunches. Too much faith is placed on opinion instead of carefully gathered evidence.

Your initial assessment revealed that Rory's vital signs are all within normal limits; however, as you reflect on your observations and review the PD NMS questionnaire that Rory has completed with the help of his wife, you identify a number of cues that require careful attention.

From your understanding of Parkinson's disease, answer the following questions to identify what Rory's signs and symptoms could indicate.

Q1 Dyskinesia is:

a Rigidity
b Anxiety about having Parkinson's disease
c A result of long-term use (5 yrs +) of levodopa
d A common Parkinson's symptom
e Absence of movement

Q2 Anosmia is:

a Loss of sense of smell—a non-motor symptom of Parkinson's
b Incompetent cardiac sphincter with gastric acid aspiration
c Post-nasal drip
d Dust-mite allergy

Q3 A sense of urgency to pass urine is:

a A non-motor symptom associated with the nervous system affecting bladder function
b Caused by fear of not getting to the toilet in time
c Due to an enlarged prostate
d A side effect of medication

Q4 Disturbed sleep may be related to:

a Non-motor symptoms adversely impacting on quality of life
b Side effects of medication
c Depression, anxiety and pain
d Daytime sleepiness
e All of the options

Note: It is common for health professionals to underestimate and dismiss the impact of symptoms that are not perceived to be life-threatening.

(b) Discriminate

Q From the list below, select four cues that you believe are the *most troubling* to Rory at this time.

a Increasing off periods (decreased ability to move)
b Problems associated with his bladder function
c His psychological wellbeing
d Carer fatigue experienced by Rory's wife Marie
e Problems with his voice and difficulties communicating with others effectively
f He's unable to play his guitar and sing in the band

(c) Relate

Q Which of the following statements are *true*?

a Rory is unaware that his wife is affected by his inability to care for himself and to help with their property.
b Rory has lost his sense of smell due to a recent influenza infection.
c Rory's declining cognitive functioning may be the result of severe sleep disturbance.
d Rory's increasing immobility is the result of lack of exercise.
e Rory's dyskinesia is likely related to long-term use of levodopa.
f Rory's difficulties with bladder functioning are severely disrupting his sleep.
g Rory's communication difficulties are increasing his need to have his wife's support in social interactions.
h Rory's psychological state is affected by the deterioration in his physical functioning.

(d) Infer and (e) Match

Q From what you know about Rory's history, his long-term health problems, and signs and symptoms (as well as your knowledge of Parkinson's disease), identify the *correct* inferences from the following. (Select the three that apply.)

Do you know the difference between bradykinesia and dyskinesia?

a Rory's PD is progressing.
b Rory's cognitive decline is to be expected because he worries too much about his condition.
c Rory has medication induced movement difficulties (dyskinesia).
d Rory's speech difficulties are indicative of a previous stroke.
e Rory has a number of non-motor symptoms consistent with PD.

(f) Predict

Q If you do not provide Rory with the appropriate referrals, information and education to assist him to manage his symptoms, what may happen? (Select the *one incorrect* response from the list below.)

a An avoidable admission to hospital as a result of unaddressed mobility issues leading to fracture following a fall.
b Adverse impacts of his current medication regimen will reduce Rory's willingness to take his medication as prescribed.
c Caregiver exhaustion will lead to relationship difficulties.
d Rory will have increasing difficulties with concentration and memory as a result of ongoing sleep disturbance.
e Increasing problems with constipation will affect the absorption of Rory's Parkinson's medications and contribute to his fluctuating level of motor and non-motor symptoms.
f Rory may attribute the changes in his symptoms to the normal ageing process and not seek help and assistance from his treating GP.

4. IDENTIFY THE PROBLEM/ISSUE

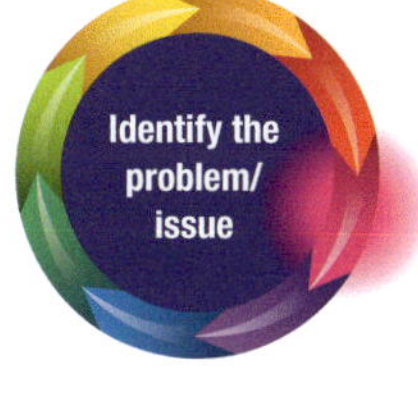

Q1 From the following list, select the nursing diagnosis that is *not* correct for Rory.

- a Impaired mobility, evidenced by slow, shuffling gait, dragging left leg
- b Medication side effects related to the long-term use of levodopa, evidenced by movement fluctuations and dyskinesia
- c Impaired sleep pattern related to bladder dysfunction, evidenced by daytime sleepiness and fatigue
- d Risk of ineffective self-care related to a lack of knowledge about PD
- e Failure to adequately attend to his self-care, evidenced by poor hygiene and unshaven face

Q2 List some of the factors that you think could have led to inadequate management of Rory's symptoms to date.

5. ESTABLISH GOALS

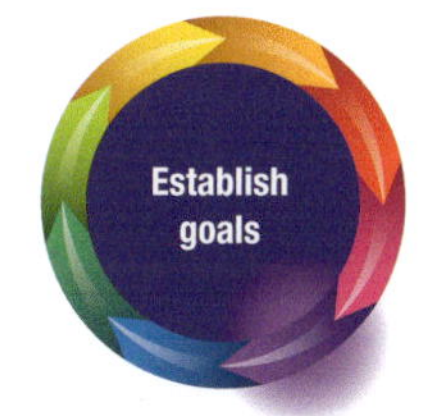

You have identified multiple issues that require attention. Rory and his wife were not aware of the supports available through the National Disability Insurance Scheme (NDIS) and other agencies. They have had limited information about Parkinson's disease. Although Rory had travelled several times to a support group for younger people with Parkinson's disease, he was not aware of the services available in his location.

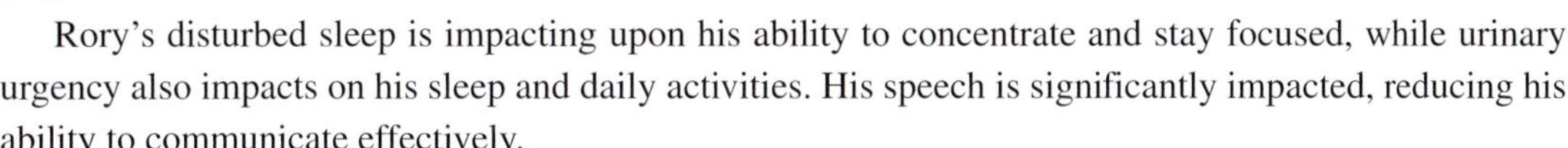

Rory's disturbed sleep is impacting upon his ability to concentrate and stay focused, while urinary urgency also impacts on his sleep and daily activities. His speech is significantly impacted, reducing his ability to communicate effectively.

Before implementing any actions to provide symptomatic relief for Rory, it is important to clearly specify what you want to happen and when.

Q From the list below, choose three *short-term* goals that are both relevant and achievable to support Rory at this time.

- a Review by specialist Parkinson's nurse for a comprehensive Parkinson's disease assessment and individualised recommendations to incorporate into Rory's care plan
- b For Rory and his wife to commence the process of an application to the NDIS to access the support and services needed to maintain his independence and ability to remain in his own home
- c Review by neurological physiotherapist or exercise physiologist to assess his mobility and to develop an exercise program to improve his mobility and level of physical fitness
- d Book the first available appointment with the GP to initiate an enhanced primary care plan (EPC), to enable Rory to access the services of healthcare professionals, a physiotherapist, an exercise physiologist and a speech pathologist
- e For Rory to link in with Parkinson's peak body (PNSW if living in NSW), for the local Parkinson's support group and social activities
- f For Rory and his wife to learn more about managing his non-motor symptoms

Nursing and Midwifery Board of Australia (NMBA) *Registered Nurse Standards for Practice* The NMBA's *Registered Nurse Standards for Practice* (2016) state that registered nurses must provide comprehensive, safe, quality practice to achieve agreed goals and outcomes that are responsive to the nursing needs of people.

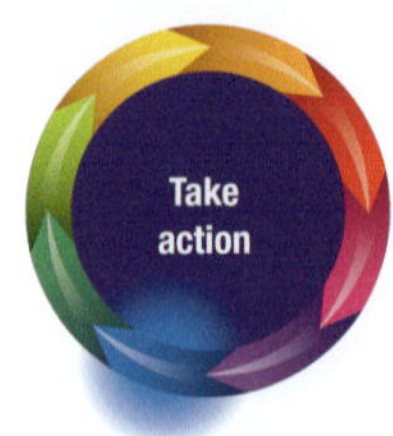

6. TAKE ACTION

You sit with Rory and Marie to review the actions you would like to initiate. They are both eager to access additional PD services and support.

Q Number the following list according to the order in which you would undertake the activities.

a Arrange a referral for Rory to be reviewed by the specialist Parkinson's nurse.

b Schedule a further, longer appointment (30 minutes) with a GP to prepare an enhanced care plan, to enable access to allied health professionals.

c Arrange a follow-up phone call in two weeks to review the outcome of the referral to the specialist Parkinson's nurse.

d Provide Rory and Marie with information about the NDIS and encourage them to access the application documents.

Something to think about . . .

Information sheets for people with Parkinson's disease and their carers are available from The International Parkinson and Movement Disorder Society:

https://www.movementdisorders.org/MDS/Resources/Patient-Education.htm and Parkinson's[UK]

https://www.parkinsons.org.uk/information-and-support

Find the contact details for the Parkinson's organisation in your state or territory.

Something to think about . . .

The National Disability Insurance Scheme (NDIS) is available for people aged between 7 and 65 years who are born with or develop a permanent disability that impacts significantly on their ability to undertake everyday activities.

Access the comprehensive NDIS website (https://www.ndis.gov.au) which will help you give accurate and timely information to people experiencing significant disability because of PD.

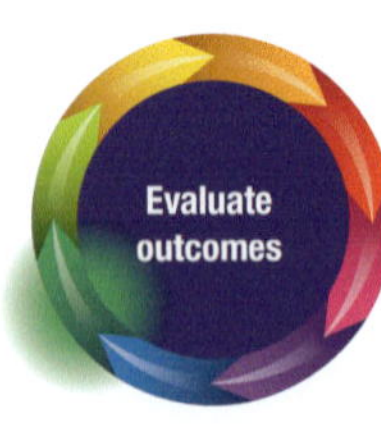

7. EVALUATE

You arrange to contact Rory in two weeks to follow up on the referral that you initiated, and to check for any further actions and support needed.

Q From the information that Rory reports when you contact him, rate the following as *completed, underway* or *waiting further follow-up*.

Limited knowledge of Parkinson's and local support services	Specialist Parkinson's nurse has begun focused education and introduced Rory and Marie to the local Parkinson's support group
Limited knowledge of Parkinson's medications	Review by specialist Parkinson's nurse has provided individualised information and enabled medication review with neurologist via Telehealth
Limited access to support services	GP has initiated enhanced access care plan Application for NDIS now underway with the support of Parkinson's NSW
Disturbed sleep	Referral initiated by neurologist; now waiting for an appointment for sleep studies

Urinary urgency	Appointment arranged for urologist review next month Provide information on financial support for continence aids https://www.health.gov.au/initiatives-and-programs/continence-aids-payment-scheme-caps#who-is-eligible
Speech and swallowing problems	Specialist Parkinson's nurse arranged an initial assessment with speech pathologist, who has provided safe swallowing strategies and enrolment in group sessions of Lee Silverman Voice Training (available via Zoom and face-to-face locally) (McDonnell et al., 2017).
Reduced mobility	Waiting for a home assessment with an occupational therapist and review by a neurological physiotherapist or exercise physiologist.

8. REFLECT

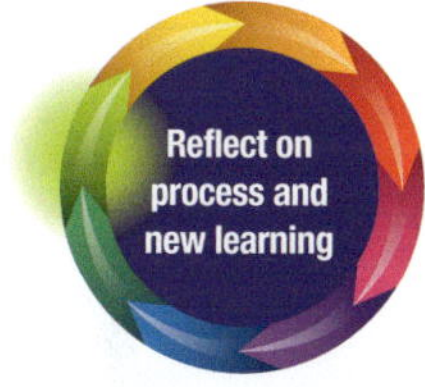

Reflect on your learning from this scenario and consider the following questions.

Q1 What are three of the most important things that you have learnt from this scenario that will inform your future practice?

Q2 What have you learnt about the importance of effective and person-centred long-term chronic disease management?

Q3 What have you learnt about the importance of active engagement with family and carers when providing care for a person with Parkinson's disease?

National Safety and Quality Health Service (NSQHS) Standards

Partnering with consumers standard

The NSQHS Standards highlight the importance of shared decision making when developing a comprehensive and individualised plan of care that addresses the significance and complexity of the person's health issues, and agreed goals for treatment and care (ACSQHC, 2021).

SCENARIO 12.2 The continuing impact of living with Parkinson's disease

CHANGING THE SCENE

For the past two and a half years you have regularly reviewed Rory's care plan and, in consultation with the specialist Parkinson's nurse, facilitated additional support for Rory and his family.

Rory is now a regular member of the local Parkinson's support group and regularly meets socially with the younger members of the group. This has provided social interaction with others experiencing similar symptoms and monthly contact with the specialist nurse. He has taken seriously the evidence that engagement in regular exercise can attenuate the motor symptoms of PD (Rawson et al., 2019; van der Kolk et al., 2019). Rory attends a Parkinson's specific weekly exercise group, PD boxing and voice training classes. Nevertheless, Rory's level of functioning continues to deteriorate with increasing motor fluctuations. Occasionally, Rory has spoken about the specialist nurse's suggestion that he consider advanced (assisted-device) therapies to assist in reducing his symptoms and the extreme motor fluctuations associated with taking oral levodopa (Alshehri, 2017; Hitti et al., 2019; Katzenschlager et al., 2018).

To learn more about DBS and the post-surgical care required for Rory, explore the following resources.

Queensland Brain Institute: What is deep brain stimulation? https://qbi.uq.edu.au/brain/brain-functions/what-deep-brain-stimulation

Brain & Spine Centre's *DBS (Deep Brain Stimulation) Surgery for Parkinson's Disease*

http://www.brainspinecentre.com.au/dbs-surgery-for-parkinsons-disease.html

Information sheet: http://www.brainspinecentre.com.au/pdf/dbs.pdf

Rory minimised his deteriorating health for two years, and continued taking his Parkinson's medications on time, avoiding constipation and exercising regularly. However, his wife and children have spoken with you several times about their sadness and grief as they witnessed the impact of PD on the previously energetic and vibrant man they love. Marie also expressed concern about Rory's increasing levels of anxiety, and he has spoken of feeling down and uncertain about his future.

After two years, Rory decided to seek a second neurologist's opinion about his suitability for advanced therapies and, in particular, deep brain stimulation (DBS) as the option he was most interested in. Five months ago, he was assessed as a suitable candidate for this intervention.

1. CONSIDER THE PATIENT SITUATION

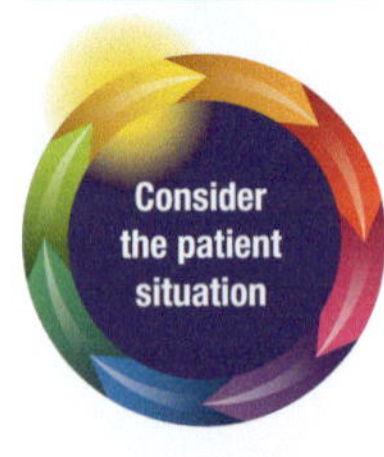

This is the first time you have seen Rory since he underwent the surgery to insert a lead into the carefully selected part of his brain and place the neurostimulator device under the skin below his collarbone.

Rory's wife requested an urgent appointment today as she is concerned that Rory seems unwell and is somewhat agitated this morning. Rory and Marie are reluctant to go to Sydney and preferred a check with you and his GP first.

2. COLLECT CUES/INFORMATION

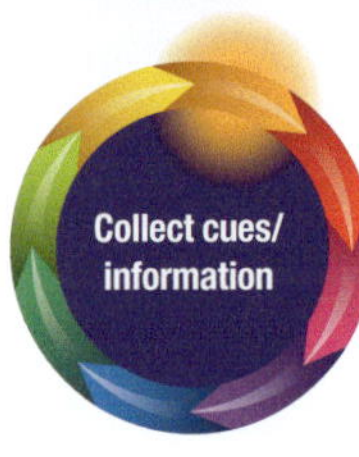

(a) Review current information

Rory and Marie sit down in your office. Rory has always been slight of build and you can now easily observe through his shirt the raised area where the stimulator has been inserted on the left-hand side of his chest. Rory has a dressing on his head covering the site where the leads were inserted. The back of his left hand is red and somewhat swollen. Marie tells you that Rory had been doing well post the DBS surgery until 36 hours ago, when he appeared tired, and this morning he was agitated.

Rory's vital signs are as follows:

Temperature	38.9°C
Pulse	115 beats/min
Respiratory rate	18
Blood pressure	L = 135/80, S = 130/75

(b) Gather new information

Q As a primary healthcare nurse, what additional cues do you need to collect? From the list below, select the five clinical assessments that are *most relevant* at this stage.

- a Condition of chest wound: dressing dry and intact, no ooze, no redness around the area
- b Weight: 62.5 kgs
- c Left hand (previous IV cannula site): erythema, swollen, tender to touch
- d Mini-mental assessment: N/A
- e Condition of scalp wounds: localised pain, erythema, warmth, no exudate
- f Pain: increase in tenderness (scalp wounds and cannula site) over past 24 hours
- g Agitation: onset this morning, restless
- h Constipation: normal bowel movements

Hint: Think back to what you know about possible post-surgical complications.

(c) Recall knowledge

While you have built your knowledge about PD since you first met Rory, this is the first time you have seen a person who has very recently had DBS surgery.

Q1 For people with Parkinson's disease, DBS is:

- a Recommended at the time of diagnosis
- b Suggested as a surgical intervention when motor fluctuations associated with long-term use of levodopa markedly reduce functioning
- c An experimental intervention not available in Australia
- d Described as a cure for movement disorders

Q2 Increasing redness and heat around surgical sites three weeks post-surgery may indicate:
- a An allergic response to the dressing materials
- b The inflammatory stage of wound healing
- c Infection
- d Keloid scarring

Q3 Pain is:
- a A symptom often reported by people with PD
- b Expected post-surgery, especially at incision sites
- c Related to post-op anxiety and agitation
- d Often indicative of infection when accompanied by fever, tachycardia and redness

Q4 Possible complications of DBS surgery include:
- a Bleeding
- b Infection
- c Brain damage
- d Stroke
- e All of the options

Q5 Possible sites of infection post DBS surgery are:
- a Incision sites on the scalp where the electrodes have been inserted
- b Neurostimulator implant site on chest wall
- c Sites where IV canula/s have been in situ
- d All of the options

Q6 Sudden onset of increased anxiety and agitation post DBS surgery:
- a Is to be expected as anxiety is a common symptom in PD
- b Is an indication that the person is worrying that the surgery was unsuccessful.
- c May indicate a developing infection
- d Should be discussed with the neurosurgeon at the next review visit

3. PROCESS INFORMATION

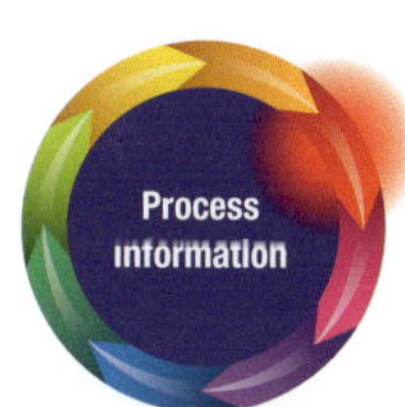

(a) Interpret (b) Discriminate and (c) Relate

When a person has a pre-existing condition such as a neurodegenerative disorder, be aware of the risk of attributing any new symptoms and signs to the disease. Compare normal cues with abnormal cues to build your understanding of Rory's signs and symptoms.

Q1 Which of the following are considered to be within normal parameters for Rory?
- a Temperature: 38.9°C
- b Heart rate: 115 beats/min
- c Respiratory rate: 18
- d Blood pressure: L = 135/80, S = 130/75

Q2 Rory often experienced anxiety in the years prior to his surgery. Anxiety is a frequently reported non-motor symptom of PD. This sudden increase in agitation with extreme restlessness this morning is normal post DBS surgery for PD.
- a True
- b False

> Unfortunately, it is not unusual for busy healthcare professionals to make a diagnosis on the basis of limited information without asking additional questions or seeking further cues to confirm the diagnosis (Blissett & Sibbald, 2017; Krupat et al., 2017). This is a form of premature closure bias.

Q3 It is important to cluster cues together and identify relationships between them (based on the information you have collected so far). Label the following as *true* or *false*.
- a Rory is afebrile and normotensive.
- b Rory is tachycardic and febrile.
- c Rory is hypotensive and bradycardic.
- d Rory is normotensive and tachypnoeic.
- e Rory is febrile and normotensive.

(d) Infer

Q From your knowledge of possible complications of neurosurgery and the patient information that Rory and Marie have brought with them, which *five* of the following factors might indicate a post-surgical infection?

a Fever
b Redness and heat around surgical sites
c Increased constipation
d Change in mood
e Tachycardia
f Increased agitation and anxiety
g Pain

(e) Predict

Q If you do not respond rapidly to Rory's signs and symptoms what may happen? (Select the *three* that apply.)

a Rory's symptoms will gradually resolve over the next few days.
b Untreated infection may result in removal of some or all of the DBS hardware.
c Delayed detection of infection may result in an intracranial infection.
d Signs and symptoms of infection will increase, with possible purulent discharge and/or breakdown of the surgical incision/s.

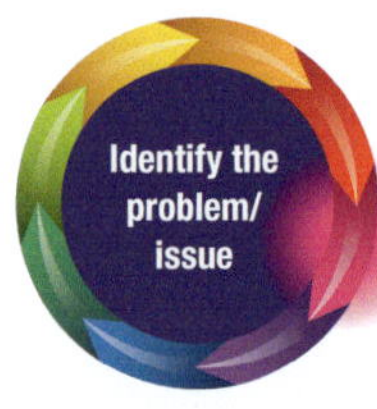

4. IDENTIFY THE PROBLEM/ISSUE

Q Select from the following list, the three *most correct* nursing diagnoses for Rory.

a Infection related to disruption in skin integrity manifested by heat, tenderness to touch and swelling
b Fever related to the systemic effects of infection
c Constipation related to lack of exercise, decreased food intake and effects of medications, evidenced by difficulty opening bowels
d Behavioural changes related to neurosurgery, evidenced by a rapid onset of agitation with restlessness
e Limited knowledge related to cognitive impairment, evidenced by inappropriate behaviour

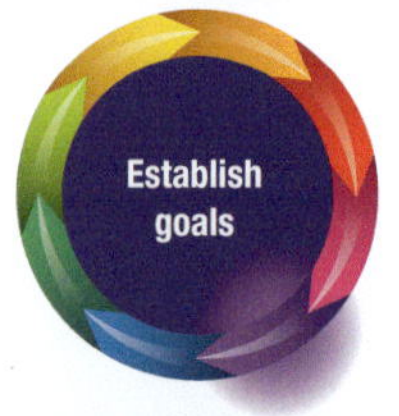

5. ESTABLISH GOALS

You recognise the potential seriousness of Rory's situation and the limitations of your regional location. Before you implement any action, it is important to clearly specify what you want to happen and when.

Q What would your priority goals be for Rory's management at this time?

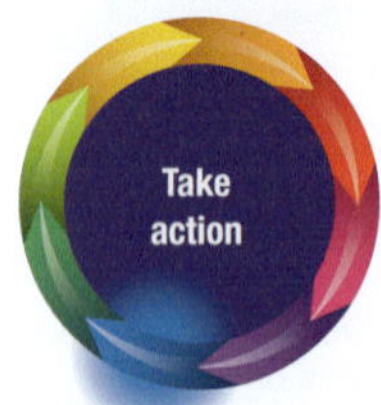

6. TAKE ACTION

National Safety and Quality Health Service (NSQHS) Standards

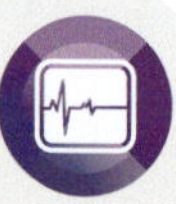

Recognising and responding to acute deterioration standard

The NSQHS Standards highlight the importance of recognising and responding to warning signs that are indicative of possible clinical deterioration. This standard identifies attributing symptoms to a pre-existing condition as a factor that can contribute to failure to recognise and respond in a timely manner. (ACSQHC, 2021).

Q1 From the list below, place the following actions in order of priority.

a Arrange an immediate review with Rory's GP.

b Discuss with Rory and Marie the need to organise a medical review.

c If no GP is available, request permission from Rory to make direct contact with his neurosurgeon.

d If travel is required, avoid a delay in initiating treatment.

e Ask the practice manager to identify a spare room where Rory and Marie can wait while you make the necessary phone calls.

You talk with Rory and Marie and emphasise how wise they were to seek a review this morning, explaining the importance of an immediate medical review. They agree to you contacting Rory's GP. Communicating your concerns about Rory's presentation to the GP, who you know has a full schedule of patients for the day, requires confidence in your knowledge, assessment skills and clinical reasoning abilities.

Q2 How would you use ISBAR to convey to the GP the importance of immediately reviewing Rory?

The GP fits Rory in between his next two appointments and calls the neurosurgeon to discuss treatment options. Rory is commenced on an oral antibiotic in combination with regular paracetamol for pain and fever.

7. EVALUATE

Evaluate outcomes

You arrange to see Rory and Marie after the review with the GP.

Q1 What will you put in place to ensure that Rory's condition is carefully monitored over the next week?

Q2 What changes in Rory's signs and symptoms might you expect to see if his infection is resolving?

8. REFLECT

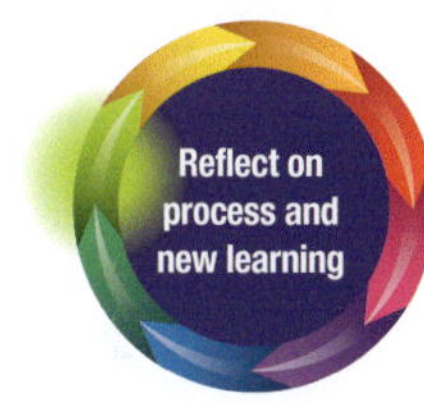

Reflect on your learning from this scenario and consider the following questions.

Q1 What are three of the most important things that you have learnt from this scenario?

Q2 When caring for someone with Parkinson's disease who has undergone neurosurgery, what nursing actions are needed to respond to post-surgical complications?

Q3 What actions will you take in clinical practice as a result of your learning from this scenario?

EPILOGUE

Rory has returned with his wife for a revised chronic disease management plan. His needs have changed since you first initiated a care plan shortly after you began working as a primary healthcare nurse at the GP clinic. This is the first time you have seen Rory since his infection after the surgery and you are surprised at the marked change in his mobility. He suggests that the impact has exceeded his expectations, although it is early days yet.

Rory is staying active with bike riding and long walks with his wife, and is now able to undertake farming duties on his property. His non-motor symptoms have improved, he is sleeping well and urinary urgency has improved markedly (down from 20 times/day to 8 times/day; nocturia from 5 times/night to once only). Overall, Rory is doing well with good motor function and is less dependent on his wife, enabling her to focus on her business. Rory reports that, at his last occupational therapy review, there was a remarkable 85 per cent improvement in his function since surgery. Only two weeks ago he walked his daughter down the aisle at her wedding—an exciting event which prior to deep brain stimulation would not have been possible.

FURTHER READING

Eggers, C., Dano, R., Schill, J., Fink, G. R., Hellmich, M., Timmermann, L. & on behalf of the CPN study group. (2018). Patient-centered integrated healthcare improves quality of life in Parkinson's disease patients: A randomized controlled trial. *Journal of Neurology, 265*(4), 764–73. doi.org/10.1007/s00415-018-8761-7

Pontone, G. M. & Weiss, H. D. (2018). Mental health and Parkinson's disease: Assessing and addressing mental health in patients and care partners improves quality of life. *Practical Neurology.* Retrieved from: https://practicalneurology.com/articles/2018-may/mental-health-and-parkinsons-disease

REFERENCES

Alshehri, A. (2017). Parkinson's disease: An overview of diagnosis and ongoing management. *International Journal of Pharmaceutical Research & Allied Sciences*, *6*(2), 163–70.

Arky, A., et al. (2020). What matters most to individuals with Parkinson's disease: Results from qualitative interviews. *Movement Disorders*, *35*.

Australian Commission on Safety and Quality in Health Care (ACSQHC). (2021). *National Safety and Quality Health Service Standards* (2nd edn). Sydney, Australia.

Australian Government Department of Health. (2018). Fact Sheet: Primary Health Care. 18 June. Retrieved: https://www1.health.gov.au/internet/main/publishing.nsf/Content/Fact-Sheet-Primary-Health-Care

Australian Nursing and Midwifery Federation Standards. (2014). *National Practice Standards for Nurses in General Practice.* Melbourne, Australian Nursing and Midwifery Federation—Federal Office.

Australian Primary Health Care Nurses Association (APNA). (2012). *Definition of Primary Health Care Nursing.* APNA, 1–4.

Ayton, D., Ayton, S., Barker, A. L., Bush, A. & Warren N. (2019). Parkinson's disease prevalence and the association with rurality and agricultural determinants. *Parkinsonism Related Disorders*, *61*, 198–202.

Bäckström, D., Granåsen, G., Domellöf, M. E., Linder, J., Jakobson Mo, S., Riklund, K., Zetterberg, H., Blennow, K. & Forsgren, L. (2018). Early predictors of mortality in parkinsonism and Parkinson disease. *Neurology*, *91*(22), e2045.

Blissett, S. & Sibbald, M. (2017). Closing in on premature closure bias. *Medical Education*, *51*(11), 1095–96.

Borgemeester, R. W. K., Drent, M. & van Laar, T. (2016). Motor and non-motor outcomes of continuous apomorphine infusion in 125 Parkinson's disease patients. *Parkinsonism & Related Disorders*, *23*, 17–22.

Bramble, M., Carroll, V. & Rossiter, R. (2018). *Evidence based models that support best practice nursing services for people with Parkinson's disease in regional NSW: An integrative literature review.* Charles Sturt University: Australia.

Chaudhuri, K. R., Rizos, A. & Sethi, K. D. (2013). Motor and nonmotor complications in Parkinson's disease: An argument for continuous drug delivery? *Journal of Neural Transmission*, *120*(9), 1305–20.

Dashtipour, K., Tafreshi, A., Lee, J. & Crawley, B. K. (2018). Speech disorders in Parkinson's disease: Pathophysiology, medical management and surgical approaches. *Neurodegenerative Disease Management*, 8(5), 337–48.

Deloitte Access Economics. (2011). *Living with Parkinson's Disease: Update (commissioned by Parkinson's Australia*). Deloitte: Canberrra, ACT.

Deloitte Access Economics (2015). *Living with Parkinson's Disease: An Updated Economic Analysis 2014 (commissioned by Parkinson's Australia Inc*). Deloitte: Canberrra, ACT.

Dementia Australia. (2021). *Dementia Statistics: Key Facts and Statistics*. January 2021. Retrieved from: https://www.dementia.org.au/statistics

Dommershuijsen, L. J., Heshmatollah, A., Darweesh, S. K. L., Koudstaal, P. J., Ikram, M. A. & Ikram, M. K. (2020). Life expectancy of parkinsonism patients in the general population. *Parkinsonism & Related Disorders*, *77*, 94–99.

Eatough, V. & Shaw, K. (2019). 'It's like having an evil twin': An interpretative phenomenological analysis of the lifeworld of a person with Parkinson's disease. *Journal of Research in Nursing*, *24*(1–2), 49–58.

Edwards, M. J., Stamelou, M., Quinn, N. & Bhatia, K. P. (2016) *Parkinson's Disease and Other Movement Disorders* (2nd edn). Oxford: Oxford University Press, Inc.

Gibson, G. (2016). 'Signposts on the journey'; medication adherence and the lived body in men with Parkinson's disease. *Social Science & Medicine*, *152*, 27–34.

Gibson, G. & Kierans, C. (2017). Ageing, masculinity and Parkinson's disease: Embodied perspectives. *Sociology of Health & Illness*, *39*(4), 532–46.

Hitti, F. L., Ramayya, A. G., McShane, B. J., Yang, A. I, Vaughan, K. A. & Baltuch, G. H. (2019). Long-term outcomes following deep brain stimulation for Parkinson's disease. *Journal of Neurosurgery*, 132(1), 1–6.

JPND Research. (2019). *What is Neurodegenerative Disease?* JPND Research. Retrieved from: https://www.neurodegenerationresearch.eu/what

Katzenschlager, R., Poewe, W., Rascol, O., Trenkwalder, C., Deuschl, G., Chaudhuri, … Lees, A. (2018). Apomorphine subcutaneous infusion in patients with Parkinson's disease with persistent motor fluctuations (TOLEDO): A multicentre, double-blind, randomised, placebo-controlled trial. *Lancet Neurology*, *17*(9), 749–59.

Kouli, A., Torsney, K. M. & Kuan, W. L. (2018). Parkinson's Disease: Etiology, Neuropathology, and Pathogenesis. In T. B. Stoker & J. C. Greenland (Eds), *Parkinson's Disease: Pathogenesis and Clinical Aspects*. Brisbane: Codon Publications.

Krupat, E., Wormwood, J., Schwartzstein, R. & Richards, J. B. (2017). Avoiding premature closure and reaching diagnostic accuracy: Some key predictive factors. *Medical Education*, *51*(11), 1127–37.

Lawson, R. A., Colleton, D., Taylor, J.-P., Burn, D. J. & Brittain, K. R. (2018). Coping with cognitive impairment in people with Parkinson's disease and their carers: A qualitative study. *Parkinson's Disease*, April 8, 2018, 1362053.

Levett-Jones, T., Dwyer, T., Reid-Searl, K., Heaton, L., Flenady, T., Applegarth, J., Guinea, S. & Andersen, P. (2017). *Patient Safety Competency Framework (PSCF) for Nursing Students*.Retrieved from: http://psframework.wpengine.com/wp-content/uploads/2018/01/PSCF_Brochure_UTS-version_FA2-Screen.pdf

Liu, Z., Heffernan, C. & Tan, J. (2020). Caregiver burden: A concept analysis. *International Journal of Nursing Sciences,* *7*(4), 438–45.

Logroscino, G., Piccininni, M., Marin, B., Nichols, E., Abd-Allah, F., Abdelalim, … Murray, C. J. L. (Collaborators) . (2018). Global, regional, and national burden of motor neuron diseases 1990–2016: A systematic analysis for the Global Burden of Disease Study 2016. *The Lancet Neurology*, *17*(12), 1083–97.

MacMahon, D. G. & Thomas, S. (1998). Practical approach to quality of life in Parkinson's disease: The nurse's role. *Journal of Neurology*, 1998. *245*(1), S19–22.

Magrinelli, F., Picelli, A., Tocco, P., Federico, A., Roncari, L., Smania, N., Zanette, G. & Tamburin, S. (2016). Pathophysiology of motor dysfunction in Parkinson's disease as the rationale for drug treatment and rehabilitation. *Parkinson's Disease*, 2016, 9832839.

McDonnell, M. N.,Rischbieth, B., Schammer, T. T., Seaforth, C., Shaw, A. J. & Phillips, A. C. (2017). Lee Silverman Voice Treatment (LSVT)-BIG to improve motor function in people with Parkinson's disease: A systematic review and meta-analysis. *Clinical Rehabilitation*, *32*(5), 607–18.

Merola, A., Espay, A. J., Romagnolo, A., Bernardini, A., Rizzi, L., Rosso, M., … Lopiano, L. (2016). Advanced therapies in Parkinson's disease: Long-term retrospective study. *Parkinsonism & Related Disorders*, *29*, 104–08.

National Institute of Environmental Health Sciences. (2019). *Neurodegenerative Diseases*. Retrieved from: https://www.niehs.nih.gov/research/supported/health/neurodegenerative/index.cfm

Nicoletti, A., Mostile, G., Stocchi, F., Abbruzzese, G., Ceravolo, R., Cortelli, P., … Zappia, M. (2017). Factors influencing psychological well-being in patients with Parkinson's disease. *PLOS ONE*, *12*(12), e0189682–e0189682.

Nursing and Midwifery Board of Australia (NMBA). (2016). *Registered Nurse Standards for Practice*. https://www.nursingmidwiferyboard.gov.au/codes-guidelines-statements/professional-standards/registered-nurse-standards-for-practice.aspx

NSW Health. (2020). *Management of Medication for Patients with Parkinson Disease*. NSW Ministry of Health, Safety Alert Broadcast System (SABS).

Parkinson's NSW. (2019). *Parkinson's NSW—In This Together—About Parkinson's Disease*. Retrieved from: https://www.parkinsonsnsw.org.au/about-parkinsons-disease/parkinsons-disease

Pontone, G. M. & Weiss, H. D. (2018). Mental health and Parkinson's disease: Assessing and addressing mental health in patients and care partners improves quality of life. *Practical Neurology*, May 2018.

Rawlins, M. D., Wexler, A. R., Tabrizi, S. J., Douglas, I., Evans, S. J. & Smeeth, L. (2016). The prevalence of Huntington's disease. *Neuroepidemiology*, *46*(2), 144–53.

Rawson, K. S., McNeely, M. E., Duncan, R. P., Pickett, K. A., Perlmutter, J. S. & Earhart, G. M. (2019). Exercise and Parkinson disease: Comparing tango, treadmill, and stretching. *Journal of Neurologic Physical Therapy*, *43*(1), 26–32.

Schapira, A. H. V., Chaudhuri, K. R. & Jenner, P. (2017). Non-motor features of Parkinson disease. *Nature Reviews Neuroscience*, *18*(7), 435–50.

Sjödahl Hammarlund, C., Westergren, A., Åström, I., Edberg, A. & Hagell, P. (2018). The impact of living with Parkinson's disease: Balancing within a web of needs and demands. *Parkinson's Disease*, *2018*, 4598651.

Soh, S., McGinley, J. L., Watts, J. J., Iansek, R. & Morris, M. E. (2012). Rural living and health-related quality of life in Australians with Parkinson's disease. *Rural and Remote Health*, *12*(4), 1–9.

Tel, B. C. & Yalçin Çakmakli, G. (2017). Parkinson's disease. In Y. Gürsoy-Özdemir, S. Bozdağ-Pehlivan & E. Sekerdag (Eds), *Nanotechnology Methods for Neurological Diseases and Brain Tumors*. London: Academic Press.

Tenison, E., Smink, A., Redwood, S., Darweesh, S., Cottle, H., van Halteren, A., … Henderson, E. (2020). Proactive and integrated management and empowerment in Parkinson's disease: Designing a new model of care. *Parkinson's Disease*, *2020*, 8673087. doi: 10.1155/2020/8673087

UK Parkinson's Excellence Network. (2019). *2019 UK Parkinson's Audit Patient management: Elderly Care & Neurology—Standards and Guidance*. Parkinson's UK.

van der Kolk, N. M., de Vries, N. M., Kessels, R. P. C., Joosten, H., Zwinderman, A. H., Post, B. & Bloem, B. R. (2019). Effectiveness of home-based and remotely supervised aerobic exercise in Parkinson's disease: A double-blind, randomised controlled trial. *The Lancet Neurology*, *18*(11), 998–1008.

van Halteren, A. D., Munneke, M., Smit, E., Thomas, S., Bloem, B. R. & Darweesh, S. K. L. (2020). Personalized care management for persons with Parkinson's disease. *Journal of Parkinson's Disease*, *10*, S11–S20.

Webster, F., Rice, K., Bhattacharyya, O., Katz, J., Oosenbrug, E. & Upshur, R. (2019). The mismeasurement of complexity: Provider narratives of patients with complex needs in primary care settings. *International Journal for Equity in Health*, *18*(1), 107.

Chapter 13

Caring for a person experiencing an acute psychotic episode

ANNA TRELOAR and PETER ROSS

LEARNING OUTCOMES

Completion of the activities in this chapter will enable you to:

- define the terms 'psychosis' and 'mental state examination' (**gather information, interpret** and **discriminate**)
- explain why an understanding of psychosis is essential to competent nursing practice (**recall** and **apply**)
- outline the clinical manifestations of psychosis that will guide your collection of appropriate cues (**gather information, interpret** and **discriminate**)
- identify possible causes of psychosis (**match** and **predict**)
- review clinical information to identify the main nursing diagnoses for a patient experiencing a psychotic episode (**synthesise**)
- describe the priorities of care for the management of a person experiencing psychosis (**setting goals** and **taking action**)
- identify clinical criteria for determining the effectiveness of nursing actions taken to manage a person experiencing psychosis (**evaluate**)
- consider how inaccurate information may interfere with person-centred care (**reflect**)
- reflect on personal reactions to people experiencing psychosis and identify appropriate management strategies (**reflect**).

INTRODUCTION

The two scenarios in this chapter focus on the care of Jando, a young man with undiagnosed psychosis who has recently been incarcerated. People who enter the prison system are often from vulnerable groups and have poor mental and physical health. Although they are entitled to the same standard of healthcare as anybody else in the community, they don't always receive it, and significant healthcare problems can be overlooked. In Jando's case, it is particularly difficult to ascertain the true nature of his problem due to situational and contextual factors that influence accurate assessment and diagnosis. Despite the challenges, nurses who work in the prison system are well positioned to provide expert clinical care. For this reason, skills in clinical reasoning are fundamental to the management of the health and wellbeing of people such as Jando.

KEY CONCEPTS

psychosis
mental state examination
co-morbidity
recovery model

SUGGESTED READINGS

P. LeMone, G. Bauldoff, P. Gubrud-Howe, M.-A. Carno, T. Levett-Jones, … D. Stanley (Eds). (2020). LeMone and Burke's Medical-Surgical Nursing: Critical Thinking for Person-Centred Care (4th edn). Pearson Australia.

Chapter 50: Mental healthcare in the Australian context

British Psychological Society, Division of Clinical Psychology. (2014). *Understanding Psychosis and Schizophrenia. Why People Sometimes Hear Voices, Believe Things that Others Find Strange, or Appear Out of Touch with Reality, and What Can Help.* Edited by Anne Cook. Canterbury: Christ Church University. Retrieved from: www.bps.org.uk.

A. Treloar. (2015). Sicoko. *Australian Nursing and Midwifery Journal, 22*(8), 46. Retrieved from: www.anmf.org.au.

SCENARIO 13.1 Establishing a therapeutic relationship with a person who has a psychotic illness

SETTING THE SCENE

It is Friday night and a new prisoner is escorted into the cell complex of the police station at the coastal resort town of Melaleuca. The prisoner's name is Jando, he is 18 years old and this is his first experience of the adult corrections system. After being assessed by the prison officers who manage the cells, and after having lodgement forms completed, Jando is escorted into a shared cell. There is a concrete block base for a bed, a plastic covered mattress, a grey blanket and no pillow or sheets. The floor is concrete and there is no window. There is a shower outlet on the wall, a stainless steel toilet with no seat, a water bubbler just above the cistern and a television mounted in a metal cage high up on the wall in a corner of the cell. There is nothing else. All personal belongings are kept by the officers and locked up. Jando is scheduled to receive a comprehensive health check on Monday afternoon by the registered nurse who works from 4 pm till 8 pm, Monday to Friday.

The epidemiology of psychosis

The psychotic disorders feature delusions, hallucinations, disorganised thinking and behaviour, and negative symptoms (American Psychiatric Association, 2013). The second national Australian psychosis survey (Survey of High Impact Psychosis) found that in 2010 the estimated treated prevalence of psychotic disorders in a one-month period for people aged 18 to 64 was 3.5 per 1000 population and that the most common disorder was schizophrenia. The onset of illness was under 25 years for 64.8 per cent of people surveyed, and for most the onset was insidious (Morgan et al., 2012).

If you are not sure what all these terms mean, access this site: https://www.sane.org/information-stories/facts-and-guides/psychosis

The aetiology and pathogenesis of psychosis

Many possible causes of psychosis have been put forward over the years, particularly for schizophrenia. It is helpful to consider the aetiology of psychosis as multifactorial, with genetic predisposition, prenatal influences, life events and drug use all implicated. Zubin and Spring (1977) developed the stress-diathesis model, which suggests that everybody has some vulnerability to psychosis—a kind of psychosis threshold—and when this is crossed, psychosis may be triggered. This vulnerability may be increased by a variety of genetic, gestational, infectious and nutritional factors; and those with this vulnerability may have an increased susceptibility, not only to psychosis, but also to other mental illnesses, including substance misuse (Ksir & Hart, 2016). Psychological pathways can include early experience of adversity (Beards & Fisher, 2014). Essock (2017) noted that extremes of social and environmental adversity greatly increase the risk of schizophrenia. Writing of a personal lived experience of schizophrenia, MacPherson (2009) highlights a very confused sense of self as a cause, but a study of non-psychiatric doctors found that most viewed the causes of schizophrenia as a combination of biogenetic and psychosocial factors with biological predominating (Magliano, Citarelli & Reid, 2020). There may be a range of subtle premorbid developmental deficits and exposure to risks in the time from before birth to early adolescence (Laurens et al., 2015). Schizophrenia may be related to three interacting pathophysiological processes—dysregulation of the dopamine system, disturbed glutamatergic neurotransmission and an increase in the proinflammatory status of the brain (Kahn & Sommer, 2015). Developments in neuroscience and the identification of biomarkers may change the way psychosis is diagnosed in the future (Keshavan et al., 2013).

Person-centred care

Jando has grown up in a quiet coastal village in NSW with his father, mother and sister. His father moved overseas with his new partner when Jando was in Year 10, saying to Jando before he left, 'You're the man of the house now.' Jando took this responsibility very seriously, along with his commitment to studying (to attain good marks in the higher school certificate [HSC]) and working with his local Landcare group to protect the dunes. He has two good friends from school and attends a small church regularly with a girl from his street. He hopes to work in environmental science one day.

1. CONSIDER THE PATIENT SITUATION

Monday 4 pm

Jonathon is the only registered nurse (RN) working at the Melaleuca police cell complex. When he arrives for work, he is told that Jando has spent the whole weekend in the cells after being taken into custody late on Friday night. Jonathon decides to see Jando first as he is new to the corrections system. The prison officer brings him into the clinic. 'Had to give him a couple of Panadol at lunchtime,' says one officer. 'For a headache . . . that's what he said anyway. Apart from that he hasn't said a thing since he was arrested.' No further information is provided about Jando. There are no medication orders; however, the prison officers keep a box of paracetamol in their office and can supply two tablets if a prisoner complains of pain. This medication is not recorded anywhere.

Jonathon recognises that Jando is now part of a vulnerable population and so access to healthcare can become an ethical issue. He knows that he needs to work in partnership with Jando as far as possible given the constraints of the custodial setting; and that, although the prison officers are not healthcare workers, he also needs to work in partnership with them to achieve the best outcomes for Jando (Levett-Jones et al., 2017).

Prisoners are identified only by their MIN (master index number), not by first or last names. Therefore, part of their experience of being taken into custody is loss of individual identity. How could Jonathon overcome this to provide person-centred care?

Tuesday 4 pm

On arrival at work the following day, Jonathon finds that, instead of attending court as he was meant to, Jando is on his way back to the cells from the local emergency department (ED). 'What happened?' Jonathon asks. 'Not too sure,' one of the officers says. 'Seems he fell over on his way into the courthouse and hit his head on the concrete. I didn't see it happen myself. I reckon one of the others could have tripped him up or given him a shove. There was a bit of an argument over food before they all left this morning. We wouldn't have worried about ED except he was talking rubbish after he fell over—kept saying something about a lease.' The prisoners in the main cell complex, usually so ready to volunteer 'helpful information', are strangely silent today.

2. COLLECT CUES/INFORMATION

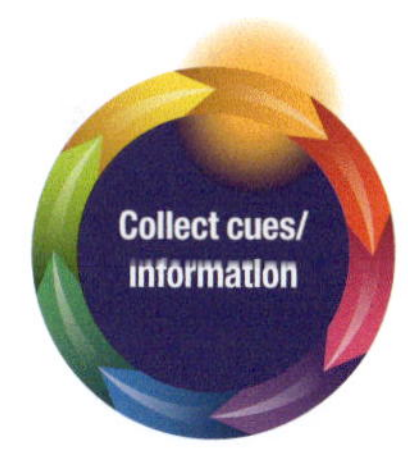

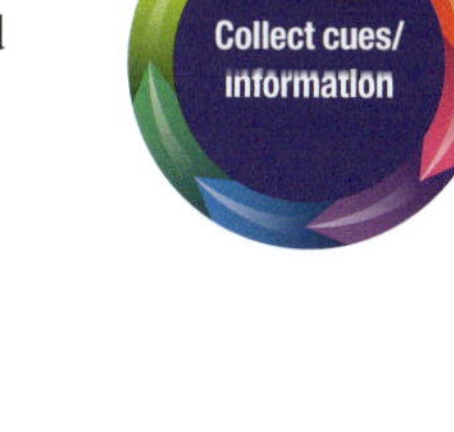

Jonathon wants to check Jando's head wound, so he asks an officer to let him into the cell where he is lying on the bed. Two steri-strips are on the laceration on his forehead. 'Nurse, they came after me and punished me,' he says sadly. 'I wish to be released but it can never happen.'

Q If Jonathon were to ignore the report from the local ED and fail to check Jando's head wound, because he believes he already knows what the problem is, which three cognitive biases would this illustrate?

a Anchoring
b Ascertainment bias
c Confirmation bias
d Fundamental attribution error
e Psych-out error
f Unpacking principle

National Safety and Quality Health Service (NSQH) Standards

Preventing and controlling healthcare-associated infection standard

The NSQHS Standards emphasise the importance of infection control measures. In prison environments, cleaning standards are less strict than in hospitals, and there is constant prisoner turnover (some having undiagnosed infections), crowded living conditions and a lack of fresh air. Therefore, strict vigilance from Jonathon is required when conducting wound assessments (ACSQHC, 2021).

'Seems so quiet, doesn't he?' says the officer. 'Hard to believe the charges.' 'What did he do?' asks Jonathon. 'Assault—quite a history apparently. Thumped his mum for no reason, then a few weeks later his sister, out of the blue. The reason he's here is because he decked a total stranger in the street. Just went up and punched him.'

(a) Review current information

Jonathon has access to limited information about Jando's health status. He is the only RN working in this prison cell complex, so he does not receive a shift handover. The prison officers have no health training and provide few details about Jando's condition. Jonathon's observations of Jando's behaviour and his ability to establish a therapeutic relationship and gain his trust are, therefore, critical to being able to gather the information needed for a comprehensive health assessment.

Nursing and Midwifery Board of Australia (NMBA) *Registered Nurse Standards for Practice* The NMBA's *Registered Nurse Standards for Practice* (2016) state that nurses must work in partnership with patients and use a range of assessment techniques. Jonathon cannot collect all the information he needs if Jando does not trust him.

Before reading the next part of the scenario, consider how Jonathon can best proceed with undertaking a comprehensive health assessment of Jando. How might he ascertain how Jando has behaved over the weekend when he has no access to the records kept by the prison officers and Jando seems reluctant to say much?

Q1 How reliable will information provided by the prison officers be?

Q2 What should Jonathon's priorities be when seeking information about Jando?

(b) Gather new information

The standard health assessment form used in the prison health service is divided into four sections: medical and surgical history; alcohol and other drug use (to predict potential for withdrawal); previous psychiatric history; and risk assessment (dealing with self-harm and suicidal ideation). Jando answers Jonathon's questions as he works through the health assessment, but volunteers little additional information and most of his replies are monosyllabic. Sometimes when he does offer more information, he seems to stop mid-sentence and lose his train of thought. Jando states that he doesn't have a regular general practitioner (GP) as he prefers to attend the ED at his local hospital for any health problems. He admits to 'some' cannabis use, but can't quantify the amount; he denies using any alcohol or other drugs. When Jonathon asks him how his head feels, Jando smiles and says, 'I have been released.' When Jando is questioned, he doesn't mention any mental health issues or previous psychiatric treatment.

Poor physical health is common among people who have mental health issues (Martin, 2016). For more information about the health and wellbeing of young people who are incarcerated, access *Young People in Custody Health Survey (YPiCHS)* at this site: http://www.juvenile.justice.nsw.gov.au/Pages/youth-justice/research/research.aspx#YoungPeopleinCustodyHealthSurvey(YPiCHS). This includes information about a current research project into stages of psychosis among incarcerated young people. The website name will shortly change to *Youth Justice*.

Q1 Why might Jando be unwilling or unable to answer Jonathon's questions about mental illness? (There is more than one correct answer.)

a Jando did not understand what Jonathon was talking about.

b Jando has never had any previous psychiatric treatment.

c Jando doesn't want the other prisoners to know anything about his health status.

d Jando doesn't want the prison officers to think he is a 'spinner'. (This is the prison slang for a person with a mental health problem.)

Jonathon proceeds to check Jando's vital signs and blood glucose level. Review the information provided below:

Temperature	36.3°C
Pulse rate	60
Respiratory rate	18

Blood pressure	110/70
Blood glucose level	6.1 mmol/L
Pain score	0/10 (However, this may not be accurate as Jando seemed unable to concentrate when Jonathon asked him to rate his pain using a numerical rating scale, where 10 is the worst pain ever experienced and 0 represents no pain.)

One of Jonathon's roles is to undertake a risk assessment of all prisoners.

Q2 What types of risk assessment might be relevant in Jando's situation?

National Safety and Quality Health Service (NSQH) Standards

Comprehensive care standard

The NSQHS Standards refer to the provision of comprehensive care and the management of risk. In Jando's situation, this will include consideration of unpredictable behaviours, such as self-harm and suicide, and aggression and violence (ACSQHC, 2021).

Q3 Which of the following statements are true in regards to risk assessments undertaken in a prison context?

a Risk assessment is never static—it changes depending on the person's mood, level of psychosocial support, situation and circumstances.
b Risk assessment is a definitive way to predict whether a person is going to attempt self-harm.
c Risk assessment only needs to be undertaken once during the person's time in the healthcare setting.
d Risk assessment is unnecessary when the person is in a cell with closed-circuit cameras monitoring behaviour around the clock.

3. PROCESS INFORMATION

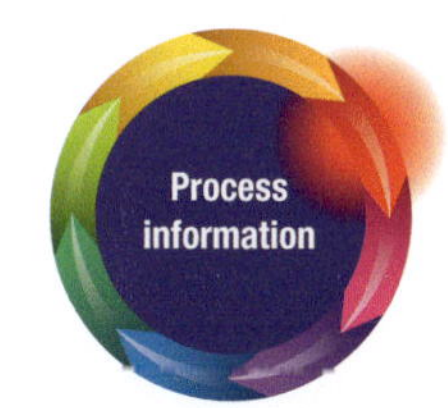

(a) Interpret

Q1 Which of Jando's vital signs are within normal parameters?

a Temperature: 36.3°C
b Pulse rate: 60
c Respiratory rate: 18
d Blood pressure: 110/70
e Blood glucose level: 6.1 mmol/L
f All of the options

Q2 Jonathon's assessment does not focus solely on the possibility of an undiagnosed mental illness. What other problems does he need to rule out?

Q3 Jando's vital signs suggest that:

a He is a physically fit young man and needs no further observations recorded at this stage.
b He is unlikely to experience any withdrawal state while in custody.
c He is highly anxious.
d He is in acute pain.

Nurses working in the prison system must undertake an assessment of potential substance withdrawal for all inmates and must be familiar with relevant signs and symptoms.

You can find information about withdrawal from legal and illegal drugs at: https://adf.org.au/reducing-risk/withdrawal

Q4 If Jonathon assumes that Jando's speech and behaviour are due to a withdrawal state, simply because many prisoners do have substance misuse problems, this is an example of:

a Anchoring
b Ascertainment bias
c Confirmation bias

- d Fundamental attribution error
- e Psych-out error
- f Unpacking principle

Q5 Signs and symptoms of alcohol withdrawal include:
- a Sweating, tremor, nausea, raised blood pressure and anxiety
- b Irritability, abdominal pain, anxiety and anorexia
- c Mydriasis, piloerection, muscle aches, rhinorrhoea and intestinal cramping
- d Extreme tiredness, hunger, mood swings and depression

Q6 Signs and symptoms of withdrawal from cannabis include:
- a Sweating, tremor, nausea, raised blood pressure and anxiety
- b Irritability, abdominal pain, anxiety and anorexia
- c Mydriasis, piloerection, muscle aches, rhinorrhoea and intestinal cramping
- d Extreme tiredness, hunger, mood swings and depression

Q7 Signs and symptoms of withdrawal from opioids include:
- a Sweating, tremor, nausea, raised blood pressure and anxiety
- b Irritability, abdominal pain, anxiety and anorexia
- c Mydriasis, piloerection, muscle aches, rhinorrhoea and intestinal cramping
- d Extreme tiredness, hunger, mood swings and depression

Q8 Signs and symptoms of withdrawal from methamphetamine include:
- a Sweating, tremor, nausea, raised blood pressure and anxiety
- b Irritability, abdominal pain, anxiety and anorexia
- c Mydriasis, piloerection, muscle aches, rhinorrhoea and intestinal cramping
- d Extreme tiredness, hunger, mood swings and depression

(b) Discriminate and (c) Relate

Q Which of the following observations might cause Jonathon to be concerned about Jando's mental health? (There are *four* correct answers.)
- a Jando doesn't talk much.
- b Jando is polite to everybody.
- c Jando doesn't laugh and joke with the other prisoners in his cell.
- d Jando eats the meals provided for him.
- e Jando often goes to the water bubbler for a drink of water.
- f Jando spends a lot of time wrapped in the grey blanket issued to him on arrival in the cell, often with his face obscured.
- g Jando passes urine at least twice a day.
- h Jando's facial expression rarely changes and most of the time he looks rather flat.

(d) Infer

Q Based on the information you now have about Jando, which of the following inferences are most likely to be *true*?
- a Jando is annoyed about being locked up, so he has decided not to co-operate with any interview or assessment process.
- b Jando is in an environment where he has no privacy and no personal space, so he tries to create it for himself by wrapping himself in his grey blanket.
- c Jando is not sleeping very well, so he looks tired during the day.
- d Jando has an alteration in his affect.

(e) Match

Think back to anybody with a psychiatric diagnosis whom you have known personally or cared for during a clinical placement. Have you seen behaviours that are similar to Jando's before? Was speech or behaviour immediately indicative of a mental health problem?

(f) Predict

Jonathon has limited time available and many other duties to attend to during his four-hour shifts. However, he also knows that he needs to communicate effectively with Jando in every way he can, with frequent interactions and persistence, particularly in this untherapeutic setting.

Patient Safety Competency Framework (PSCF)

Domain 2–Therapeutic communication

The PSCF specifies that nurses must demonstrate the ability to use verbal and non-verbal communication skills to convey respect and empathy, and to encourage the person to express their feelings and needs, while at the same time maintaining professional boundaries.

Source: *The Patient Safety Competency Framework for Nursing Students*, https://patientsafetyfornursingstudents.org

Q If Jonathon doesn't take the appropriate actions at this time, what could happen to Jando? (There is more than one correct answer.)
- a Jando might go to court and his possible mental health issue not be recognised during the hearing.
- b Jando could be remanded and moved to a large jail without further health assessment because the receiving nurse at the jail sees that it has already been completed in the prison cell complex.
- c Jando's mental state might worsen.
- d Jando's mental state might improve.
- e Jando's time on remand is made more difficult because he has an undiagnosed and untreated mental illness.

4. IDENTIFY THE PROBLEM/ISSUE

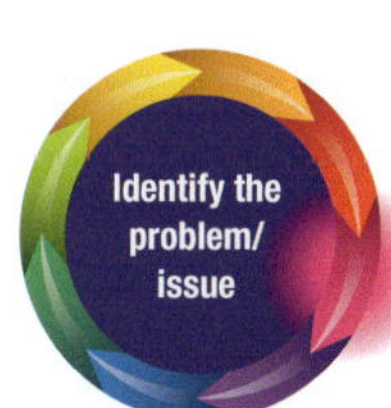

Q With the limited information Jonathon has been able to collect so far, which of the following are potential nursing diagnoses for Jando?
- a Risk of self-harm related to suicidal ideation
- b Risk of harm to others related to delusional beliefs
- c Ineffective communication related to thought disorder, evidenced by thought blocking, poverty of ideation and possible perseveration
- d Impaired therapeutic engagement with RN caused by delusional beliefs, incarceration, fear, social isolation and lack of privacy, evidenced by limited response to questions and reluctance to disclose freely

5. ESTABLISH GOALS

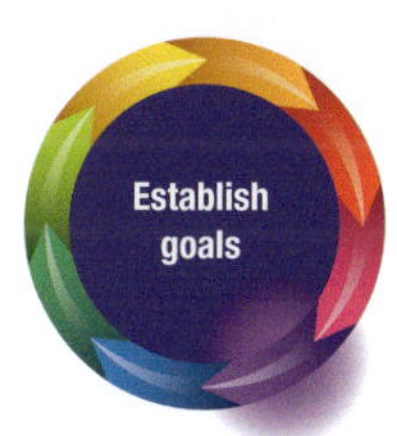

Q Which of the following are *not* priority goals for Jando's care at this time?
- a To establish a therapeutic relationship
- b To conduct regular physical assessments
- c To ensure Jando's safety
- d To begin to educate Jando about psychosis and its treatment
- e To challenge Jando's delusional beliefs and assure him that the auditory and visual hallucinations he is experiencing are not based in reality
- f To discuss the side effects of cannabis use

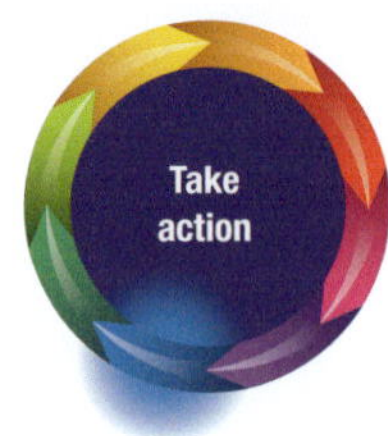

6. TAKE ACTION

Jonathon needs to gain Jando's trust, in spite of the contextual challenges. Without this trust, there is little possibility that Jando will disclose more information about himself. It is particularly difficult for a nurse to gain the trust of a prisoner because of the culture of the correctional setting and because prisoners may assume that the nurse is employed by the corrections system, not by the health service. Jonathon needs to provide physical care, as well as convey an atmosphere of safety and security, a sense of protection and a feeling of companionship (Hawamdeh & Fakhry, 2014). He also wants to be a recovery-focused nurse, even in such a challenging setting and, as such, 'holds hope for the client when the client is without hope' (Dalum et al., 2015). Recovery involves the person building a meaningful and satisfying life (even with some residual symptoms). For young people, it includes a dynamic interplay between personal and environmental processes (Rayner, Thielking & Lough, 2018).

Nursing and Midwifery Board of Australia (NMBA) *Registered Nurse Standards for Practice* The NMBA's *Registered Nurse Standards for Practice* (2016) stipulate that RNs must communicate effectively, act as patient advocates and differentiate between personal and professional relationships. Therefore, Jonathon needs to establish a therapeutic relationship and maintain confidentiality, while advocating for Jando's need for mental healthcare.

Q1 Which two of the following statements are *not* correct? A therapeutic relationship:

- a Is the same as any social relationship
- b Is not necessary at this time because Jando is locked up and now being dealt with by the legal system
- c Has defined boundaries to protect both nurses and patients
- d Is based on trust
- e Respects a person's rights
- f Adheres to confidentiality
- g Must always be open to scrutiny.

Q2 Match the correct action to its related rationale in the table below.

Action

- Undertake regular risk assessments
- Observe, engage and continue to assess Jando's mental state
- Provide simple education about psychosis
- Develop a therapeutic relationship

Action	Rationale
	A mental state examination should be done every shift, as mental state can change rapidly.
	Although risk assessments cannot ensure safety, they provide early warning of possible risks, allowing staff to take preventive action.
	Without a strong therapeutic relationship, assessments and treatment will be more difficult to undertake.
	Jando does not understand that his experiences are caused by a psychotic illness; therefore, he may not accept treatment.

7. EVALUATE

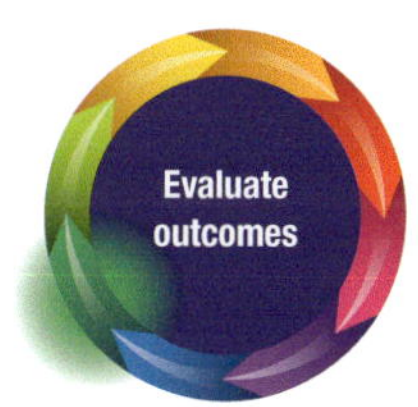

Jonathon is confident that Jando is safe because he has no means to harm himself; his cell is monitored round the clock on CCTV and he has shown no sign of harming his fellow prisoners in their shared cell during his time in custody. Jando's vital signs do not suggest any physical illness and, while he doesn't say much, there is nothing so far to suggest an acute confusional state. When Jonathon walks past the cells, Jando looks up and says hello. This suggests to Jonathon that there is some therapeutic engagement, with the beginning of trust and the possibility of further development towards a therapeutic relationship.

Jando sometimes seems unaware of what is happening around him and, when the other prisoners in his cell are chatting among themselves or watching television, he occasionally seems to be whispering to somebody when there is nobody close by him.

Q What might these observations about Jando indicate? Identify the two correct answers from the options below.

a Jando is responding to internal stimuli.
b Jando is lonely, so he is talking to himself.
c Jando is reciting a poem to help pass the time as he doesn't enjoy television.
d Jando is confused and thinks he is talking to his mother on his mobile which the prison officers removed on his arrival.
e Jando has influenza which has caused a sore throat, so he cannot speak loudly without pain.
f Jonathon is beginning to establish some rapport with Jando.

8. REFLECT

Jonathon knows that people experiencing their first psychotic episode are likely to feel 'scared, lost and alone' (Lamph, 2010, p. 38) even without being taken into custody. His role is to reach out, establish contact, and offer and start treatment and care (Sebergsen, Norbert & Talseth, 2014).

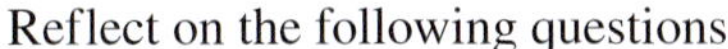

Reflect on the following questions.

Q1 Why is there a health service in the prison setting?

Q2 What is the best way to provide effective healthcare in the prison setting, and who should be involved?

Q3 If there is no health service in the prison system, what might be the effects on the community as a whole once prisoners are released?

Something to think about . . .

Your responses to these questions may help you to reflect on, and to understand, equity and access in healthcare (Baum, 2016), and your future role as a registered nurse. Your responses may also reveal certain attitudes or beliefs in relation to your future role which you may not have realised you hold.

SCENARIO 13.2 Not just an unprovoked aggressive outburst

CHANGING THE SCENE

The following day is Wednesday and when Jonathon gets to work one of Jando's cellmates calls out to him: 'Hey, chief! You better take a look at Jando. He's hanging out real bad. He needs something now.' There is a muffled laugh from the other men in Jando's cell. Jonathon is surprised as there have been no objective signs of withdrawal from any drugs or alcohol during Jando's five days in the cells. Jando is brought into the clinic and seems puzzled, almost perplexed. Jonathon asks him if he uses any drug at all on a regular basis. He doesn't reply, so Jonathon repeats the question and, at last, Jando seems able to focus. 'No, not at all,' he says. He then repeats this statement, 'No, not at all! No, not at all!' Jonathon concludes that the cellmates are joking, or perhaps trying to secure some diazepam for Jando in the hope that he will divert it to them. Still, just before Jonathon goes off duty, he looks in on Jando once again. He is lying on his bed, facing the wall; his lips are moving, and occasionally he shakes his head and seems to be pushing something away from him.

Although it is after the end of Jonathon's shift, he takes Jando back to the clinic. Jonathon thinks back over what Jando had said about 'being released,' which he had assumed referred to being released from custody, and which the officers had misinterpreted as being a mention of 'a lease'. Jonathon wonders about the reason for Jando's unprovoked assaults. He remembers Jando's look of perplexity when asked about drug use, and how he had been slow to respond to the questions. There was also the mention of using cannabis 'sometimes' at his initial assessment. So Jonathon asks Jando what he was doing when he was lying on his bunk immediately before being brought back to the clinic.

'They came back, nurse,' Jando tells him sadly. 'They will not release me.' Jonathon asks who 'they' are and Jando calmly explains that 'they' are the seven devils, who have been with him for a year or more now. Sometimes he looks into people's eyes and he knows that the seven devils are in them too. When he saw them in his mother, he hit her to drive them out and save her from them. It was the same with his sister. And later in the street, he tried to protect a stranger from them too. That was when he was arrested and brought to the cells. Tonight, he says, they have been coming very close to him in the cell which is very frightening, so he has been praying and trying to push them away. He can hear them whispering to him and telling him he is lost forever now and will never be released from them. He says in a very small voice to Jonathon that he only wants to save his mother and sister from the power of the seven devils, and he no longer expects to survive himself.

Jonathon continues to talk with Jando, using the framework of the full mental status examination to gather more information. There is no family history of mental illness, but this episode does coincide with Jando's regular use of cannabis in order to relax from the pressures of Year 12 and the HSC. Jando had not liked to say too much about this during his initial assessment on Monday as he feared further charges related to the use of an illegal drug.

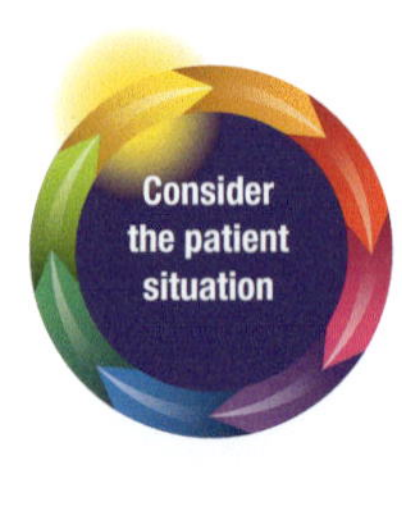

1. CONSIDER THE PATIENT SITUATION

Jonathon has been collecting cues since he first met Jando on Monday. His initial concerns have been validated and his preliminary assessment that Jando might have a mental illness has been confirmed. He must now undertake a comprehensive mental health assessment and ensure that Jando is referred to the appropriate services, whether he is released from Court on Friday or remanded in custody. He needs to further develop the therapeutic relationship he has established with Jando, and provide some very simple education about what Jando's experiences mean and what can be done to help him recover.

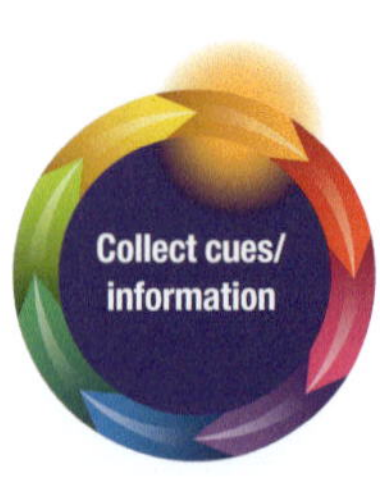

2. COLLECT CUES/INFORMATION

(a) Review current information

Jonathon organises the cues and information he has collected so far in the form of a mental state examination.

What is the difference between the MSE (mental state examination) and the MMSE (mini mental state examination)?

Appearance: Slim, fit-looking, young Caucasian male with short blonde hair; clean-shaven, wearing prison green tracksuit, no body odour, no visible lacerations on hands, laceration on right temporal area with two steri-strips, clean and dry, no sign of infection

Behaviour: Initially reserved, apparently shy or fearful, but now engaging better and able to give some account of himself; limited eye contact

Speech: Soft voice, somewhat hesitant

Mood: States 4/10 on self-report, using the Self-Report Scale where 0 is 'worst have ever felt' and 10 is 'best have ever felt'

Affect: Blunted

Thought content: Delusional—believes he can see the seven devils in people's eyes; believes they intend to harm his mother and sister as well as a stranger in the street; believes he will never be 'released' from them; and does not expect to survive; however, does deny intent to harm himself or any suicidal ideation, as well as denying having a plan or means for suicide; denies any thought of harming any other person
Thought form: Thought blocking, possible perseveration, poverty of ideation
Perceptual disturbances: Says he can hear the seven devils whispering; feels them coming close to him at times and pushes them away; he also sees them in people's eyes
Insight and judgment: Does not yet understand that his experiences are related to a diagnosable mental illness; however, is amenable to nursing assistance, explanations, education and referrals
Orientation: Knows that he is in Melaleuca Police Station; unsure of day or date; knows month; knows year
Sleep: Usually sleeps well, but has not been able to sleep well since being taken into custody
Appetite: Says he knows he should try to fast to drive the devils away but adds that sometimes he does get very hungry, so he eats all that is provided
Anhedonia: Not able to comprehend question relating to this; just says he does not deserve to enjoy anything because he has allowed the devils to come too close to his mother and sister when he should have been protecting them.

Can you identify some other disorders of thought form?

Insight and judgment are usually recorded together in the MSE. Do you know how judgment should be formally assessed?

Jonathon also performs a brief alcohol and other drug assessment, and this time Jando opens up to Jonathon because of the rapport that has been established, and because Jonathon explained that health information is not made available to the police so that he will not be charged with illegal drug use. Jando acknowledges that through Year 12 he used to smoke 'a couple of cones, or sometimes more, each day' to help him cope with the stress of the HSC. He denies any other drug use at all, both legal and illegal, since completing the HSC last November, and says he ceased cannabis use when the HSC results came out about six weeks ago. Jonathon is aware that there is a statistical association between cannabis use and the incidence of psychotic disorders (Ksir & Hart, 2016), though it may not play a key part in the development of psychosis in high-risk groups.

(b) Gather new information

Jonathon is now confident that he has made an accurate assessment of Jando's mental state, but he also needs to gather some corroborative evidence from others who know Jando well. Jando has no GP, and the summary from his presentation to the local ED after he fell over only notes that he was observed for four hours, all observations were normal and two steri-strips were applied to a laceration on his right temporal area. The prison officers have not observed much that is of relevance to the mental state assessment, and they view Jando as 'a good inmate' because he makes no demands and causes no trouble. Jonathon asks Jando if he may ring Jando's mother to ask how she sees things. Jando agrees and, although he is not allowed to speak to his mother himself, he does sit next to Jonathon while Jonathon makes the call.

Jando's mother is tearful when Jonathon explains who he is and why he is ringing. She has not been able to visit Jando and has only had a single call from him, which is routine for a person newly taken into custody. She tells Jonathon that Jando is always quiet but 'a lovely boy'—very thoughtful and considerate, and very concerned for his 12-year-old sister's safety and wellbeing since their father left and moved overseas with a new partner. Jando is very helpful to his mother and a good student. He enjoys sport, has two good friends and recently became close to a girl from his street whom he met at the church. He has twice visited her at the university where she is enrolled.

Jando himself has elected to take a gap year during which he is doing voluntary work with a landcare group, as the environment and its proper management is very important to him. At school, his teachers did not see him as 'the academic type' but the creative arts department found he had real talent. Jando's mother continues to explain that she hasn't noticed anything very different since he finished the HSC, only that he seems to be even quieter, spends more time in his room listening to music and writing in his journal, and seems to stay up very late—sometimes even all night. Occasionally, she has come into a room and found Jando apparently talking to somebody but when she asked about this, he mumbled something and left the room. At other times, she has noticed that he seems 'lost for words', as if he has got stuck in the middle of a sentence. In Year 11, Jando used to joke with his sister and play games with her a lot but she says in the past year he has rarely smiled. When she asked whether he was okay, Jando replied that he was saving the world and was thankful for that opportunity.

Jando's mother knows of no mental health issues on either side of the family and was not aware that Jando had been using cannabis for the past year. The attack on his sister was entirely unexpected and occurred one Saturday afternoon when she was watching a DVD with her mother. Similarly, the attack on his mother was also unexpected and occurred when she asked him if he had had a good day. In both cases, he had shouted loudly, 'NO!', and tried to push his sister and his mother to one side. Neither was injured. Jando's mother was surprised but concluded that he was overtired. She did not discuss these incidents with anybody and never mentioned them to Jando's father on the rare occasions when she did email him. Sounding rather uncertain, she does add that she thinks Jando's paternal uncle may have spent a long period in 'an asylum' during his twenties but that her ex-husband's family were reluctant to discuss the details.

Jonathon now has an account of prodromal symptoms including social withdrawal, decline in functioning, strange behaviours, sleep disturbance and unusual beliefs (Holt, 2013).

Q How can you be sure you have collected accurate information when the witnesses to the events either have no nursing knowledge or are unreliable historians, and the person for whom you are caring may not be able to give you a full account of what happened?

(c) Recall knowledge

Q1 Which three of the following statements are *not* accurate?

- a Cannabis does not cause psychosis but is associated with it.
- b A substance-induced psychotic disorder may resolve with appropriate treatment or may progress to become a chronic condition like schizophrenia.
- c People with psychosis never attempt suicide.
- d Illegal drugs are always involved if a person develops a psychosis.
- e There are many causes of psychosis.
- f People with psychosis have no hope of recovery.
- g Metabolic monitoring is now part of the mental health nurse's role in caring for a person taking second-generation antipsychotics.

Q2 Co-morbidity refers to a person who has:

- a Both a substance dependence and a mental health problem
- b Both anxiety and depression
- c Both a mental health problem and a legal issue
- d Both schizophrenia and delirium

Q3 The recovery model emphasises which of the following?

- a People who have experienced a psychotic episode will never get better.
- b People who have experienced a psychotic episode will need somebody to tell them what to do for the rest of their lives.
- c People who have experienced a psychotic episode shouldn't be expected to work or study, and usually end up on the disability support pension.
- d People who have experienced a psychotic episode choose their recovery pathway and who will assist them to travel this pathway, so they can achieve the life they want and the outcomes they desire.

The recovery model is a holistic and person-centred approach to the care of people with a mental illness that is premised on the understanding that it is possible to recover from a mental health condition. For further information see: https://www.verywellmind.com/what-is-the-recovery-model-2509979

3. PROCESS INFORMATION

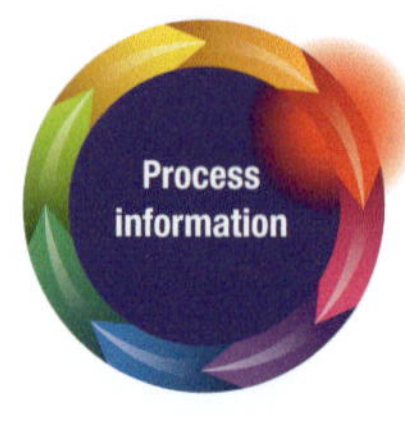

(a) Interpret

Jonathon knows that Jando needs a period of observation and assessment before a final diagnosis can be made. The case formulation table shows what Jonathon knows about Jando at this time.

	Predisposing factors	Precipitating factors	Perpetuating factors	Prognostic indicators, including protective
Biological	Genetic predisposition?		Not known at this time–continued cannabis misuse could perpetuate	Has ceased cannabis use six weeks ago
Psychological		Stress from HSC and possibly from father's departure	Incarceration, if lengthy	
Social				Stable home Supportive mother Voluntary employment

(b) Discriminate

Jonathon is happy with this formulation but knows that at this stage Jando's prognosis is still uncertain. He considers risk factors for relapse or for the development of a chronic psychotic disorder.

Q Based on what Jonathon already knows about Jando, which *three* of the following could be significant risk factors for future relapse?

- a Continued cannabis misuse
- b Additional use of other illegal substances such as methamphetamine
- c Insufficient income
- d Provision of community mental health support
- e Regular GP contact
- f Working or studying
- g Not taking medication if prescribed
- h Stigma

(c) Relate and (d) Infer

Q What do you see as most important in contributing to Jando's current mental state?

- a His use of cannabis in the preceding year
- b His unexpected incarceration
- c His head wound

(f) Predict

Q1 What might happen to Jando if he is remanded to a major city jail and if the receiving RN does not look at his health assessment?

Q2 Based on all the information you now have available, which two of the following statements are the *most* accurate predictions for Jando?

- a Jando may have a genetic predisposition to psychosis.
- b Jando's cannabis misuse may have contributed to his psychotic episode.
- c Jando's mother is not interested in him and this has caused all his problems.
- d Jando's involvement with his church has confused his thinking.
- e Jando will never recover and now can't go to university or get a job.
- f Jando should not have children.

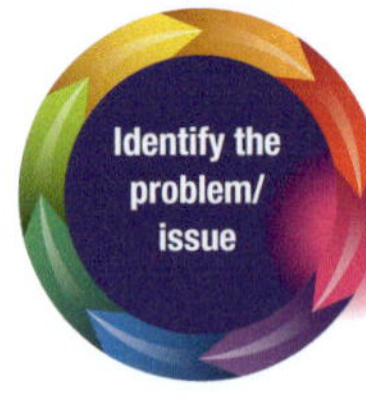

4. IDENTIFY THE PROBLEM/ISSUE

Q1 Now that Jonathon has been able to discover much more about Jando, what are the most likely nursing diagnoses?

- a Risk of self-harm related to suicidal ideation
- b Risk of harm to others related to delusional beliefs
- c Problems in effective communication caused by thought disorder, evidenced by thought blocking, poverty of ideation and possible perseveration
- d A problem in establishing a therapeutic relationship with Jonathon, caused by delusional beliefs, incarceration, fear, misunderstanding of reason for his current situation, social isolation and lack of privacy, evidenced by limited response to Jonathon's questions and reluctance to disclose freely

Q2 What do you think might be the most likely final psychiatric diagnoses for Jando?

- a Psychotic episode
- b Substance-induced psychotic disorder
- c Cannabis misuse
- d Cannabis withdrawal
- e Major depressive disorder
- f Generalised anxiety disorder
- g Adjustment disorder

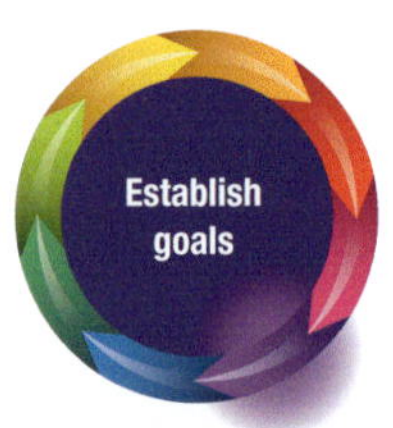

5. ESTABLISH GOALS

Q At this time, what are the most important goals in relation to Jando's nursing diagnoses?

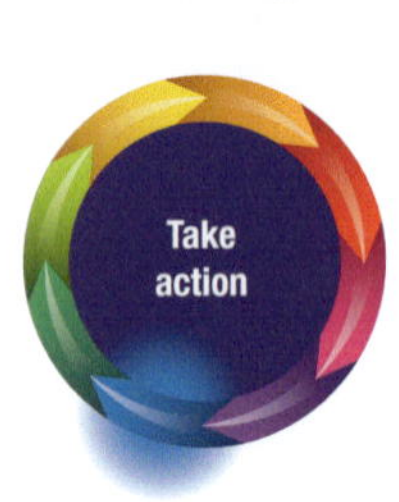

6. TAKE ACTION

Jonathon is obliged to discuss his concerns about Jando's condition with the duty doctor on call at the main jail in Sydney.

Q1 How would you use ISBAR over the phone to inform the duty doctor (who is hundreds of kilometres away from Jonathon and Jando, and will never meet either of them) of Jando's most urgent needs at this time?

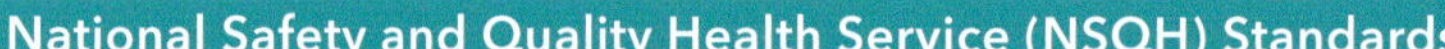

National Safety and Quality Health Service (NSQH) Standards

Communicating for safety standard

The NSQHS Standards outline the importance of a comprehensive and accurate clinical handover, with communication of critical information and careful documentation of updates or alterations to planned care. This is particularly important in this situation, as the duty doctor must rely solely on what Jonathon tells him in order to prescribe appropriate treatments (ACSQHC, 2021).

Jonathon receives a faxed medication order from the doctor for an antipsychotic to be commenced tonight. He also needs to educate Jando about the reason for the medication, how it works and possible side effects.

Patient Safety Competency Framework (PSCF)

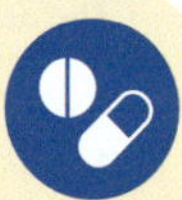

Domain 9—Medication safety

The PSCF specifies that competent nurses provide appropriate patient education about medication use, side-effects, storage and disposal.

Source: *The Patient Safety Competency Framework for Nursing Students*, https://patientsafetyfornursingstudents.org

Jando's safety, now and in the future, is Jonathon's main priority. He informs the prison officers of his assessment and flags Jando as a person with a mental illness (without breaching confidentiality).

Jonathon wants to ensure that when Jando appears in court on Friday, either he is admitted to an inpatient mental health unit or, if he is remanded in custody, on arrival at his jail of placement he is lodged in an area which is staffed by mental health nurses who can provide a supportive environment for him. Jonathon also needs to explain the need for a mental health admission to both Jando's solicitor and the court liaison nurse.

Q2 Each of the actions above require a specific rationale. In the table below, match the action to the related rationale.

Action

- Provide information to prison officers to enable them to manage Jando in custody as a person with a mental illness.
- Begin psychoeducation with Jando.
- Describe how Jando presents and summarise assessment data to the duty doctor.
- Notify Jando's solicitor and/or the court liaison nurse of his mental illness.

Action	Rationale
	Jando requires treatment and this cannot be commenced effectively without antipsychotic medication.
	Because Jando is experiencing a psychotic episode, he needs close observation and appropriate management.
	Until Jando understands that his experiences are not based in reality, he cannot begin to develop insight into his mental illness or to begin his recovery.
	If the solicitor is not aware of Jando's psychosis, he will be unable to ensure that the magistrate makes the most appropriate decision when Jando appears in court.

7. EVALUATE

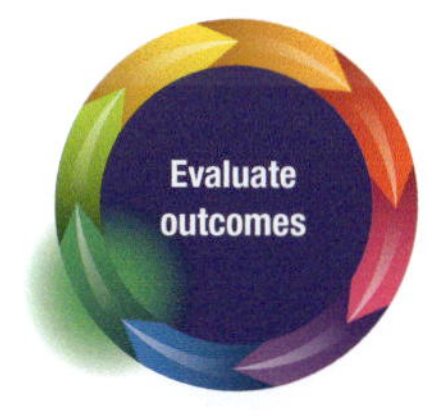

Jonathon's role requires him to provide healthcare that meets the complex physical and psychosocial needs of people who are incarcerated, many of whom have substance abuse and psychiatric problems. How would Jonathon know that his actions in caring for Jando have been effective?

8. REFLECT

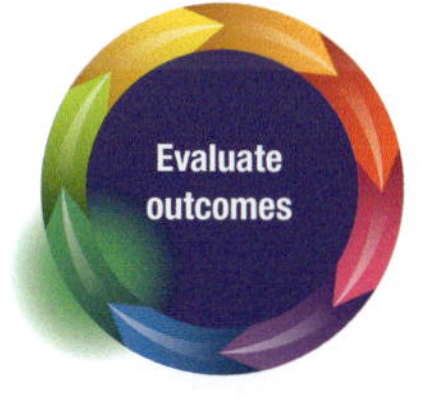

Prior to being incarcerated, Jando had been developing mental illness for over a year, while still attending school and spending time with friends and family.

Q1 Why do you think nobody noticed what was happening to Jando?

Q2 Who could have intervened if they had concerns about Jando's mental health?

Q3 What might those people have done to support Jando?

Q4 What sources of help were available to Jando that he might have accessed himself?

Q5 How could he have found out more about help-seeking, support and recovery?

Something to think about . . .

Many students are anxious about working with people who have a mental illness. This may be related to several issues: the stigma surrounding mental illness in the community, the sensational press coverage of incidents involving people with a mental illness, a belief that people with a mental illness are always violent, or personal or family experiences. These flawed perceptions can undermine the quality and safety of the care provided to this vulnerable population.

EPILOGUE

Jando accepted the medication which was prescribed for him, but he had trouble understanding that his distressing experiences are symptoms of a mental illness. He also found it difficult to believe that he could recover and his distressing symptoms would pass.

When Jando presented at court, the magistrate considered all the information available to him, including Jando's statement that he regrets shoving the man in the street and that he only intended to protect him from the seven devils. The magistrate directed that he be released from custody and taken to the local mental health inpatient unit, where Jonathon had organised a bed.

Jando gained a lot from the ward program, the antipsychotic medication was effective and he experienced no major side effects. He was introduced to his community case manager and found him easy to talk to and confide in. Jando's landcare group visited him in hospital and said that they were looking forward to his return, as the bitou was getting out of control down at the dunes. Some of his friends visited regularly and expressed their regret for not asking 'RUOK?' when they noticed Jando's unusual behaviour. When his friend from church visited, she brought him a Wollemi pine which he had always wanted.

Jando's mother and sister attended a support group where they were given a lot of information about psychosis, and their church group provided support and reassurance that Jando is well regarded in the church community.

A month later, Jando was discharged home with community support and regular appointments with the community psychiatrist. Jando was referred to a GP to monitor his overall health status. The first thing he did when he got home was to apply for an environmental science degree at the university where his friends were studying. Jando recovered and took his place back in the community where he belonged. He was no longer confused, scared, embarrassed or worried about disclosure (van Dusseldorp, Goossens & van Achterberg, 2011).

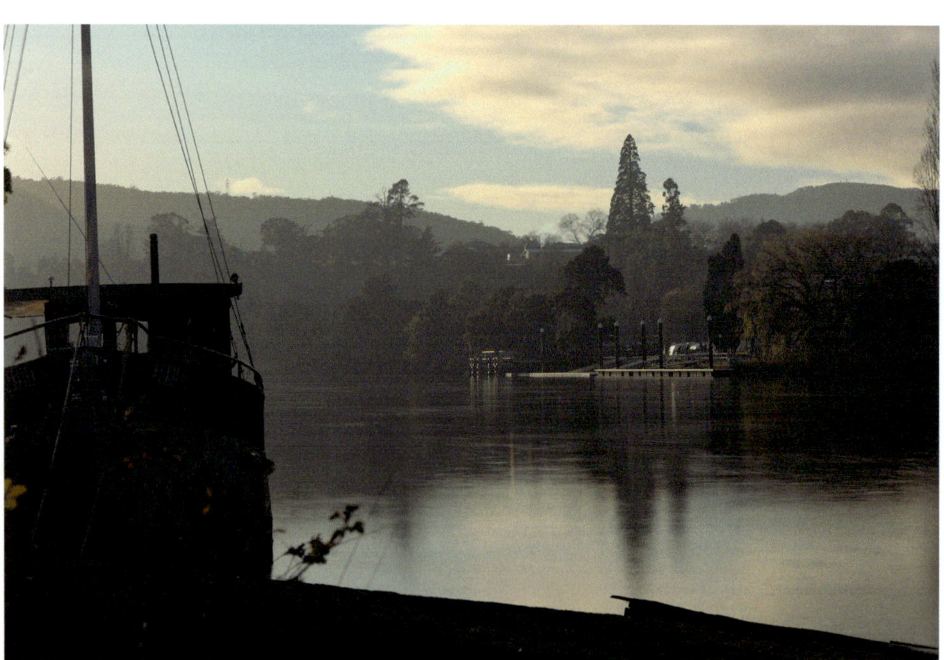

Jando grew up in a small coastal town
James Ross, student studying Bachelor of Media at UTAS

Something to think about...

If you are worried about a friend's mental health, you can:

Ask, 'RUOK?'

Listen without judging.

Assist with some very simple problem solving.

Suggest you go with your friend to see a GP.

Suggest your friend contacts the local community mental health team.

Advise your friend that, in crisis, the nearest ED will be able to access mental health support.

Tell your friend about websites that are reputable, and can provide information and support. For example, https://www.previousnext.com.au/case-studies/mind-health-connect and www.mindspot.org.au

Make sure your friend has the Lifeline phone number: 131114.

Let somebody else know if your friend is not amenable to any of your suggestions and you are still very concerned.

FURTHER READING

Cavanaugh, S. (2014). Recovery-oriented practice. *Canadian Nurse, 110*(6), 28–30. Retrieved from: www.canadian-nurse.com

Phillips, N. (2010). *Lost in a Mind Field: Schizophrenia and Other Psychoses*. Concord West: Shrink-Rap Press andFinger Lime Books. Retrieved from: https://shrinkrap.com.au

REFERENCES

American Psychiatric Association. (2013). *Diagnostic and Statistical Manual of Mental Disorders* (5th edn). Arlington, VA: American Psychiatric Association.

Australian Commission on Safety and Quality in Health Care (ACSQHC). (2021). *National Safety and Quality Health Service Standards* (2nd edn). Sydney, Australia.

Baum, F. (2016). Medical and health service interventions. In *The New Public Health* (4th edn). Melbourne: Oxford University Press.

Beards, S. & Fisher, H. (2014). The journey to psychosis: An exploration of specific psychological pathways. *Social Psychiatry and Psychiatric Epidemiology*, *49*, 1541–44.

Dalum, H., Pedersen, I., Cunningham, H. & Eplov, L. (2015). From recovery programs to recovery-oriented practice? A qualitative study of mental health professionals' experiences when facilitating a recovery-oriented rehabilitation program. *Archives of Psychiatric Nursing*, *29*, 419–25.

Essock, S. (2017). When social and environmental adversity causes schizophrenia. *American Journal of Psychiatry, 174*(2), 89–90.

Hawamdeh, S. & Fakhry, R. (2014). Therapeutic relationships from the psychiatric nurses' perspectives: An interpretative phenomenological study. *Perspectives in Psychiatric Care, 50*, 178–85.

Holt, L. (2013). Recognising psychosis. *Healthcare Counselling and Psychotherapy Journal*, *13*(3), 14–17.

Kahn, R. & Sommer, I. (2015). The neurobiology and treatment of first-episode schizophrenia. *Molecular Psychiatry*, *20*, 84–97.

Keshavan, M., Clementz, B., Pearlson, G., Sweeney, J. & Tamminga, C. (2013). Reimagining psychoses: An agnostic approach to diagnosis. *Schizophrenia Research*, *146*, 10–16.

Ksir, C. & Hart, C. (2016). Cannabis and psychosis: A critical overview of the relationship. *Current Psychiatry Reports, 18*(12), 1–11.

Lamph, G. (2010). Early psychosis: Raising awareness among non-mental health nurses. *Nursing Standard*, *24*(47), 35–40.

Laurens, K., Luming, L., Matheson, S., Carr, V., Raudino, A., Harris, F. & Green, M. (2015). Common or distinct pathways to psychosis? A systematic review of evidence from prospective studies for developmental risk factors and antecedents for the schizophrenia spectrum disorders and affective psychoses. *BMC Psychiatry, 15*(205).

Levett-Jones, T. Dwyer, T., Reid-Searl, K., Heaton, L., Flenady, T., Applegarth, J., Guinea, S. & Andersen, P. (2017). *Patient Safety Competency Framework (PSCF) for Nursing Students*. Sydney, NSW.

MacPherson, M. (2009). Psychological causes of schizophrenia. *Schizophrenia Bulletin, 35* (2), 284–86.

Magliano, L., Citarelli, G. & Read, J. (2020). The beliefs of non-psychiatric doctors about the causes, treatments and prognosis of schizophrenia. *Psychology and Psychotherapy: Theory, Research and Practice, 93*(4), 674–89.

Martin, C. (2016). The value of physical examination in mental health nursing. *Nurse Education in Practice*, *17*, 91–96.

Morgan, V., Waterreus, A., Jablensky, A., Mackinnon, A., McGrath, J., Carr, V.,... Saw, S. (2012). People living with psychotic illness in 2010: The second Australian national survey of psychosis. *Australian and New Zealand Journal of Psychiatry*, *46*(8), 735–52.

Nursing and Midwifery Board of Australia (NMBA). (2016). *Registered Nurse Standards for Practice*. Melbourne: NMBA.

Rayner, S., Thielking, M. & Lough, R. (2018). A new paradigm of youth recovery: Implications for youth mental health service provision. *Australian Journal of Psychology*, *70*, 330–40.

Sebergsen, K., Norberg, A. & Talseth, A. (2014). Being in a process of transition to psychosis, as narrated by adults with psychotic illnesses acutely admitted to hospital. *Journal of Psychiatric and Mental Health Nursing*, *21*, 896–905.

van Dusseldorp, L., Goossens, P. & van Achterberg, T. (2011). Mental health nursing and first episode psychosis. *Issues in Mental Health Nursing*, *32*, 2–19.

Zubin, J. & Spring, B. (1977). Vulnerability—A new view of schizophrenia. *Journal of Abnormal Psychology*, *86*(2), 103–26.

Chapter 14

Caring for an older person with altered cognition

SHARYN HUNTER and JAMIE GILLS

LEARNING OUTCOMES

Completion of the activities in this chapter will enable you to:

- explain why an understanding of cognitive decline, dementia, delirium, depression (the 4Ds) and mild cognitive impairment are essential to competent practice (**recall** and **application**)
- identify the clinical manifestations of mild cognitive impairment, dementia, delirium and depression that will guide the collection and interpretation of appropriate cues (**gather, review, interpret, discriminate, relate** and **infer**)
- identify risk factors for older people experiencing mild cognitive impairment, dementia, delirium and depression (**match** and **predict**)
- review clinical information to identify the main nursing diagnoses for a person experiencing dementia, delirium and depression (**synthesise**)
- describe the priorities of care for a person experiencing dementia, delirium and depression (**goal setting** and **taking action**)
- identify clinical criteria for determining the effectiveness of nursing actions taken to manage dementia, delirium or depression (**evaluate**)
- transfer what you have learnt about cognitive decline, mild cognitive impairment, dementia, delirium and depression to new clinical situations (**reflect** and **translate**).

INTRODUCTION

This chapter focuses on the care of Mr Dang Tien, an older person who experiences an alteration in cognition. Although nurses often use the term 'confusion' to describe this phenomenon, confusion is an ambiguous term and does not adequately describe the dimensions of this health breakdown condition. When nurses encounter older people with changes in their cognition, it is essential that they have knowledge and understanding of the related pathophysiological and psychosocial issues. A thorough assessment must be conducted as it will assist in determining the cause and type of cognitive change presenting. Further, it is important to distinguish between the different types of cognitive changes, as this will determine the appropriate actions required by the healthcare team.

There are four types of altered cognition associated with the older person (Hunter & Miller, 2016; Insel & Bager, 2002). They are: cognitive **d**ecline, **d**ementia, **d**elirium and **d**epression, often referred to as the 4Ds. Each type has specific features and, when the nurse engages in clinical reasoning, the type of altered cognition can be appropriately identified and assessed, the causes determined and the correct interventions implemented. Clinical reasoning skills allow for early recognition and management of the 4Ds, with the aim of preventing complications and further decline. Person-centred care and the development of a therapeutic relationship with the older person are integral to this process.

KEY CONCEPTS

cognitive decline
delirium
dementia
depression
mild cognitive impairment

SUGGESTED READINGS

K. Insel & T. Bager. (2002). Deciphering the 4Ds: Cognitive decline, delirium, depression and dementia: A review. *Journal of Advanced Nursing, 38*(4), 360–68.

P. LeMone, G. Bauldoff, P. Gubrud-Howe, M.-A. Carno, T. Levett-Jones, … D. Stanley (Eds). (2020). *LeMone and Burke's Medical-Surgical Nursing: Critical Thinking for Person-Centred Care* (4th edn). Pearson Australia.

Chapter 40: A person-centred approach to assessment of the nervous system
Chapter 43: Nursing care of people with neurological disorders

SCENARIO 14.1 Caring for an older person with delirium

Cultural consideration: What is different about Vietnamese names and how should you address a Vietnamese person?

SETTING THE SCENE

Mr Dang Tien (Jimmy) is a 75-year-old man with a history of chronic obstructive pulmonary disease (COPD), transient ischemic attacks (TIAs) and hypertension. He also has mild osteoarthritis in his hands and knees.

THE AETIOLOGY AND PATHOGENESIS OF THE 4DS

Cognitive decline

During normal ageing, the speed at which individuals acquire information gradually declines, but their ability to recall information remains intact (Insel & Bager, 2002). These changes are referred to as cognitive decline and they are unrelated to disease processes. Mild cognitive impairment (MCI) is a syndrome that is characterised by cognitive decline which is different from normal ageing, but does not meet the criteria for mild dementia (Patel & Holland, 2012). The key difference between normal ageing and MCI is that the older person with MCI has little or no recognition of memory loss. A cognitive assessment may reveal no significant impairment and there may be no noteworthy changes in instrumental activities of daily living. Currently, it is difficult to differentiate MCI from cognitive decline. Importantly though, MCI can progress to dementia (Patel & Holland, 2012).

Dementia

Dementia refers to a group of diseases, each with a different cause and a unique combination of manifestations. It is a gradual, progressive, irreversible deterioration of cerebral function which results in disturbance of many higher cortical functions, including memory, thinking and judgment (American Psychiatric Association, 2013). Impairment in cerebral function is commonly accompanied, and occasionally preceded, by deterioration in emotional control, social behaviour or motivation. This deterioration leads to a decreased ability to independently perform activities of daily living (American Psychiatric Association, 2013).

Types and causes of dementia

- **Alzheimer's disease**—causes mostly unknown, but in some cases there is a genetic link
- **Vascular dementia**—chronic decrease in cerebral blood flow, usually related to strokes and hypertension
- **Lewy body disease**—causes mostly unknown, but people with Parkinson's disease develop similar symptoms
- **Creutzfeldt-Jakob disease (CJD)**—may be related to a protein called a Prion
- **Fronto-temporal dementia**—causes mostly unknown, but there is a genetic link in some cases
- **Korsakoff syndrome**—caused by vitamin B1 deficiency; usually resulting from alcohol misuse.

Delirium

Delirium is described as an acute, reversible, clinical syndrome of cognitive function, characterised by an acute decline that impairs cognitive and physical function (Inouye, 2006). Delirium occurs as a result of a change in the health status of the older person (Fick, Agostini & Inouye, 2002). It is an important early indicator of a deteriorating patient and it may be the only signal of a developing illness or the exacerbation of a chronic disease.

National Safety and Quality Health Service (NSQH) Standards

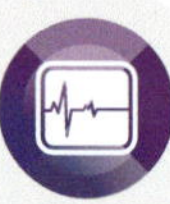

Recognising and responding to acute deterioration standard

The NSQHS Standards emphasise the importance of recognising and responding to acute deterioration. Prompt recognition of the older person's acute changes in cognition leads to appropriate care and the prevention of adverse outcomes (ACSQHC, 2021).

When an older person develops delirium, they will have an acute alteration in attention, and may have changes in perception (visual hallucinations), memory, thinking (delusions usually persecutory), orientation, sleep/wake cycle and (increased/decreased) psychomotor activity (Inouye, 2006). The course of delirium is dynamic and the symptoms may vary and fluctuate.

Delirium can result from the interaction between predisposing factors and precipitating factors, which increases a person's vulnerability and contributes to delirium. Predisposing factors include: advanced age, dementia, depression, functional dependency and a number of medications. Precipitating factors include: surgery, infections, serious illness, pain and physical restraints (Inouye, 2006).

Healthcare professionals frequently under-recognise delirium in older people or confuse it with other conditions such as dementia (Australian Commission on Safety and Quality in Health Care [ACSQHC], 2016). Failure to correctly recognise delirium in its early stages often produces poor outcomes for older people. Episodes of delirium increase the risk of falls, pressure areas, injury, cognitive and functional decline, dehydration, incontinence, malnutrition and mortality (Inouye, 2006).

There are three types of delirium: hyperactive, hypoactive and mixed (ACSQHC, 2016). Hyperactive delirium is characterised by an increased response to stimuli and psychomotor activity, while hypoactive delirium is characterised by a reduced alertness and psychomotor activity, and is commonly known as the 'quiet' delirium. The mixed type has features of both hyperactive and hypoactive delirium.

Depression

Depression in older people is often missed as its signs and symptoms can be attributed to the ageing process, dementia or poor health (Baldwin, 2008). In older people, depression often manifests with vague physical symptoms, memory loss and various behavioural changes. Affective changes also can occur and these include anxiety, irritability, diminished self-esteem and negative feelings about self. The presence of both anxiety and depression has been shown to be associated with increased cognitive impairment (Beaudreau & O'Hara, 2009). Genetics, personality and life experiences are probable causes if the older person has a previous history of depression; however, if the depression is experienced for the first time when older, physical health problems or losses may be the cause.

THE EPIDEMIOLOGY OF THE 4DS

The epidemiology of the 4Ds varies. It is widely accepted that cognitive decline occurs in all people as they age. However, dementia is not a natural part of ageing, even though most people with dementia are older. After the age of 65, the likelihood of living with dementia doubles every five years. Approximately 1 in 10 people over 65 have dementia and this increases to 3 in 10 people over the age of 85 (Dementia Australia, 2021). Currently, there is no cure for dementia and it is the second leading cause of death in Australia (Dementia Australia, 2021).

Delirium affects up to 18 per cent of older people admitted into Australian hospitals with between 2 and 8 per cent of people developing delirium during hospitalisation (ACSQHC, 2016). One Australian study found that 9.7 per cent of patients 70 years and over admitted to hospitals in Queensland had delirium at admission while a further 7.6 per cent developed delirium during hospitalisation (Travers et al., 2013). Currently, there is no data about the prevalence of delirium among Aboriginal and Torres Strait Islander peoples; however, it is thought to be higher in this population than in other Australians (ACSQHC, 2016).

The prevalence of depression in older people is estimated to be between 10 and 15 per cent (National Ageing Research Institute [NARI], 2009).

Access this link to learn more about dementia in older people from culturally and linguistically diverse (CALD) backgrounds: https://fecca.org.au/resources/database-of-research-on-ageing

Continuing with our scenario, Mr Dang Tien is currently receiving a visit from the community nurse for medication monitoring, as the dose of his antihypertensive medication was increased last week. The community nurse visits on Monday, Wednesday and Friday and reviews his blood pressure.

Mr Tien's medication regimen

- atenolol (Tenormin): 100 mg once daily (increased from 50 mg)
- fluticasone propionate (Seretide): twice daily
- salbutamol (Ventolin): two puffs PRN

Today is Friday and when Kristy, the community nurse, arrives she immediately notices that Mr Tien has a moist cough and he looks exhausted. Kristy asks him how he is feeling and he replies, 'Not too bad.' As they go into the kitchen, Kristy observes that Mr Tien's medicines are in disarray. Usually, he has his medications arranged in an orderly way, just like he used to keep his workplace. He takes a seat and Kristy begins assessing him.

Kristy is able to compare the current observations with those she has previously recorded for Mr Tien, as follows:

Current observations	**Normal for Mr Tien**
Temperature: 36.9°C	Temperature: 36.4°C
Pulse rate: 100 beats/min	Pulse rate: 85 beats/min
Respiratory rate: 28 breaths/min	Respiratory rate: 22 breaths/min
Blood pressure (sitting): 180/90	Blood pressure (sitting): 130/85
O_2 sats: 89%	O_2 sats: 96%
Bilateral crackles in both lung bases	No crackles in lung bases
Urinalysis: NAD	Urinalysis: NAD

During Kristy's visit, Mr Tien's daughter Nguyen Qui arrives. She always comes home to have lunch with her father. She asks her father why he is still in his night clothes as he is always up, showered and dressed when Kristy visits. His breakfast is still on the table, too.

Kristy makes the decision to transfer Mr Tien to the local hospital emergency department (ED) and he is subsequently admitted with pneumonia. While in the ED, blood and sputum are collected for pathology testing.

Q Mr Tien has pneumonia but is afebrile. Why is this?

Person-centred care

The goal of person-centred care is to interact with the patient as a person. Collecting personal information, using the person's past life and history in care, respecting the person's choices and focusing on what the person *can* do, as well as their disabilities, are all part of person-centred care (Edvardsson & Nay, 2010).

National Safety and Quality Health Service (NSQH) Standards

Partnering with consumers standard

The NSQHS standards state that people receiving care are to be considered partners in planning, design and delivery of care (ACSQHC, 2021). Being person-centred enables nurses to partner with consumers in a meaningful way.

Q What factors might contribute to the risk of older people not being recognised as cognitively competent?

Mr Tien's life story

Mr Dang Tien arrived in Sydney from Vietnam in 1975 with his wife, Dang Doh, and their three children aged 18, 15 and 12. He was 39 years old and his wife was 38. He left Vietnam when the communist regime from North Vietnam moved into Ho Chi Minh City (formerly Saigon). Mr Tien was a respected professional and a Catholic, and he was unable to stay in Vietnam under the communist regime. Mr Tien had good friends in Australia and they were able to assist him and his family to escape. He worked as an engineer prior to his move to Australia, and spoke fluent French as well as Vietnamese. He was able to speak in English but not write it.

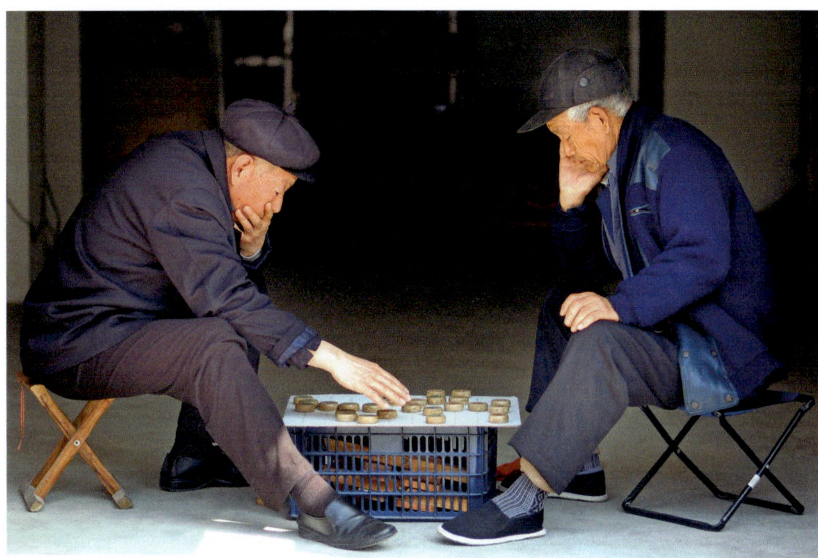

Mr Tien playing Chinese chess with a friend
© zhuda/Shutterstock

When he arrived in Sydney, Mr Tien went to work in a factory as a maintenance engineer, where he was given the nickname 'Jimmy' by his workmates. He worked long hours and saved to buy his own business. In 1990, Mr Tien purchased a dry-cleaning shop and his eldest son and daughter joined him in this business. Mrs Tien had always stayed at home and looked after her husband, her children and then the grandchildren when they came along.

Mr Tien retired from the business four years ago because he was unable to physically cope with the work due to his COPD. Since then, his eldest son, Dang Lu, and his son-in-law have run the business. Mr Tien's wife died two years ago from breast cancer and he moved to his daughter's home, where he lives with her, her husband and his two grandsons. His eldest son moved into the family home when his father moved out; it is around the corner from Nguyen Qui's home.

Despite Mr Tien being regarded as a quiet, gentle man, he has always been very sociable, enjoying his days at the shop and the company of his friends and neighbours. He usually speaks Vietnamese at home with the family and English outside the home. Mr Tien plays Chinese chess on Tuesdays and Fridays at the local seniors centre.

With some assistance from his daughter and son-in-law, Mr Tien still manages to grow the Asian vegetables that they eat daily. He loves Vietnamese food, which his wife always cooked, but he does eat Western food occasionally. He prefers to eat with chopsticks.

When Mr Tien was diagnosed with COPD, he stopped smoking. He had started when he was a teenager and it became a habit. The progression of the disease has been relatively slow since he stopped smoking and because he is very health conscious.

Mr Tien regularly visits the acupuncturist and the Chinese herbalist for minor ailments. He is not one to complain about his illnesses or the loss of his wife. He feels he is ageing well, as he has a good appetite, is still able to do the things he enjoys, has a good relationship with his children and sleeps about six hours a night, only waking once or twice to go to the toilet. Mr Tien has never been hospitalised.

Cultural consideration: Why is it not appropriate for the night nurse to call Mr Tien 'Jimmy'? Hint: Refer to this web page: www.diversicare.com.au/wp-content/uploads/2015/10/Vietnamese.pdf

Patient Safety Competency Framework (PSCF)

Domain 3–Cultural competence

The PSCF states that being culturally competent is an essential skill required by all nurses. Nurses must demonstrate respect for each person's cultural values, beliefs, life experiences and health practices.

Source: *The Patient Safety Competency Framework for Nursing Students*, https://patientsafetyfornursingstudents.org

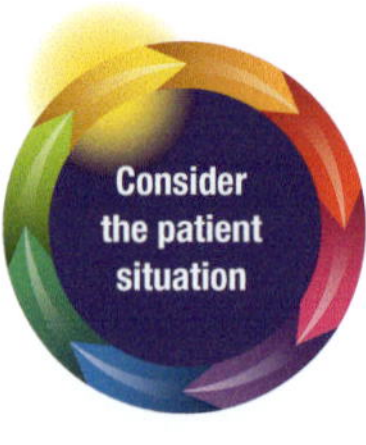

1. CONSIDER THE PATIENT SITUATION

It is now Friday night in the respiratory unit and, while answering a call bell, the night duty nurse notices that Mr Tien is out of bed and urinating in the sink near his bed. She says sharply, 'Jimmy, that's not a toilet. That's the sink!' Mr Tien goes back to his bed and the nurse puts the bed rails up. During the night, he is restless and incontinent, and continually pulls off his nasal prongs.

National Safety and Quality Health Service (NSQH) Standards

Communicating for safety standard

The NSQHS Standards state that clinical handover should be structured to effectively communicate the healthcare requirements of people. ISBAR is one example of a structured communication tool that can be used to guide clinical handovers (ACSQHC, 2021).

Morning handover report (0700)

Mr Tien behaved inappropriately during the night, using the sink as a toilet. Do not use the sink until it has been cleaned. We are an acute respiratory ward—why do we get the confused oldies? I put his bed rails up, so he couldn't get out again and he didn't. But I had to keep an eye on him because he didn't sleep much and he was incontinent of urine. He doesn't talk much, just yells in gibberish . . . though he could have been speaking Vietnamese, I wouldn't know. He doesn't speak English, although in handover last night they said he did. I think he's demented and will need placement. Just what we need—another bed blocker.

Clinical reasoning errors: The comment about Mr Tien being demented is an example of both anchoring and ascertainment bias.

His obs are stable; he is putting out urine in good amounts (all over the bed). I think he needs an IDC. His bowels haven't opened. He was tossing and turning all night. He's still coughing. I spent the whole night putting his nasal prongs back on and keeping him from getting tangled up in his IV. I am exhausted, what a night ...

Something to think about ...

Bed rails are considered a form of restraint. According to best practice guidelines, bed rails should only be used: as a last resort; after a thorough assessment of the older person's needs; after other alternatives have been trialed and failed; when appropriate consent is obtained; when it is the only practical, least restrictive and safest strategy available. When bed rails are used, the person being restrained should be closely monitored. Always review your organisation's policies and procedures before considering the use of bed rails.

What questions should Tricia ask the night duty nurse about Mr Tien?

Tricia, a new graduate nurse, is allocated to the care of Mr Tien for the morning shift.

Quick Quiz!

Before progressing to the next stage of the clinical reasoning cycle, test your understanding of some of the terms used so far. Select the correct response for each of the following statements.

Q1 COPD is:
- a A disease of the bronchioles
- b An acute disease of the small and large airways
- c A chronic airway disease

Q2 Seretide and Ventolin are used to:
- a Increase airway diameter and reduce inflammation of the bronchioles
- b Reduce swelling and inflammation of the lungs
- c Increase airway diameter and moisture in the bronchioles

Q3 'Bed blocker' is a disparaging term used to describe which of the following?
- a A patient who is always getting out of bed and blocking nurses' movement
- b A bed that is raised on blocks so that patients with respiratory problems can breathe more easily
- c A patient whose hospitalisation extends beyond the standard period of admission, preventing new admissions

Q4 Urinary incontinence is a term typically used to describe:
- a An episode of urination that did not occur in a toilet
- b An inability to control urination
- c A controlled ability to urinate

2. COLLECT CUES/INFORMATION

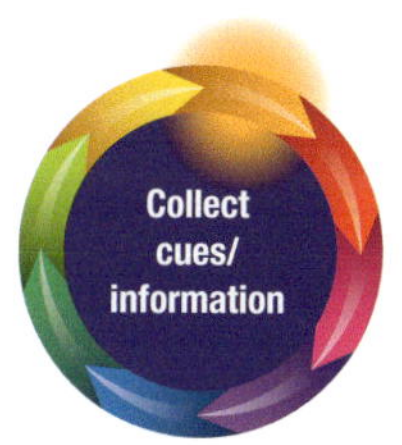

(a) Review current information

Now that you have some understanding of Mr Tien's situation, the next stage of the clinical reasoning cycle is to collect relevant cues and information. Tricia has the following information about Mr Tien:

1. His previous level of functional abilities
2. Details of current medications and medical history
3. His usual sleep pattern
4. His usual bowel and bladder function
5. Results from his admission urinalysis.

Q Can you identify another five important cues that need to be reviewed by Tricia?

(b) Gather new information

At 0800 hours, Tricia goes to Mr Tien's room. The bed rails are still up and Mr Tien's nasal prongs are around his neck. Tricia notices that no water has been drunk from his water jug and his cup is empty on the bedside locker. Mr Tien's breakfast of porridge, tea and toast has not been eaten and he has been incontinent of urine.

Tricia takes Mr Tien's vital signs and completes a respiratory assessment. She also conducts an abbreviated mental test score (AMTS) and a confusion assessment method (CAM).

The AMTS is a cognitive assessment tool that can be used to quickly assess an older person. It takes five minutes to complete and includes 10 questions. The maximum score is 10 and a score of less than 7 is suggestive of cognitive impairment. The AMTS can identify cognitive impairment but it is not reliable in identifying delirium.

For more information about AMTS, access: https://academic.oup.com/ageing/article/44/6/1000/80740

The CAM is a valid 'gold standard' delirium diagnostic tool. It also takes about five minutes to complete.

For more information about the CAM, access: https://www.ncbi.nlm.nih.gov/pmc/articles/PMC2585541

Currently, the CAM is commonly used in nursing practice. However, another tool, the 4AT, is increasingly replacing the CAM in the hospital setting. The 4AT has been shown to be simple, quick and with a high degree of accuracy in detecting delirium (Tieges, et al., 2021). Another advantage of the 4AT is that it can be included in electronic medical records.

A copy of the 4AT tool is available at: https://www.the4at.com

Tricia finds it difficult to complete these assessments as Mr Tien is only able to tell her his age, address and the year he first arrived in Australia. She can't understand some of Mr Tien's responses, as his English is mixed up with Vietnamese. Some of the questions Mr Tien doesn't attempt to answer—he just stares at Tricia's hands.

More information about cognition and hosptialised older people can be found at Victorian State Government Department of Health and Human Services, *Older people in hospital*, available at: https://www2.health.vic.gov.au/hospitals-and-health-services/patient-care/older-people

Q Identify two relevant cues that you believe Tricia should collect at this stage to help her understand the care Mr Tien requires:

a. Level of consciousness and orientation
b. Urinalysis
c. Level of psychomotor activity
d. Bowel pattern
e. Mr Tien's mood, speech and conversation ability
f. Skin assessment
g. Fluid balance status
h. Falls status

(c) Recall knowledge

Tricia begins to recall what she knows about the causes of altered cognition in older people.

Q1 See how much you know about the 4Ds by matching the alteration in cognition to the correct symptoms.

Hint: Reading K. Insel & T. Bager. (2002). Deciphering the 4Ds: Cognitive decline, delirium, depression and dementia: A review. *Journal of Advanced Nursing, 38*(4), 360–68 will help you complete the table: doi.org/10.1046/j.1365-2648.2002.02196.x

Alteration in cognition

- Delirium
- Dementia
- Depression
- Cognitive decline

Alteration in cognition	Onset	Level of consciousness	Mood	Self-awareness	Activities of daily living
		Alert		Unaware of deficits	
	Acute, hours-days		Fluctuates	Fluctuates	May be intact or impaired
		Drowsy		Aware of cognitive change	
	Chronic, months-years	Alert	No change		No change

Q2 Which of Mr Tien's medical conditions may alter his cognitive status?
  a COPD
  b TIAs
  c Pneumonia
  d All of these options

Q3 How might TIAs contribute to altering Mr Tien's current cognitive status?
  a A TIA can cause cerebral hypoxia and cell death, which can lead to the development of delirium.
  b A TIA can cause confusion, which can lead to the development of depression.
  c TIAs can cause cerebral ischaemia and cell death, which can lead to the development of dementia.

Q4 How might pneumonia contribute to altering Mr Tien's cognitive status?
  a Infections may trigger an episode of delirium in older people.
  b Pneumonia causes hypoxia, which leads to dementia in older people.
  c Pneumonia causes hyperthermia, which triggers an episode of delirium in older people.
  d Pneumonia causes severe fatigue, which predisposes the older person to the development of depression.

What is the difference between hypoactive and hyperactive delirium?

Q5 How might COPD contribute to altering Mr Tien's cognitive status?
  a COPD can cause cerebral hypoxia and cell death, which can lead to the development of dementia.
  b COPD can cause confusion which can lead to the development of depression.
  c COPD can cause cerebral hypoxia which can lead to the development of delirium.

Something to think about ...

Healthcare issues can arise when nursing older migrants as they often follow their original culture (Queensland Health, 2011). Tricia would need to consider a number of aspects of Vietnamese culture when nursing Mr Tien.

Q6 Review the information you have about Mr Tien and describe how each cultural aspect relates to him:

If you need help, refer to this web page: www.diversicare.com.au/wp-content/uploads/2015/10/Vietnamese.pdf

Cultural aspect	Mr Tien
Example: Language	Speaks Vietnamese, English and French. Usually speaks Vietnamese with family and English outside the home.
Food and diet	
Attitudes to illness and pain	
Cultural beliefs	
Family (living arrangements)	
Religion	

3. PROCESS INFORMATION

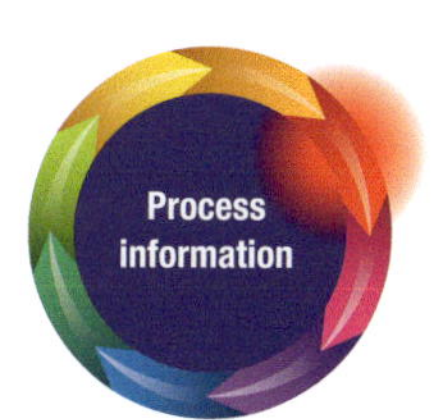

(a) Interpret

Q Which of the following are within normal parameters for Mr Tien?

a Temperature: 36.9°C

b Pulse rate: 95 beats/min

c Respiratory rate: 28 breaths/min

d Blood pressure: 175/90

e SaO_2: 90% (room air)

f Lung sounds: crackles in left lower lung bases

(b) Discriminate

Q1 From the information that you know about Mr Tien and the cues that have been collected by Tricia, which three cues are *most relevant* to determine Mr Tien's cognitive status *at this time*?

a Vital signs

b Level of confusion

c SaO_2 level

d CAM positive result (acute change, easily distracted, rambling and unclear conversation, alert)

e AMTS result 3/10

f Breathlessness

g Urinalysis NAD on admission

h Mr Tien's cognition has not been assessed prior to admission.

i Mr Tien plays chess on Tuesdays and Fridays at the local seniors hall.

Hint: A score of less than 6 for the AMTS suggests cognitive impairment but it does not screen for delirium.

Q2 From the list below, what information is *unnecessary* for Tricia to consider in order to make any inferences about Mr Tien? (Select three responses.)

a Mr Tien normally sleeps for six hours and is up to the toilet at least once every night.

b His bowels opened yesterday.

c No significant abnormalities were noted in urea and electrolytes (U&Es).

d Mr Tien usually speaks Vietnamese at home with the family and English outside the home.

e Mr Tien lives at home with his daughter.

f Mr Tien is a quiet, gentle man.

g Mr Tien enjoys living with his daughter and son-in-law.

h Mr Tien manages, with assistance from his daughter and son-in-law, to grow the Asian vegetables they eat daily.

i Mr Tien has not had any previous hospitalisations.

j Mr Tien loves Vietnamese food. He will eat Western food occasionally. He prefers to eat with chopsticks.

Q3 There are many myths about alterations in the cognition of older people. Which of the following statements is *true*?

a All older people will develop dementia.

b When people become older, they can expect to feel depressed.

c Older people are at increased risk of developing delirium when they experience acute physiological changes.

d All older people will lose their short-term memory.

e As people age, they cannot learn new information.

f Some level of confusion is experienced by all older people.

Q4 Why is it important for Tricia to have knowledge of the myths associated with ageing and cognition?

(c) Relate and (d) Infer

It is important to cluster the cues together and to identify relationships between them (based on the information you have collected so far). From this, you can make inferences about Mr Tien's condition.

Whether Mr Tien has dementia, depression and/or delirium will be ultimately determined by the medical officer. The role of the nurse is to work collaboratively with the healthcare team and to report their nursing diagnoses to the team, so they can make an informed and accurate medical diagnosis.

Q1 Are the following statements *true, false* or a *possibility*.

- a Mr Tien is incontinent because the bed rails prevent him from getting out of bed to go to the toilet.
- b Mr Tien is incontinent because he has dementia.
- c Mr Tien is depressed because he has COPD and is hospitalised.
- d Mr Tien has language difficulties because he has dementia.
- e Mr Tien did not eat his breakfast because he does not eat porridge or toast, or drink white tea.
- f Mr Tien has not been drinking because he is experiencing delirium.
- g Mr Tien is confused because he is an older person.
- h Mr Tien is in a delirium because he is older and ill with pneumonia.
- i Mr Tien has impaired communication because he is experiencing delirium.

Q2 Can an older person be diagnosed with dementia as well as depression or delirium, or with all three?

Hint: Think about the causes and risk factors for an older person developing delirium. See *Delirium Clinical Care Standard* (ACSQHC, 2021) at: https://www.safetyandquality.gov.au/our-work/clinical-care-standards/delirium-clinical-care-standard

Q3 Identify three factors that have led to Mr Tien's cognitive alteration.

- a Advancing age
- b History of hypertension
- c Pneumonia
- d Hospitalisation
- e Intravenous therapy
- f Antibiotic therapy

(e) Match

Q Have you ever cared for someone with cognitive alteration? In what way were their presenting signs and symptoms the same as, or different from, Mr Tien's?

NSW Health has adopted the CHOPs (Care of confused hospitalised older persons) program which provides six principles of care for an older person experiencing an alteration in cognition unassociated with normal ageing. For more details, visit: www.aci.health.nsw.gov.au/chops.

(f) Predict

Q If Tricia does not take the appropriate and timely actions regarding his altered cognition, what could happen to Mr Tien? (Select the four correct responses.)

- a He could have a stroke.
- b He could be diagnosed with dementia.
- c He could become hypoxic.
- d He could become septic.
- e He could fall.
- f He could become dehydrated.
- g He could become suicidal.
- h He could develop a pressure sore.

4. IDENTIFY THE PROBLEM/ISSUE

Identify the problem/ issue

Now is the time for you to bring together (synthesise) all of the information collected and inferences you've made to identify the key nursing diagnoses for Mr Tien.

Q Select from the following list, the *incorrect* nursing diagnosis for Mr Tien.

- a Functional incontinence related to acute confusional state, evidenced by Mr Tien using the sink to urinate and incontinent of urine in the bed once bed rails raised
- b Impaired communication related to acute confusional state, evidenced by Mr Tien yelling in 'gibberish', not speaking English and AMTS assessment findings
- c Pneumonia, evidenced by AMTS 3/10, CAM positive result and communication difficulties
- d Impaired memory related to pneumonia, evidenced by communication difficulties, AMTS and CAM results, and using the sink as a toilet

e Impaired oxygenation and breathing related to pneumonia, evidenced by respiratory rate 28, SaO_2 90% (room air) and crackles in left lower lung bases
f Sleep/wake alteration related to acute confusional state, evidenced by night nurse's report
g Risk of falls related to acute confusional state
h Risk of skin breakdown related to age, acute confusional state and pneumonia

5. ESTABLISH GOALS

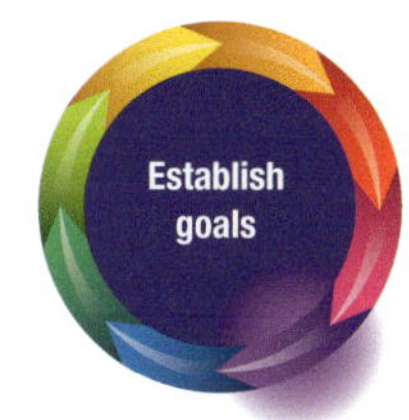

Q From the list below, choose the most important *short-term* goals (within 24 hours) for Mr Tien's management.

a For Mr Tien to be orientated and alert
b For Mr Tien to be able to communicate his needs and wants
c For Mr Tien to return home
d For Mr Tien's language skills to return to baseline
e For Mr Tien to be more interactive with staff
f For Mr Tien to stop using the sink as a toilet
g For Mr Tien to be placed in a residential aged-care facility
h For Mr Tien to eat three-quarters of the food presented at meal times
i For Mr Tien not to fall
j For Mr Tien's oral intake to be 1000 mL/24 hrs
k For Mr Tien's oxygen saturation level to remain above 95% and respiratory rate below 22 breaths/min

6. TAKE ACTION

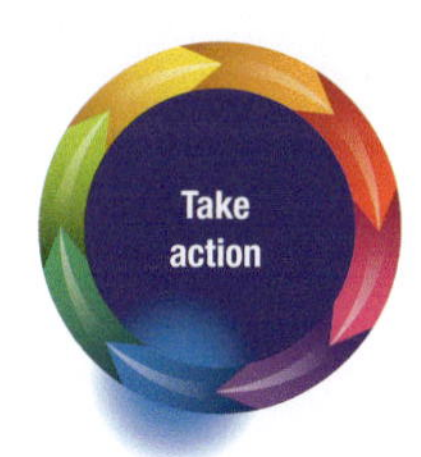

Q1 All of the actions below are appropriate, however some must be performed *immediately*. Reorder the nursing actions in the table into immediate priorities and non-immediate priorities.

Immediate priorities	Non-immediate priorities
Move Mr Tien to an area where he can be closely observed	Monitor Mr Tien's vital signs and oxygen saturation level
Maintain Mr Tien's fluid balance chart	Notify Mr Tien's doctor of his condition
Communicate via phone with Mr Tien's daughter	Engage the interpreter service to assist with communication strategies
Lower the bed rails on Mr Tien's bed	Ensure Mr Tien is wearing his nasal prongs
Regularly orientate Mr Tien to the hospital environment	Check that the IV cannula is patent

Q2 In the tables below, match the rationales for care to the corresponding nursing action.

Airway, breathing and circulation

Rationale

- To ensure adequate oxygen delivery
- To ensure clear, accurate and timely communication of Mr Tien's vital signs
- To ensure adequate fluid intake and prevent dehydration

Nursing action	Rationale
Monitor oxygen saturation levels	
Document all nursing observations and actions accurately and contemporaneously	
Prompt and assist Mr Tien with oral fluids	

Disability

Rationale

- To determine Mr Tien's level of cognition
- Restlessness and lethargy are indicators of continuing acute confusional state.
- To identify the progress of delirium
- To assist with communication, to improve safety and provide comfort for Mr Tien
- To prevent pressure areas due to reduced mobility
- To prevent episodes of incontinence

Nursing action	Rationale
Reassess using the CAM	
Engage interpreter service to assist with the other cognitive assessments	
Prompt and assist Mr Tien with toileting	
Monitor psychomotor activity	
Encourage family to stay with Mr Tien	
Communicate Mr Tien's progress to his family	
Encourage gentle ambulation and regular position change	

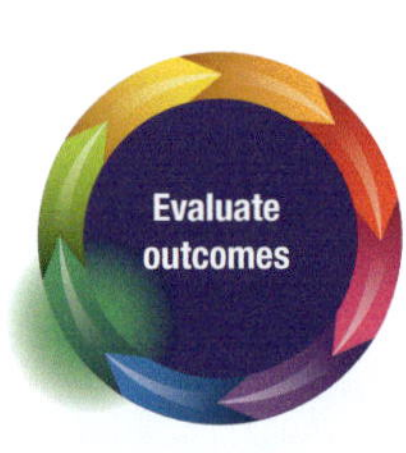

7. EVALUATE

It is 1430 hrs and the end of Tricia's shift. Mr Tien's current signs and symptoms provide cues that will allow her to make a determination of whether or not her interventions have been effective and his condition is improving.

Q Rate each of the following signs and symptoms as *unchanged, improving, deteriorating* or *fluctuating*.

a Language ability: not speaking
b Psychomotor activity: lethargic
c Mood: withdrawn
d Pulse: 90
e BP: 150/85
f Respirations: 24
g SaO_2: 94% (via nasal prongs)
h Urinary continence: using a urinal with prompting and assistance
i Oral intake: eating and drinking food brought in by daughter and with her assistance

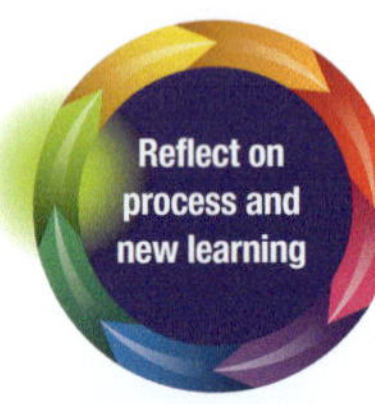

8. REFLECT

Reflect on your learning from this scenario.

Q1 What have you learnt that you can apply to your future nursing practice?

Q2 What actions might the night duty nurse have taken to better manage Mr Tien?

Q3 If you suspect that an older person has an alteration in cognition, what three actions would you take and why would you take them?

Q4 Imagine you overheard one of the nurses calling Mr Tien, 'Sweetheart'. What would your reaction be and why?

If unsure about the answer to Q4, read Gardner et al. (2001), *'Don't call me sweetie!' Patients differ from nurses in their perceptions of caring:* doi: 10.1016/s1322-7696(08)60020-7. PMID: 15484648

SCENARIO 14.2 Caring for an older person with dementia

CHANGING THE SCENE

Mr Tien's condition improves and, after five days, he is discharged and returned home with his daughter, Mrs Nguyen Qui. He has made a good recovery from his pneumonia and delirium but has not returned to his normal level of cognitive or physical functioning. Mr Tien and his family are told by the nurse and medical officer at the hospital that it may take several weeks before he will start to feel strong and clear-headed again.

1. CONSIDER THE PATIENT SITUATION

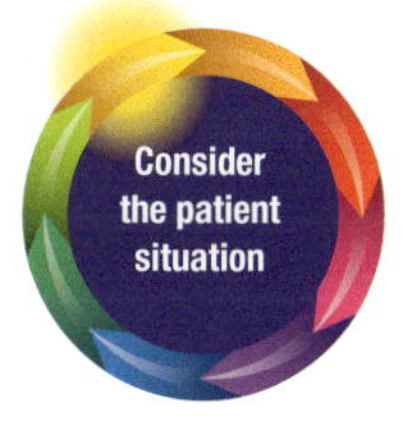

Three weeks following discharge, Kristy, the community nurse, is visiting Mr Tien. His daughter Mrs Qui answers the door and immediately says: 'I'm worried. Dad isn't getting any better and he is more forgetful. Some days he forgets to eat breakfast, doesn't shower or shave, and keeps putting on the same clothes. When I get home, I try to get him to change or bathe but he gets upset and tells me to leave him alone. He tells me I'm not a good daughter, that a good daughter would not question her father. I can't leave him alone all day like this. And he hasn't been going to his chess days since his return from hospital. I am so worried about him.'

Kristy then visits Mr Tien in the next room. He smiles when she enters and nods his head in greeting. Kristy asks him how he is feeling and he replies, 'I'm okay, but my daughter keeps telling me what to do.'

2. COLLECT CUES/INFORMATION

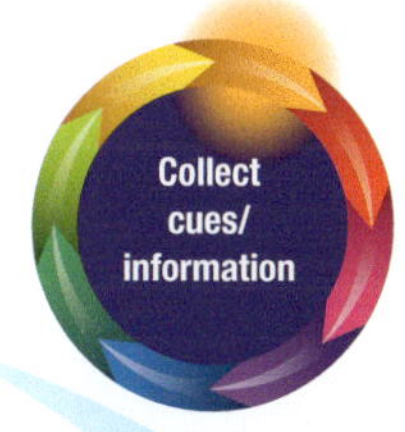

(a) Review current information

Q From the list below, identify the five pieces of information that are *most important* for Kristy's review of Mr Tien at this stage?

- a Current cognitive abilities
- b Details of current medications
- c History of vascular risk factors
- d History of sleep pattern
- e History of bowel and bladder function
- f Mr Tien's past life in Vietnam
- g Medical history
- h Hydration/nutritional status
- i Current level of functional abilities
- j The fact that Mr Tien has not been to his chess sessions since discharge

Hint: Think back to all that you know about Mr Tien and his situation.

(b) Gather new information

Q1 What new information should Kristy gather that would assist her in understanding Mr Tien's current condition more fully?

Q2 Which assessment instruments could Kristy consider using to help her come to a deeper understanding of Mr Tien's current level of cognition?

- a Glasgow Coma Scale (GCS)
- b Mini Mental Status Examination (MMSE)
- c Depression, Anxiety, Stress Scales (DASS21)
- d Abbreviated Mental Test Score (AMTS)
- e Confusion Assessment Method Instrument (CAM)

See the following for more information on these instruments.

GCS: https://www.glasgowcomascale.org/

MMSE: www.ihpa.gov.au/sites/g/files/net636/f/publications/smmse-tool-v2.pdf

DASS21: https://maic.qld.gov.au/wp-content/uploads/2016/07/DASS-21.pdf

AMTS: https://academic.oup.com/ageing/article/44/6/1000/80740

CAM: https://www.delirium.health.qut.edu.au/identification-and-management/confusion-assessment-method

3. PROCESS INFORMATION

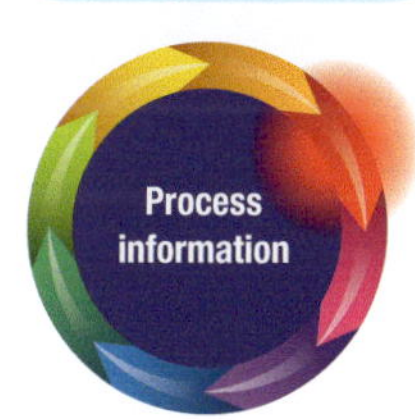

(a) Interpret

Q Which five of the following assessment findings (recorded by Kristy at 1200 hours) would *not* provide her with relevant information about what is happening to Mr Tien?

- a Temperature: 36.4°C
- b Pulse rate: 87 beats/min
- c Respiratory rate: 22 breaths/min

d Blood pressure: 170/85
e SaO_2: 96% (room air)
f Respiratory: lungs clear
g CAM: negative result
h AMTS: 5/10
i DASS21: negative for depressive symptoms but mild anxiety and stress levels
j Food and fluid intake: adequate with prompting from daughter
k Urinalysis: NAD
l Bowels: opened today
m Mood: irritable

Hint: A score of 5 for the AMTS suggests cognitive impairment.

(b) Discriminate

Q From the cues and information you now have, you need to narrow down the information to what is most important. From the list below, select the cues that you believe are *most relevant* to Mr Tien's cognitive status *at this time*.

a Vital signs
b Level of confusion
c SaO_2
d CAM negative result
e AMTS 5/10
f Urinalysis
g DASS21 results
h Mood

Kristy has also noted that Mr Tien's blood pressure is elevated and she will need to report this to Mr Tien's GP.

Patient Safety Competency Framework (PSCF)

Domain 4—Teamwork and collaborative practice

The PSCF states that nurses must collaborate and communicate effectively with members of the healthcare team in ways that facilitate mutual respect and shared decision making.

Source: *The Patient Safety Competency Framework for Nursing Students,* https://patientsafetyfornursingstudents.org

(c) Relate and (d) Infer

Q Cluster the cues together and identify relationships between them. Label the following *true, false* or a *possibility*.

a Mr Tien has cognitive decline associated with ageing.
b Mr Tien is confused because he is hypoxic.
c Mr Tien is confused because he is an older person.
d Mr Tien is depressed because he has not been able to return to his normal activities.
e Mr Tien's cognition has deteriorated because he may have experienced a cerebral vascular event.
f Mr Tien remains in a delirium because he is older and was ill with pneumonia.

(e) Predict

Q If Kristy does not take the appropriate actions regarding Mr Tien's altered cognition at this time, what could happen to Mr Tien? (Select the correct response.)

a Mr Tien could have a stroke.
b Mr Tien could develop depression.
c Mr Tien could fall.
d Mr Tien could become suicidal.
e Mr Tien could develop delirium again.
f Mr Tien's cognitive impairment may be missed.

4. IDENTIFY THE PROBLEM/ISSUE

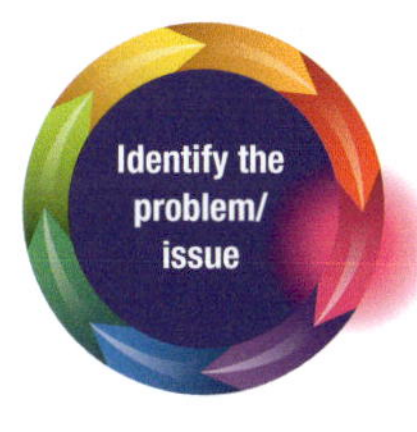

Q Select from the following list, the correct nursing diagnoses for Mr Tien.

a Impaired communication with daughter related to an alteration in cognition, evidenced by Mr Tien's saying, 'I'm okay, but my daughter keeps telling me what to do', and that Mrs Qui is 'not a good daughter'

b Mood disorder related to an alteration in cognition, evidenced by the DASS21 results and Mr Tien not going to his regular chess days

c Personal hygiene deficit related to an alteration in cognition, evidenced by Mr Tien's not bathing and shaving, and putting on the same clothes each day

d Acute confusional state related to an alteration in cognition, evidenced by Mrs Qui stating that Mr Tien is more forgetful

e Cognitive impairment related to a currently unknown pathophysiology, evidenced by Mrs Qui's statement that Mr Tien is more forgetful; CAM negative; T, PR, RR and SaO_2 normal for Mr Tien; AMTS 5/10; DASS21 results; urinalysis–NAD

f Altered nutrition/hydration intake related to an alteration in cognition, evidenced by Mr Tien forgetting to eat breakfast and needing prompting from his daughter to eat

Nursing and Midwifery Board of Australia (NMBA) *Registered Nurse Standards for Practice* The NMBA's *Registered Nurse Standards for Practice* (2016) indicate that RNs must be able to comprehensively assess patients and develop a plan of care based on their assessment findings.

5. ESTABLISH GOALS

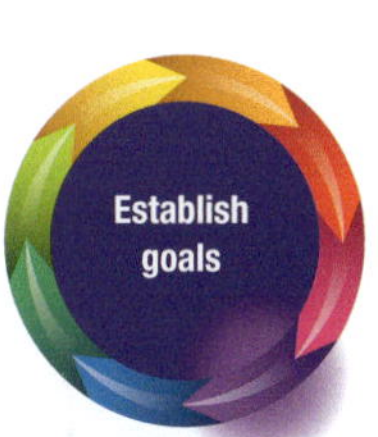

Q From the list below, choose the four most important *short-term* goals for Mr Tien's management at this time.

a For Mr Tien to be orientated and alert

b For Mr Tien to be assessed by his GP

c For Mr Tien to be assessed by ACAT for residential aged-care placement

d For Mr Tien to be showered, shaved and dressed in clean clothes daily

e For Mr Tien's cognition to be assessed by a geriatrician

f For Mr Tien to receive services from an ACAT-approved provider

g For Mr Tien not to state that his daughter is a bad daughter

h For Mr Tien to have an understanding of his cognitive change

i For Mr Tien to eat his meals and drink at least 1600 mL/day

An assessment by ACAT (Aged Care Assessment Team) is required before placement into a residential aged-care facility can occur.

6. TAKE ACTION

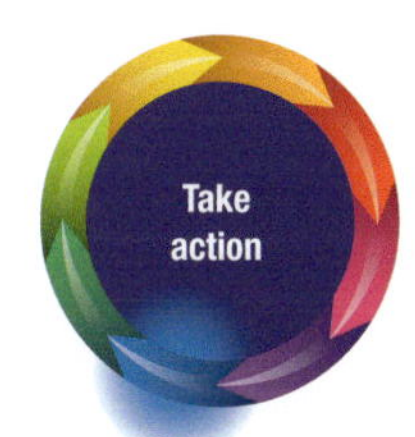

Q Select the nursing actions that must be performed before Kristy concludes her visit with Mr Tien and label these actions with a 1; label the actions that Kristy will perform once she returns to the office with a 2; and label the incorrect actions with a 3.

a Ring Mr Tien's eldest son.

b Discuss the results of the assessments with Mrs Qui.

c Explain to Mr Tien that he is not to speak to his daughter in a negative way.

d Suggest some strategies for Mrs Qui to help with Mr Tien's personal hygiene.

e Plan for readmission to hospital.

f Make a referral to ACAT.

g Arrange for Mr Tien to receive Meals on Wheels.

h Suggest some communication strategies to help Mrs Qui receive positive responses from Mr Tien.

i Discuss the need to organise Mr Tien's admission to a residential aged-care facility in the near future.

j Suggest some strategies that Mrs Qui can use to ensure Mr Tien is eating and drinking adequately.

k Notify Mr Tien's GP of his condition.

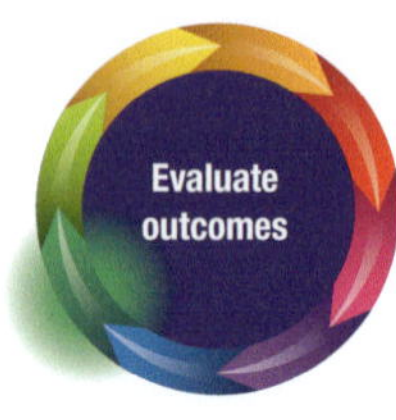

7. EVALUATE

It is now one week later and Kristy is visiting Mr Tien and his daughter. Mr Tien's signs and symptoms provide you with data to make a determination about whether the above interventions have been effective, and if Mr Tien's condition is improving.

Q Rate each of the following signs and symptoms as *unchanged, improving* or *deteriorating*.

AMTS	5/10
CAM	Negative result
Mood	Calm
Pulse	87
Blood pressure	140/75
Respirations	20
SaO_2	96%
DASS 21	No depressive, anxiety or stress symptoms
Personal hygiene	Mr Tien's son, grandsons or son-in-law assist Mr Tien with his showering, shaving and dressing daily.
Communication	Mrs Qui has not been called a bad daughter since Kristy explained what was happening and Mrs Qui has not been bathing him.
Nutrition/hydration	Mrs Qui reports that Mr Tien is eating and drinking as he would usually do.

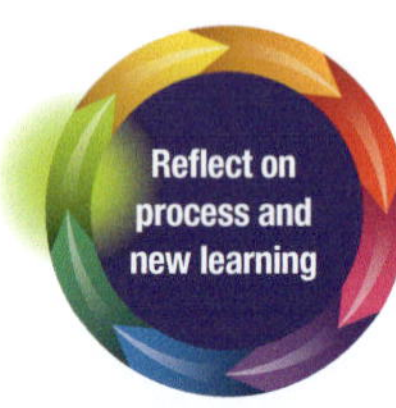

8. REFLECT

Reflect on your learning from this scenario.

Q1 What are three of the most important things that you have learnt from this scenario?

Q2 What three actions will you take in clinical practice as a result of your learning from this scenario?

Q3 What have you learnt about cultural awareness from this scenario that you can apply to your practice?

EPILOGUE

Following further assessment by Mr Tien's GP, he was diagnosed with vascular dementia. The doctor suggested that Mr Tien probably suffered a vascular event triggered by his hypertension during or after hospitalisation. Mr Tien continues to live with his daughter and his family is very supportive. They prefer to care for him at home, with help from community services. Mr Tien is enjoying spending more time with his son and grandsons. He does not attend his chess sessions anymore, but some of his close friends come over for lunch once a month. Mr Tien still works in his garden.

FURTHER READING

Australian Commission on Safety and Quality in Health Care (ACSQHC). (2021). *Delirium Clinical Care Standard*. Sydney: ACSQHC. Retrieved from: https://www.safetyandquality.gov.au/our-work/clinical-care-standards/delirium-clinical-care-standard

Calley, C. T. G., Womack, K., Moore, P., Hart, J. & Kraut, M. (2010). Subjective report of word-finding and memory deficits in normal aging and dementia. *Cognitive Behavioural Neurology, 23*(3), 158–91.

Smith, K., Flicker, L., Shadforth, G., Carroll, E., Ralph, E., Atkinson, D, … LoGiudice, D. (2011). Original research, 'Gotta be sit down and worked out together': Views of Aboriginal caregivers and service providers on ways to improve dementia care for Aboriginal Australians. *Rural and Remote Health: The International Electronic Journal of Rural and Remote Health Research, Education, Practice and Policy, 11*(1650), 1–14.

REFERENCES

American Psychiatric Association. (2013). *Diagnostic and Statistical Manual of Mental Disorders* (5th edn). Arlington, VA: American Psychiatric Association.

Australian Commission on Safety and Quality in Health Care. (2021). *Delirium Clinical Care Standard*. Sydney: ACSQHC.

Australian Commission on Safety and Quality in Health Care. (2021*). National Safety and Quality Health Service Standards* (2nd edn). Sydney: ACSQHC.

Baldwin, R. (2008). Mood disorders: Depressive disorders. In R. Jacoby, C. Oppenheimer, T. Dening & A. Thomas (Eds), *Oxford Textbook of Old Age Psychiatry*. Oxford: Oxford University Press.

Beaudreau, S. A. & O'Hara, R. (2009). The association of anxiety and depressive symptoms with cognitive performance in community-dwelling older adults. *Psychology and Aging*. 24, 507–12.

Dementia Australia. (2021). *Key Facts and Statistics 2021*. Retrieved from: at www. https://www.dementia.org.au/statistics

Edvardsson, D. & Nay, R. (2010). Acute care and older people: Challenges and ways forward. *Australian Journal of Advanced Nursing*, *27*(2), 63–68.

Fick, D. M., Agostini, J. V. & Inouye, S. K. (2002). Delirium superimposed on dementia: A systematic review. *Journal of the American Geriatrics Society*, *50*(10), 1723–32.

Gardner, A., Goodsell, J., Duggen, T., Murtha, B., Peck, C. & Williams, J. (2001). 'Don't call me sweetie!' Patients differ from nurses in their perceptions of caring, *Collegian*, *8*(3), 32–38.

Hunter, S. & Miller, C. (2016). *Miller's Nursing for Wellness in Older Adults*. Sydney: Lippincott Williams & Wilkins Pty Ltd (Chapters 11–15).

Inouye, S. K. (2006). Delirium in older persons. *New England Journal of Medicine*, *354*(11), 1157–65.

Insel, K. & Bager, T. (2002). Deciphering the 4Ds: Cognitive decline, delirium, depression and dementia: A review. *Journal of Advanced Nursing*, *38*(4), 360–68.

Levett-Jones, T. Dwyer, T., Reid-Searl, K., Heaton, L., Flenady, T., Applegarth, J., Guinea, S. & Andersen, P. (2017). *The Patient Safety Competency Framework for Nursing Students*. Retrieved from: http://psframework.wpengine.com/wp-content/uploads/2018/01/PSCF_Brochure_UTS-version_FA2-Screen.pdf

National Ageing Research Institute (NARI). (2009). *Depression in Older Age: A Scoping Study—Final Report*. Retrieved from: www.beyondblue.org.au/docs/default-source/research-project-files/bw0143nari-2009-full-reportminus-appendices.pdf?sfvrsn4

Nursing and Midwifery Board of Australia (NMBA). (2016). *Registered Nurse Standards for Practice*. Retrieved from: www.nursingmidwiferyboard.gov.au/Codes-Guidelines-Statements/Professional-standards.aspx

Patel, B. B. & Holland, N. W. (2012). Mild cognitive impairment: Hope for stability, plan for progression. *Cleveland Clinic Journal of Medicine*, *79*(12), 857–64.

Queensland Health (2011). *Vietnamese Australians*. Retrieved from: https://www.health.qld.gov.au/__data/assets/pdf_file/0029/157439/vietnamese2011.pdf

Tieges, Z. Maclullich, A. M. J., Anand, A., Brookes, C., Cassarino, M., O'Connor, M., … Galvin, R. (2021). Diagnostic accuracy of the 4AT for delirium detection in older adults: Systematic review and meta-analysis, *Age and Ageing, 50*(3), 733–43, doi.org/10.1093/ageing/afaa224

Travers, C. Byrne, G. J., Pachana, N. A., Klein, K. & Gray, L. (2013). Delirium in Australian hospitals: A prospective study. *Current Gerontology and Geriatrics Research*, vol. 2013, Article ID 284780, 8 pages. doi.org/10.1155/2013/284780

Chapter 15

Caring for a young person with a disability

STEPHEN GUINEA, JESSICA McKIRKLE and CHRISTINE IMMS

LEARNING OUTCOMES

Completion of the activities in this chapter will enable you to:

- describe techniques for effective therapeutic nurse/patient communication in the context of young adults with a disability (**recall** and **application**)
- explain and describe common physiological, developmental and psychosocial manifestations of cerebral palsy, particular to a young adult, that will guide the collection of cues (**gather, review, interpret, discriminate, relate** and **infer**)
- review information to identify the main nursing diagnoses for a person with a disability and their family (**synthesise**)
- describe the priorities of care for a young adult with a disability, taking into account legislation and the role of the registered nurse in advocacy for patient autonomy (**goal setting** and **taking action**)
- identify criteria for evaluating the effectiveness of nursing actions taken to enhance person-centred care (**evaluate**)
- consider potential challenges to planning and implementing person-centred care for a person with a disability (**reflection** and **translation**)
- reflect on your ability to practise person-centred care that promotes advocacy for the young adult with a disability (**reflection** and **translation**).

INTRODUCTION

The two scenarios introduced in this chapter focus on the care of a young adult with a physical disability. You will meet Amelia, a 22-year-old woman who has cerebral palsy, and explore her story of transition to an autonomous young adult. Cerebral palsy (CP) is the most common physical disability in children in Australia (Australian Cerebral Palsy Register Group [ACPRG], 2018). It is caused by non-progressive injury to the developing foetal or infant brain (Wimalasundera & Stevenson, 2016), and is a complex, permanent condition that primarily affects an individual's movement and posture. People who have cerebral palsy often have additional conditions, such as vision or hearing loss, epilepsy, communication difficulties, intellectual impairment or behavioural problems.

For teens and young adults with a chronic illness or disability, this period of their life is often characterised as one of transition: transition from paediatric to adult care, from dependence to autonomy, and interdependence or independence. In addition, entwined with this period of transition is the stigma associated with physical and intellectual disability that may accompany cerebral palsy (Myers et al., 2020; Rosenbaum & Rosenbloom, 2012). Structured social age markers, which historically have been used to define the timing of a child transitioning to adolescence and young adulthood, may be less relevant for those with a disability as these transitions may occur at later ages. Defining the timing and duration of transitions may be more effectively based on a series of decisions made by the multidisciplinary healthcare team, the individual, and their family (Furlong, 2009). The aim of the multidisciplinary healthcare team should be to minimise the negative impact on the health and wellbeing of the young adult with a disability and their carers (Brown, Higgins & MacArthur, 2019).

Person-centred care of a young adult requires an in-depth and holistic approach, respecting them as individuals, as well as members of their families and wider communities. Knowledge of the person's physical, psychosocial and cultural history and preferences is essential to person-centred care. Nurses require insight into the young adult's needs as an *autonomous person* and must respond effectively to the expert knowledge of the patient and their family, rather than as someone for whom a series of tasks needs to be completed (Brown, Higgins & MacArthur, 2019). Well-developed clinical reasoning skills can assist nurses to understand and consider different perspectives such as those portrayed in this chapter, resulting in empathic, considered and appropriate nursing care.

KEY CONCEPTS

disability
cerebral palsy
person-centred care
family-centred care
healthcare transition
interprofessional healthcare team
discharge planning

SUGGESTED READINGS

Agency for Clinical Innovation. (2014). *Key Principles for Transition of Young People from Paediatric to Adult Health Care.* Retrieved from: www.aci.health.nsw.gov.au/__data/assets/pdf_file/0011/251696/Key_Principles_for_Transition.pdf

A. Merritt & M. Boogaerts. (2014). Psychosocial care. In E. Chang & A. Johnson (Eds), *Chronic Illness & Disability: Principles for Nursing Practice* (2nd edn). Sydney: Churchill Livingstone.

D. Tasker & T. De Bortoli. (2019). Communicating with people who have communication impairment. In T. Levett-Jones (Ed.), *Critical Conversations for Patient Safety: An Essential Guide for Health Professionals* (2nd edn). Sydney: Pearson Australia.

SCENARIO 15.1 Discovering the person behind the disability

SETTING THE SCENE

Amelia Traynor is a 22-year-old woman who was admitted to hospital three days ago for treatment of aspiration pneumonia and the insertion of a percutaneous endoscopic gastrostomy (PEG) tube. Amelia has a diagnosis of cerebral palsy. She underwent the surgical insertion of the PEG tube yesterday morning. You have been allocated the care of Amelia during the morning shift. The time is 1130 hrs and you are preparing to assist Amelia with her shower.

The epidemiology of cerebral palsy

Cerebral palsy (CP) affects 1.4 in every 1,000 births in Australia (ACPRG, 2018). There are proportionally more Aboriginal and Torres Strait Islander children affected by cerebral palsy in Australia, and these children often have more severe motor and other associated impairments compared with their non-Indigenous peers. Birth prevalence of CP has declined in Australia, with the percentage of children born with moderate to severe disability decreasing (ACPRG, 2018).

For most people, the causes of CP remain unknown. However, four groups that are at statistically greater risk of CP are: males (approximately 57%); premature babies; babies of low birth weight; and children from a multiple birth (ACPRG, 2018). The financial cost of caring for a person with CP in Australia has been estimated at over $145,642 per person per year, of which the largest cost burden is borne by the person or their family (Deloitte Access Economics, 2020). It must be acknowledged that there may be significant psychosocial, emotional and physical costs to individuals and their families associated with living with CP.

The aetiology and pathogenesis of cerebral palsy

Cerebral palsy is a term that refers to a group of permanent disorders of development, movement and posture. It is caused by non-progressive disturbances to the developing brain during pregnancy or soon after birth. Cerebral palsy is a complex disability, where the manifestations are dependent on the areas of the brain affected. It can affect body movement, muscle control, muscle coordination, muscle tone, reflex, posture and balance (Wimalasundera & Stevenson, 2016). In addition to motor disorders, people living with CP often experience disturbances of sensation, perception, cognition, communication and behaviour (Wimalasundera & Stevenson, 2016).

Cerebral palsy is classified according to the part of the body affected and is defined as bilateral or unilateral. Bilateral CP affects both sides of the body. It may be further classified as diplegic where both legs are affected with the arms affected to a lesser extent, or quadraplegic where all four limbs, as well as the muscles of the trunk, face and mouth, are affected. Unilateral (or hemiplegic) CP affects the left or right side of the body only.

Cerebral palsy is also classified according to the way it affects people's movements, with each classification related to the damaged part of the brain. These are presented in Table 15.1.

Functional presentations associated with cerebral palsy

Along with understanding what part of the body is affected and the type of motor disorder, there are four important functional classification systems used for people with CP that provide a clear description of their abilities and paint a picture of the severity of the condition. In each of these classification systems, the individual's usual ability is described. The Gross Motor Function Classification System—Expanded and Revised (GMFCS-ER) provides a way of classifying the individual's ability to make self-initiated movements related to sitting and walking. The GMFCS is a five-level system as presented below (based on Palisano et al., 2008).

Level I—Walks without restrictions; limitations in more advanced gross motor skills
Level II—Walks without assistive devices; limitations walking outdoors and in the community
Level III—Walks with assistive mobility devices; limitations walking outdoors and in the community
Level IV—Self-mobility with limitations; individuals are transported or use power mobility outdoors and in the community
Level V—Self-mobility is severely limited even with the use of assistive devices.

Table 15.1 *Motor disorders associated with cerebral palsy*

Movement disorder	Prevalence (of all people living with cerebral palsy)	Aetiology	Manifestations
Spastic	70–80%	Damage to the motor cortex	Muscle tone is increased, so movements feel stiff or limbs resist movement. • Stiff, rigid muscles due to hypertonia • Stiff, jerky or absent limb movement • Difficulty controlling individual muscles or muscle groups required, e.g. when handling objects or speaking.
Dyskinetic (dyskinesia)	6% (in isolation)	Damage to the basal ganglia	Involuntary patterns of movement of groups of muscles or body parts. Dyskinesia manifests in different ways depending on the locus of damage to the basal ganglia. • Dystonia: slow twisting or repetitive movements, or abnormal posture of a limb (or digit, mouth or eyes) or the body, that may be triggered when the person attempts to move, or by excitement, startle, stress or other events. • Athetosis: slow, continuous writhing movements that are present at rest and worsened by attempts to move. Muscle tone fluctuates between hypotonia (floppy muscle tone) and hyperkinesia (extremely variable muscle tone). • Chorea: involuntary movements that are brief, abrupt, irregular and unpredictable. Chorea can affect speech and swallowing as well as limb movement, and is often worsened when attempting to move, or with anxiety or stress.
Ataxic (ataxia)	6%	Damage to the cerebellum	Ataxia is an incoordination of muscle control when a person attempts to perform voluntary muscle movements involving the arms and legs. Movements are not smooth and may appear tremulous, jerky, imprecise, unbalanced or uncoordinated.
Mixed	Common	Multiple areas of damage	Depending on the areas of brain damage, mixed motor type will involve a combination of movement disorders. Most commonly those with spasticity will also have dystonia.

Sources: Based on Cerebral Palsy Alliance. (2018). *Types of Cerebral Palsy*. Retrieved from www.cerebralpalsy.org.au/what-is-cerebral-palsy/types-of-cerebral-palsy; J. Crosbie, A. A. A. Alhusaini, C. M. Dean & R. B. Shepherd (2012). Plantarflexor muscle and spatiotemporal gait characteristics of children with hemiplegic cerebral palsy: An observational study. *Developmental Neurorehabilitation*, *15*(2), 114–18.

The Manual Ability Classification System (MACS) is designed to describe the individual's ability to handle objects in important daily activities, such as eating, dressing or at school/work. The five levels of the MACS are presented below (Eliasson et al., 2006):

Level I—Handles objects easily and successfully
Level II—Handles most objects but with somewhat reduced quality and/or speed of achievement
Level III—Handles objects with difficulty; needs help to prepare and/or modify activities
Level IV—Handles a limited selection of easily managed objects in adapted situations
Level V—Does not handle objects and has severely limited ability to perform even simple actions.

The Communication Function Classification System (CFCS) describes the individual's communication ability. The five levels of the CFCS are listed below (based on Hidecker et al., 2011):

Level I—Sends (can talk or use device) and receives (understands) with familiar and unfamiliar communication partners effectively and efficiently
Level II—Sends and/or receives with unfamiliar and/or familiar communication partners but may be slower
Level III—Sends and receives with familiar communication partners effectively but not with unfamiliar communication partners
Level IV—Inconsistently sends and receives communication even with familiar communication partners
Level V—Seldom effective sender and receiver even with familiar communication partners.

The Eating and Drinking Ability Classification System (EDACS) assists in understanding the ability individuals have with managing eating and drinking. These are the five levels of the EDACS (Sellers et al., 2014):

Level I—Eats and drinks safely and efficiently
Level II—Eats and drinks safely but with some limitation to efficiency
Level III—Eats and drinks with some limitations to safety; there may be limitations to efficiency
Level IV—Eats and drinks with significant limitations to safety
Level V—Unable to eat or drink safely; tube feeding may be considered to provide nutrition.

The Visual Function Classification System (VFCS) was published in 2020 and describes how young people with cerebral palsy use their visual abilities in daily life. The five levels of the VFCS are (summarised from Baranello et al., 2019):

Level I—Uses visual function easily and successfully
Level II—Uses visual function successfully but needs to use compensatory strategies
Level III—Uses visual function but needs some adaptations
Level IV—Uses visual function in very adapted environments but use is restricted and inconsistent
Level V—Does not use visual function even in very adapted environments.

Knowing the motor type, the distribution of the disorder and an individual's classification provides a wealth of important information about someone with CP. A person may have limited ability to walk (GMFCS Level III), good communication (CFCS Level I), adequate ability to handle objects (MACS Level II), significant difficulties managing food and drink (EDACS Level IV), and good visual function (VFCS Level I). In addition, 20–28 per cent of individuals with CP may have moderate to severe intellectual impairment (ACPRG, 2018), which can also impact on their daily functioning. As can be appreciated, no two people with cerebral palsy are the same and cannot be treated as such. Whilst the damage to the brain does not deteriorate over time, the effects of CP on the body may result in increasing impairment, especially in their musculoskeletal system. Therefore, an individualised care plan is required to meet the needs of people with this disability and those of their family.

National Safety and Quality Health Service (NSQH) Standards

Comprehensive care standard

The NSQHS Standards specify that health professionals must provide coordinated healthcare that is 'aligned with the patient's expressed goals of care and healthcare needs, considers the impact of the patient's health issues on their life and wellbeing, and is clinically appropriate' (ACSQHC, 2021).

Person-centred care

Amelia Traynor was born to Kathryn and Jim Traynor at 33 weeks gestation via caesarean section, secondary to pre-eclampsia. Her initial APGAR score at birth was 7 with no movement of limbs and 'floppy' muscle tone. This score remained unchanged at 5 and 10 minutes post-birth.

What is an APGAR test? What assessment information does it provide?

Over the coming months, Amelia failed to meet developmental milestones and subsequently underwent a number of tests, observations and evaluations.

Amelia's diagnosis of spastic quadriplegic cerebral palsy was made when she was 12 months old. Her condition has resulted in the following functional impairments:

Due to the complex nature of CP, confirming a diagnosis can take some time. When it is severe, a diagnosis may be made soon after birth, but for many children, diagnosis may take longer. Recent efforts towards early detection and intervention have reduced the time to diagnosis, and many children will be diagnosed within the first 12 months of life. Diagnosis is best made using a neuro-developmental assessment, general movements assessment, MRI, cranial ultrasound or CT scans.

- Amelia converses with people effectively; however, she has slow and slurred speech. People who don't know Amelia take about 15 minutes to get used to how she speaks—they can then usually understand what she says (CFCS Level II).
- Amelia requires a fully supported wheelchair to help her with sitting balance, and someone to push the chair (GMFCS Level V).
- Amelia has difficulty handling objects. She needs someone to set up activities and support her to do them (MACS Level III).
- Amelia does not have an intellectual impairment.

Amelia lives with her parents in a single-storey house in a metropolitan area. When Amelia was a child, her mother Kathryn stopped work to provide full-time care. Both Kathryn and Jim are central to Amelia's care and have, with considerable effort, managed to juggle the demands of work and family life through a strict routine. Typically, Jim has been responsible for Amelia's physical transfers—they have a hoist in the family home to assist with this—whilst Kathryn has managed her daughter's hygiene, nutritional and health requirements. Both parents assist with socialisation, including transporting Amelia to activities. Amelia is rarely alone, accompanied by either her parents or siblings most of the time. Both parents are active in the CP community, engaging in fundraising and community awareness programs; and Jim and Kathryn have ensured Amelia has been a central figure in these activities.

Amelia is the eldest of three children and her two siblings are Sebastian, 18 years, and Naomi, aged 15. The relationship between Amelia and Naomi is very close. In contrast, Sebastian, at times, speaks to his friends of resenting his older sister as he feels he has missed out on some of the opportunities and 'normal' life that his friends have had.

At the age of 19, Amelia completed secondary school. For Amelia, secondary school was characterised by her differences. While she was, on occasion, teased about her disability, a greater challenge to her self-concept was the ways in which accommodations were made for her disability; accommodations that

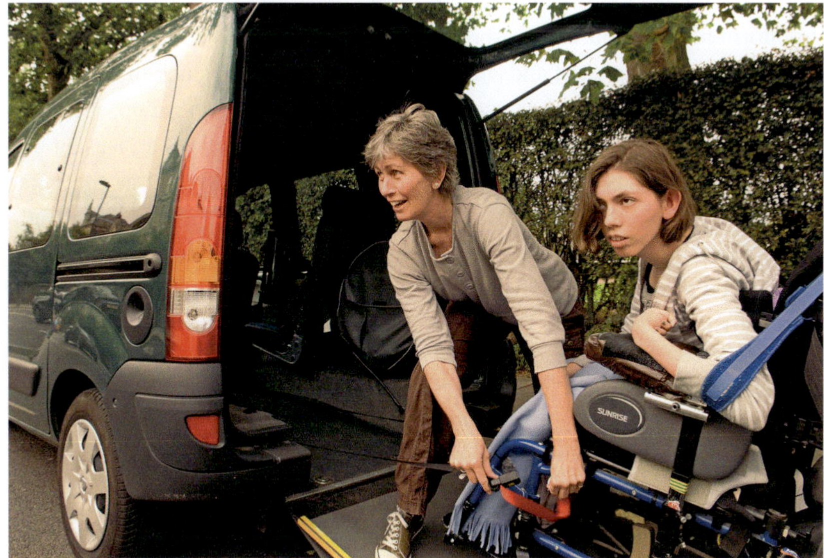

Source: Paul Doyle/Alamy Stock Photo

she did not always want. Whilst Amelia knew that people meant well, she often felt that, when people went out of their way to make her feel included, it highlighted the fact she was different. As Amelia reached her late teens, these same feelings extended towards her parents as well. Consequently, over the past two years, Amelia has been yearning for greater autonomy and more independence from her mother and father.

Key Principles for Transition of Young People from Paediatric to Adult Health Care from the Agency for Clinical Innovation and Trapeze (2014) provides useful information about planning for transition.

For children and teenagers living with disability, the transition to becoming an autonomous adult may be delayed, with parents continuing to assume a significant role in decision making on behalf of their child. Amelia feels she is ready and capable of making her own decisions in relation to who provides her care, and who she socialises with and when. Recently, Amelia has been chatting to friends online about engaging in further study. One friend in particular introduced her to a not-for-profit organisation called the Cerebral Palsy Alliance.

Amelia has explored programs offered by this organisation and has wondered if she would be eligible for assistance that would help her obtain future employment, and enable her to move out of home and into supported accommodation. Amelia tried to discuss this with her parents and, while her father appeared to consider the idea, her mother would not engage in any discussion. Amelia has had to put such ambitions on hold due to the recent deterioration in her health.

The Cerebral Palsy Alliance has a useful website: www.cerebralpalsy.org.au

While Amelia has always had some difficulty with eating and drinking (EDACS Level III), she has been able to maintain her ability to do so. Over the past six months, Kathryn noticed Amelia attempting to clear her throat and 'gurgling' much more frequently than usual when drinking. Following a series of assessments by her paediatrician and a speech pathologist, Amelia was gradually progressed to Grade 5 thickened fluids to minimise the risk of choking and aspiration, and to provide adequate nutritional intake. However, Amelia's dysphagia worsened and resulted in aspiration pneumonia, requiring hospitalisation.

On admission to hospital, Amelia was febrile with a temperature of 39.2°C. She was tachycardic, dehydrated and lethargic. A formal assessment by a speech pathologist and radiographer, comprising video fluoroscopy, found a delayed onset of laryngeal closure and aspiration into both lungs. These assessment findings concluded that Amelia was unable to clear fluids and protect her airway due to her impaired swallow and weak cough. It was recommended that Amelia undergo a surgical insertion of a PEG for enteral nutrition and remain nil-by-mouth from this time.

1. CONSIDER THE PATIENT SITUATION

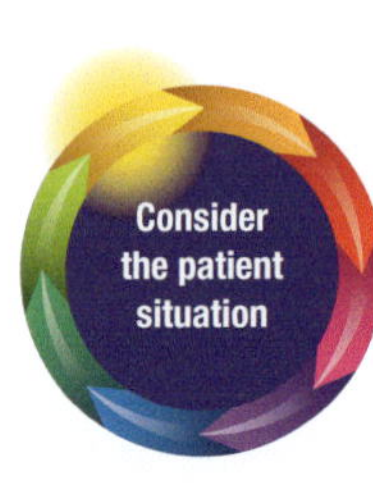

It has been a busy morning in the surgical ward; however, you are feeling like you're doing a good job today as you've provided care according to Amelia's nursing care plan. This has included: attending to Amelia's toileting needs; obtaining vital signs; administering her morning medications and enteral nutrition; assessing the PEG insertion site; and attending to pressure area care. You have just returned from your morning break and have collected the shower chair, towels, a clean hospital gown and the lifter to assist with transferring Amelia from bed to the shower chair.

You approach Amelia to inform her that you will be showering her as soon as a second nurse is able to assist with the transfer. Amelia becomes agitated and states forcibly, 'I have been stuck in this bed all morning. I never stay in bed this late. I feel sweaty and uncomfortable and I just want to get up, showered and in my chair.' You are unsettled by this outburst as it was handed over that Amelia is a pleasant and compliant patient. However, the awkwardness of responding to this outburst is avoided as the nurse arrives to assist with the transfer.

Once in the shower, you are relieved that Amelia appears more settled. You have almost finished the shower when Amelia asks, 'Can you hand me the shower head? I like the feeling of water on my face. I can do things you know.' Whilst you're drying Amelia, she begins to open up. Here is what she says:

> *What I really like is when people ask me for my opinion. I like to get up early in the morning, have a shower before breakfast and get in my chair. I don't like being in bed all day. I don't like these hospital gowns. I am not sick and would like my own clothes. Just because I have CP, people think that everything, every decision needs to be made for me. I am not a kid. I know I can do things for myself, and make decisions for myself. Even mum and dad don't understand this. I love mum and dad but they control*

every part of my life. This PEG tube is a good example. I was not really given any choice; I had to get the tube. I hate it! I was hoping to move out of home and to have carers who are my own age. I don't want to be so dependent on my parents. I know people who have CP and they are independent. I know I can be too, but the tube is going to make it even harder.

2. COLLECT CUES/INFORMATION

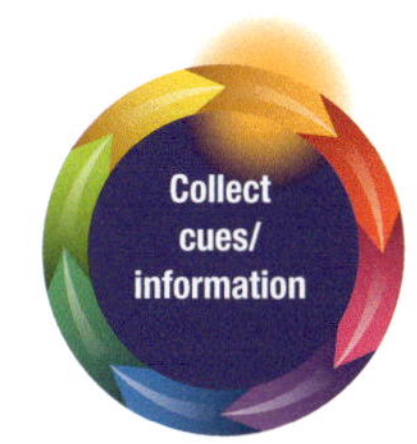

(a) Review current information

Following the shower, you reflect on the very personal information that Amelia has just shared. You realise that Amelia has a desire for autonomy—a desire that is not being met in this hospital admission, and perhaps not within the family unit. You also feel unsure about what to do in this situation. You decide to start by reviewing what you know in terms of related subjective and objective data (see Table 15.2).

Table 15.2 *Subjective and objective information about Amelia*

Subjective	Objective
Amelia states her desire to: • be asked her opinion in planning her care • be showered before breakfast • select her clothes for the day • make decisions independent of her parents • move out of home and into supported accommodation • be showered and dressed by someone her own age • not be dependent on her parents.	**Medical/surgical history:** • Elective admission to an adult surgical unit for treatment of aspiration pneumonia and insertion of PEG tube • Diagnosed with spastic quadriplegic cerebral palsy at 12 months of age • Deterioration of swallow reflex and weak cough **Vital signs at 1000 hrs:** • Temperature: 37.4°C • Pulse rate: 82 (strong and regular) • Respiratory rate: 22 • Blood pressure (at rest): 134/78 mmHg • O_2 saturations: 96% (room air) • Numeric pain scale: 4/10 **Lung auscultation:** • Late inspiratory fine crackles in bases of both lungs **Integumentary:** • Skin dry and intact **Wounds:** • PEG insertion site–clean with slight serous fluid

Q Which objective assessment findings suggest Amelia's aspiration pneumonia is improving? Why?

(b) Gather new information

Nurses are familiar with conducting health history assessments. However, engaging in conversations that focus on developmental and psychosocial issues relating to disability can be challenging. Such conversations can be particularly challenging when assessing physical, emotional and social dimensions of adolescents and young adults.

Q1 You suspect that Amelia's health history on admission has omitted some important information needed to provide person-centred care. How would you initiate a conversation with Amelia in order to conduct a more holistic assessment?

a 'Amelia, I want to discuss further what you were saying in the shower. You are visibly upset, so let's talk about this now and see if we can come up with a solution together.'

b 'Let's have an open and honest conversation about what is going on in your life. Let's invite your mum as she can give some great insight into the issues you are facing.'

c 'Amelia, thank you for opening up to me in the shower and sharing some concerns you have. I was wondering if we could talk about this some more, so we can come up with an appropriate solution together. Is now a good time?'

d 'Amelia, from what you are saying, there appears to be some urgency to this situation. I can see you're upset, but if you talk to me now I can get a routine in place to meet your needs.'

The Royal Children's Hospital Melbourne provides guidance for engaging with and assessing an adolescent, including communication style, how to convey confidentiality and requirements for consent: www.rch.org.au/clinicalguide/guideline_index/Engaging_with_and_assessing_the_adolescent_patient

Q2 Each of the questions in the following table are from different categories in the HEEADSSS assessment (The Royal Children's Hospital Melbourne, 2016). They can be used in planning person-centred care by providing useful insights to Amelia's values, beliefs and desires. Identify the corresponding focus for each set of questions in the table below.

Focus

- Safety from injury and violence
- Education and employment
- Activities
- Drugs and alcohol
- Home
- Eating and exercise
- Suicide, depression and self-harm
- Sexuality and gender

Focus	Psychosocial assessment
	Where do you live? How long have you lived where you live? Who do you live with? How do you feel about the relationships in your life? Where would you like to live? Can you tell me about the types of benefits and supports you receive?
	When did you finish school? What did you like about school? What did you dislike about school? How did you get along with your classmates? What are your thoughts about study in the future? What are your thoughts about work, now and in the future?
	How do you feel about the PEG tube? How will the PEG tube impact on your life? How do you feel the PEG will impact on how you see yourself? What does receiving fluids through your PEG feel like? What do you feel can be done to help normalise receiving nutrition via the PEG? How will you manage when you want to go to a restaurant with your friends?
	Do you spend most of your time with friends or family? Do you have a best friend or a few friends? How long have you had your friends for? Where do you meet your friends? When and where do you meet with your friends? How do you get there? What kinds of organised activities do you go to? How much time do you spend in front of the TV or a computer each day? What are your feelings about faith and spirituality?

Focus	Psychosocial assessment
	How do you feel about smoking, drinking and illicit drugs? What is the impact of cigarettes, alcohol and illicit drugs at home? When you meet your friends, how many of your friends smoke, drink and take illicit drugs? How do you pay for any drugs or alcohol you use? What would you like to change about your use of cigarettes, alcohol and/or illicit drugs?
	Have you had a previous girlfriend or boyfriend? Can you tell me about your previous sexual relationships? Have you ever used, or are you currently using, contraception? Have you had a sexual experience in the past that made you feel uncomfortable or disrespected? Do you want to have children? Have you been, or are you, pregnant? When did you last have a Pap test or breast examination? When did you last have a testicular examination?
	Do you have feelings of being down or sad? If so: • How often do you have these feelings? • What do you do when you have such feelings? Do you have trouble falling or staying asleep? Do you find yourself feeling tired or having little energy? Do you feel more vulnerable than usual? Do you feel hopeless or helpless? Have you had thoughts of hurting yourself in some way?
	What mobility devices do you use? What modes of transport do you use? Do you feel safe using these? What challenges concern you about your safety?

Source: Based on The Royal Children's Hospital, Melbourne. (2019). 'The HEEADSSS psychosocial interview for adolescents' in *Engaging with and assessing the adolescent patient*. Melbourne, Australia. Available from: https://www.rch.org.au/clinicalguide/guideline_index/Engaging_with_and_assessing_the_adolescent_patient

The HEEADSSS assessment tool can guide the process of psychosocial screening.

(c) Recall knowledge

You begin to recall what you know about the role of the nurse in promoting person-centred care.

Q1 A person-centred approach to nursing care emphasises:

- a The nurses' knowledge and experience
- b The point of view of the individual as a partner in their own care
- c The nurse as the provider of care
- d An unequal power relationship between the nurse and the individual

Q2 An essential part of a therapeutic relationship is collaborative decision making. Collaborative decision making involves:

- a The nurse and the individual agreeing on a goal
- b Negotiating the approach to achieving the goal that is most acceptable to the nurse and the individual
- c Combining the nurse's knowledge and experience with the individual's knowledge, perspectives and desires
- d All of the options

Q3 One of the most effective approaches to the management of disability is self-management. Self-management is when:

- a The person takes responsibility for the management of their own condition

b There is shared responsibility between the nurse and the person in the management of their care
c The person is independent in the management of their own care
d The person hands the responsibility for the management of their own condition over to another

Q4 Nurses contribute to person-centred care by empowering the person so that they can manage their own care. Empowerment may involve:
a Defining what the nurse will or will not do
b Defining what the person will or will not do
c Family members speaking on behalf of the person
d The nurse understanding and empathising with the person's point of view, as well as negotiating and resolving conflicting expectations relating to healthcare

Q5 A critical role of the nurse is that of an advocate for the individual. Which five of Amelia's statements indicate the need for patient advocacy?
a I feel like they (mum and dad) control every part of my life.
b What I really like is when people ask me for my opinion.
c I was not really given any choice; I had to get the (PEG) tube.
d I was hoping to move out of home.
e I like to get up early in the morning; I don't like being in bed all day.
f I was hoping to have some carers my own age.
g I was hoping to be showered and dressed by someone my own age.
h I am not sick and would like my own clothes.

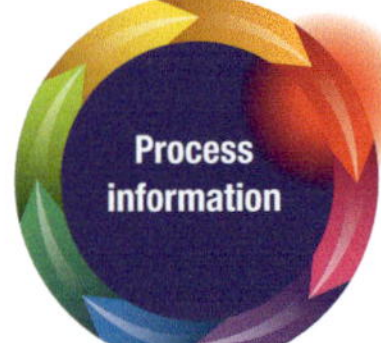

3. PROCESS INFORMATION

(a) Interpret

The next step in the clinical reasoning cycle is to interpret the data you have collected about Amelia. Interpretation of information can be more difficult when working with data that is subjective rather than objective. In such situations, our sometimes unconscious biases may inadvertently influence the way in which data is interpreted, due to one's previous life experiences or prior expectations. This is called *ascertainment bias*, with examples including stereotyping, ageism, stigmatising and gender bias. Understanding and considering different perspectives allows nurses to plan and implement empathetic, considered and appropriate person-centred care. To better understand ascertainment bias in relation to Amelia, consider the following questions:

Q1 What are your previous life experiences and prior expectations that could influence your interpretation of the information about this situation?

Q2 The situation involves differing values, beliefs and priorities. We are aware of Amelia's values, beliefs and priorities, but those of Amelia's family are not as well known. How might they affect the situation?

Nursing and Midwifery Board of Australia (NMBA) *Registered Nurse Standards for Practice* The NMBA's *Registered Nurse Standards for Practice* (2016) state that RNs must respect each person's dignity, culture, values, beliefs and rights. This means that, as nurses, we need to be aware of the ways our biases may influence our nursing practice.

(b) Discriminate

Amelia's scenario is complex. The subjective nature of the situation, the essential role of the family in Amelia's life and the complexity of this situation require the discrimination between what is achievable in the short term and what will take longer to achieve.

Q From the list below, select four cues that you believe are most troubling to Amelia at this time.

a Not being asked her preference for activities of daily living
b Her desire to move from home to supported accommodation
c Parents' involvement in the planning and implementation of Amelia's care
d Pain score of 4/10
e Temperature: 37.4°C
f The insertion of the PEG tube
g Bilateral fine crackles in the bases of both lungs

(c) Relate and (d) Infer

It is important to cluster the cues together and to identify relationships between them (based on the information you have collected so far). From these cues, you can make inferences about Amelia's situation.

Q Are the following *true* or *false*?

a Due to her cerebral palsy, Amelia cannot legally provide informed consent.
b The insertion of the PEG tube signifies for Amelia a deterioration in her condition.
c Amelia's agitation can be attributed to a temperature of 37.4°C, abnormal lung sounds and pain score of 4/10.
d Amelia's transition from adolescence to adulthood has been delayed due to her disability-related needs.
e Amelia's desire for independence from her parents is not realistic due to her disability and insufficient community services.
f Amelia requires the PEG tube as she cannot feed herself.
g Amelia's medical diagnosis of spastic cerebral palsy will result in an inability to conceive and a limited life span.

(e) Match

If this is the first time you have encountered this kind of situation, you will probably experience feelings of uncertainty towards engaging in conversations that involve negotiating the different perspectives and desires of the person and their family.

Q Think about people you have encountered in your everyday life who may have the same disability as Amelia. How do they appear to function independently?

(f) Predict

Now is the time to consider the consequences of your action or inaction by predicting potential outcomes for Amelia and her family.

Q Amelia is due to be discharged tomorrow. If there is no change initiated during this admission, what might be the consequences? Indicate whether each of the following is *highly likely, possible* or *unlikely*.

	Highly likely	Possible	Unlikely
a Amelia's mother and father will continue to manage all aspects of Amelia's life.			
b Amelia will enrol herself into an online learning program.			
c Amelia will be empowered in self-management of her activities of daily living.			
d Amelia's psychosocial issues will not be resolved.			

	Highly likely	Possible	Unlikely
e A partnership between Amelia and her mother will occur in the form of negotiating how and when nutrition will be provided.			
f Amelia will be at risk of depression or self-harm due to not 'being heard'.			

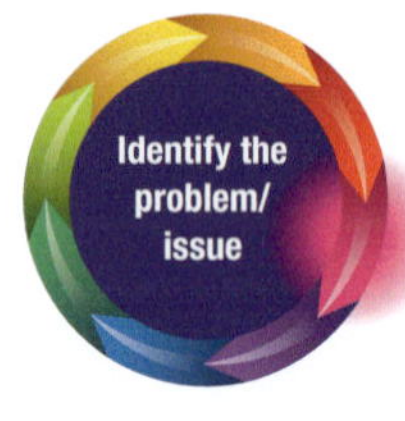

4. IDENTIFY THE PROBLEM/ISSUE

At this stage, you bring together (synthesise) all of the facts you have collected and inferences you have made to make a definitive nursing diagnosis for Amelia.

Q Select from the following list, *one* nursing diagnosis that best reflects Amelia's current situation.

a Ineffective health management related to aspiration, as evidenced by a medical diagnosis of aspiration pneumonia

b Potential for disturbed personal identity of parents related to change of roles, as evidenced by Amelia's increasing independence

c Infection related to PEG tube insertion site, as evidenced by temperature of 37.4°C

d Impeded transition to autonomous adulthood related to disability and family dynamics, as evidenced by Amelia's desire for increased independence

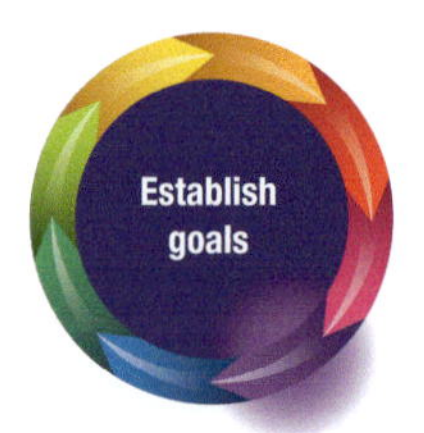

5. ESTABLISH GOALS

Q From the list below, choose the three *most important* short-term (up to one week) goals for Amelia's management at this time.

a For Amelia to be an active participant in education relating to the care of her PEG tube and enteral nutrition

b Discharge Amelia to supported accommodation for people living with disability

c To communicate Amelia's preferences in relation to her activities of daily living by documenting these in her nursing care plan

d For Amelia to demonstrate autonomy in decision making and lifestyle choices, including social relationships

e To arrange a family meeting with Amelia and her family prior to discharge, to facilitate the beginning of discussions about Amelia's desire for increased autonomy and independence

f For Amelia's parents to provide Amelia greater autonomy and independence

g For Amelia to reach the milestones that signify progression from adolescence to adulthood

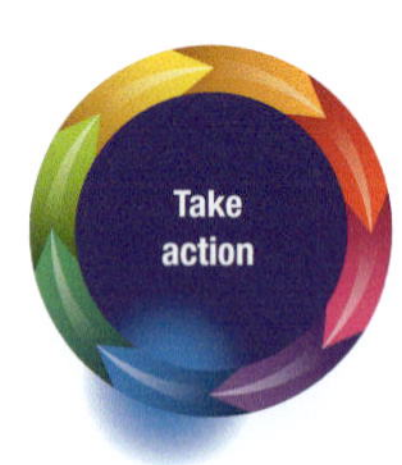

6. TAKE ACTION

You have identified three important short-term goals to be implemented prior to Amelia's discharge tomorrow. To promote person-centred care, you communicate your assessment findings from this morning and the three goals by documenting them in the (a) nursing care plan, (b) progress notes and (c) handover to the afternoon shift. You complete the notes using the SOAP format.

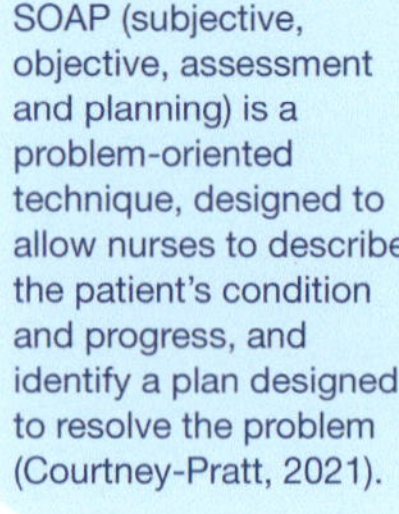

Q Complete progress notes entries according to the SOAP acronym for communicating your assessment findings and plan for Amelia.

S	
O	
A	
P	

7. EVALUATE

Evaluate outcomes

Q It is now the end of your shift. Which of the following strategies would indicate to you that you have made a positive difference to Amelia's nursing care? (Identify the three correct responses.)

a Amelia reports that her preferences for activities of daily living are being considered by the nursing staff.

b Amelia's parents are insisting that they attend to Amelia's hygiene needs as they understand her preferences.

c Nursing staff actively engage Amelia in education regarding care of the PEG tube and enteral nutrition.

d A family meeting will be planned prior to discharge.

8. REFLECT

Reflect on process and new learning

In the last stage of the clinical reasoning cycle, it is important to consider what you have learnt and how your learning will inform and shape your future practice.

Patient Safety Competency Framework (PSCF)

Domain 1–Person-centred care

The PSCF states that nurses must be able to plan and provide care that is respectful of the person's individual needs, values and life experiences.

Source: *The Patient Safety Competency Framework for Nursing Students*, https://patientsafetyfornursingstudents.org

Q1 What are the three most important things that you have learnt about planning and providing care for a young adult with a disability?

Q2 What do you see as the greatest challenges to nurses providing person-centred care when caring for someone with a disability?

Q3 What actions will you take in your future practice as a result of your learning from this scenario?

SCENARIO 15.2 Amelia's discharge

CHANGING THE SCENE

It is the morning of Amelia's discharge and you receive the handover report from the night shift:

> *In Bed 8 is Amelia Traynor, a 22-year-old female who was admitted four days ago for treatment of aspiration pneumonia and insertion of a PEG. Amelia slept really well overnight. She is afebrile for the first time this admission and her other vital signs are stable. PEG site is clean and dry. Her peripheral IV cannula has been removed and she continues on antibiotics via the PEG. No complaints of pain overnight. Amelia is being discharged home today, most likely this afternoon as it will take a while to get her organised. I am pretty sure her mum will be in soon if she is not already.*

1. CONSIDER THE PATIENT SITUATION

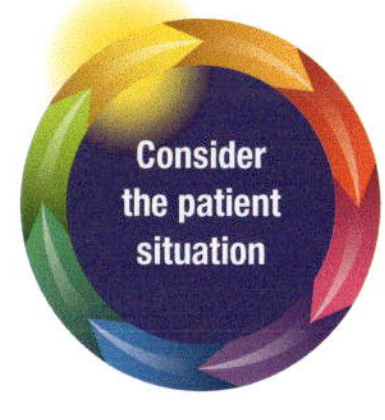

At the completion of handover, you review Amelia's discharge paperwork. You notice that there are no entries in Amelia's progress notes that respond to the issues you communicated yesterday and you are concerned that there has been no follow-up about a family meeting, as recommended in your nursing notes and your handover.

Today, on entering Amelia's room, you see that she has been showered, is dressed in her own clothes and is already in her chair. Amelia appears pleased to see you. Whilst you are assisting Amelia with her enteral nutrition, the following conversation unfolds:

You:	*The things you were talking about yesterday, you know, about wanting greater autonomy, do you still feel that way today?*
Amelia:	*Yes.*
You:	*Has anyone come to talk to you about a family meeting so that some of these issues can be discussed?*
Amelia:	*No, I haven't spoken to anyone but you since yesterday. I'm supposed to be going home today, so I guess that means nothing will happen.*
You:	*I'm not sure but leave it with me and I'll see what we can do.*

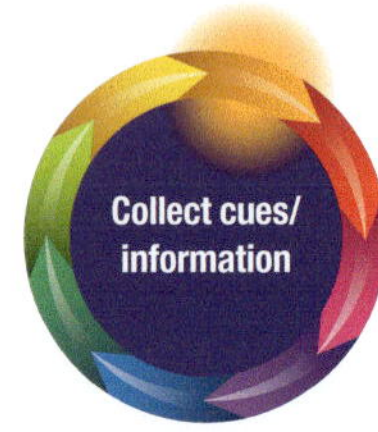

2. COLLECT CUES/INFORMATION

(a) Review current information

You acknowledge that your concern for Amelia is based on your interpretation of what Amelia has told you. You recognise a need to gather the perspectives of Amelia's family and members of the interprofessional healthcare team for the planning of effective person-centred care.

(b) Gather new information

You decide that you need more information in order to follow up on your recommendations from yesterday. You re-read Amelia's progress notes and discharge documentation, searching for any referrals to the interprofessional team. You realise that your entry in Amelia's progress notes yesterday did not propose a plan for organising a family meeting, and you did not identify who would arrange and coordinate the meeting. You start to think about what it is that you want to achieve and how to go about doing this.

Q1 What is a family meeting? How might it contribute to increasing Amelia's desire for autonomy?

Q2 What are the two *most relevant* reasons a family meeting should occur in Amelia's situation?

- a Family meetings are one way in which Amelia and her family can be involved in the process of planning for person-centred care, whilst being supported by nurses and members of the interprofessional healthcare team.
- b Family meetings are utilised only when family situations are complex or problematic.
- c Family meetings can be a proactive way of managing and planning person-centred care within inpatient, community and extended care contexts.
- d Family meetings provide an opportunity for family involvement in the planning of care, as it is the family members who understand the person's needs best.

(c) Recall knowledge

Members of the interprofessional healthcare team involved in the planning and implementation of care will differ depending on the needs of the person and, in Amelia's case, the family. You consider the healthcare professionals who would positively contribute to a family meeting for Amelia.

Q Using the following table, match the healthcare professional with their role description.

Health professional

- Patient care attendant/assistant in nursing
- Case manager
- Health technician
- Registered nurse
- Physiotherapist
- Occupational therapist
- Social worker
- Podiatrist

- Pharmacist
- Dietician
- Dentist
- Speech pathologist
- Medical officer

Health professional	Description
	Assesses a patient's health status, identifies health problems and develops and coordinates care
	Ensures that patients receive fiscally sound, appropriate care in the best setting. This role may be fulfilled by any member of the healthcare team, but usually one who is most involved in the person's care
	Diagnoses and treats dental health problems
	Has specialised knowledge regarding diets required to maintain health and treat disease
	Prepares and dispenses pharmaceuticals in the hospital and community setting
	Assists people with impaired function to gain the skills to adapt and perform activities of daily living, or modifies the environment to enable this
	A range of professionals (e.g. lab technicians/radiographers) who use specialised tests and objective data to inform the diagnosis and treatment of health problems
	Assists clients with musculoskeletal, cardiovascular or respiratory problems; services are provided in inpatient or community settings
	Responsible for health promotion and health prevention, as well as the medical diagnosis and the medical therapy required for a person with a disease or injury
	Counsels individuals and their support persons regarding finances, accommodation services and community supports–a significant role is connecting individuals and their families to government services
	Health staff who assume delegated aspects of basic care
	Diagnoses and treats foot conditions
	Has specialised knowledge in the study, diagnosis and treatment of communication and swallowing disorders

3. PROCESS INFORMATION

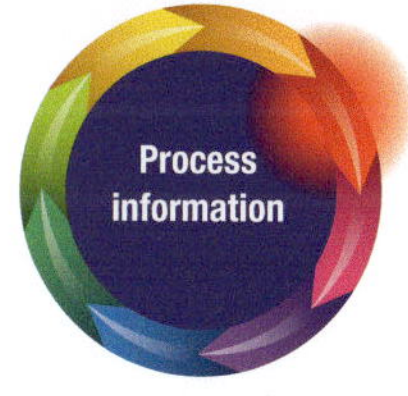

(a) Interpret and (b) Discriminate

The next step of the clinical reasoning cycle is to interpret the information that you have collected and, while applying your knowledge about Amelia, narrow down this information to what is most important.

Q1 Based on the information collected, which do you believe are the *seven* most relevant health professionals to be present at the family meeting?

a Case manager

b Dentist

c Dietitian
d Health technician
e Medical officer
f Occupational therapist
g Patient care attendant
h Pharmacist
i Physiotherapist
j Podiatrist
k Registered nurse
l Social worker
m Speech pathologist

Q2 Who would you suggest performs the role of case manager?

(c) Relate and (d) Infer

Each of the following individuals should be included in the family meeting to ensure that all of the key information is collated and the correct inferences drawn.

- The *speech pathologist* will provide information about the aetiology of Amelia's aspiration and the pathophysiology of her impaired swallow. The speech pathologist will provide exercises to enable Amelia to safely manage oral secretions. They may also assist Amelia to identify 'safe' foods for social eating or eating pleasure.
- The *social worker* will provide information about government services, not-for-profit support groups, options for supported accommodation and strategies for facilitating Amelia's transition, increasing her autonomy and independence. Importantly, the social worker will facilitate the transfer of Amelia's case to a case manager in the community.
- The *registered nurse* will provide documented evidence related to Amelia's trajectory of care during the hospitalisation, and advocate for the person by reporting Amelia's stated desire for autonomy in her healthcare decisions and greater independence.
- *Amelia* will have the opportunity to voice her perspectives, values and desires to her parents, in an environment that is supported by the interprofessional healthcare team.
- The *medical officer* will inform the meeting about Amelia's medical needs from this admission as well as options for medical support in the community.
- *Kathryn, Jim, Sebastian* and *Naomi* will be provided with an opportunity to voice their perspectives, values and desires in an environment that is supported by the interprofessional healthcare team.
- The *occupational therapist* will provide advice and support related to adaptive strategies for promoting autonomy and interdependence, either at home or in supported accommodation. This can include accessing health packages and the NDIS, and consideration of vocational preparation planning. They may also assist with designing an adaptive approach if Amelia wishes to contribute to the practical aspects of managing the administration of enteral nutrition and PEG care.
- The *case manager* will co-ordinate the meeting and ensure everyone's voice is heard. Importantly, the case manager will facilitate a process of negotiation in order to establish a plan of action that is agreed upon by all participants of the family meeting.
- The *dietitian* will provide advice about meeting nutritional requirements, frequency and timing of enteral feeds, and issues relating to infection control. This will include education and a plan for meeting daily nutritional needs, as well as follow-up requirements post discharge.

(e) Match

Q Have you ever participated in a family meeting (also known as a case conference)? If so, who was present and what did they contribute?

(f) Predict

Now is the time to consider the possible consequences for the planning process by predicting the probable outcomes of the family meeting.

Q Which of the following possible outcomes of the family meeting is the most probable?

a The concerns of each participant will be heard and resolved during the family meeting.

b The concerns of each participant will be heard and a plan comprising short-term goals will be developed.

c The concerns of each participant will be heard and a plan comprising short- and long-term goals will be developed.

d The concerns of each participant will be heard and a plan comprising long-term goals will be developed.

4. IDENTIFY THE PROBLEM/ISSUE

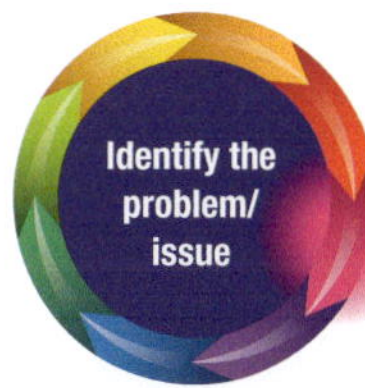

At this stage of the clinical reasoning cycle, you bring together (synthesise) all of the facts you have collected and all of the inferences you have made to make definitive nursing diagnoses for Amelia and her family.

Q From the following list, identify two nursing diagnoses that best reflect the situation confronting Amelia and her family.

a Altered family processes, and change to family roles and structure related to increased autonomy and independence, as evidenced by changes to long-standing roles and uncertainty

b Knowledge deficit (of parents) related to disability services, as evidenced by parents fulfilling role as primary carer

c Risk of self-concept disturbance (of parents) related to altered role performance and self-esteem disturbance, as evidenced by implementation of strategies to promote Amelia's autonomy

d Decisional conflict related to multiple or divergent sources of information, as evidenced by verbalised uncertainty about choices or decisions

5. ESTABLISH GOALS and 6. TAKE ACTION

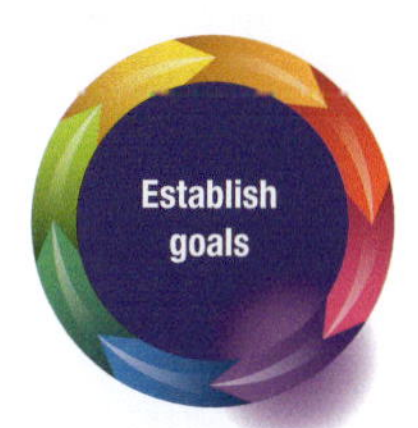

As has been seen in this chapter, young adults such as Amelia who are living with a disability encounter a number of unique challenges that can impede, hinder and delay achieving the milestones of adulthood. The primary goal of person-centred care is to support the person's rights to self-determination and autonomy, by providing them with sufficient information to participate in decision-making processes and maintain a feeling of being in control.

In relation to planning care that is person-centred, the management goals should be SMART:

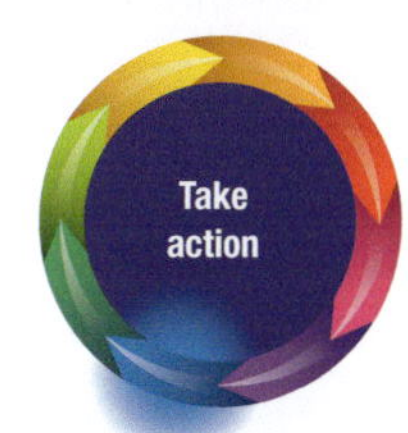

- **S**pecific
- **M**easurable
- **A**chievable
- **R**ealistic
- **T**imely

It is important to begin the process of planning care by asking Amelia and her family to identify three goals: one short-term (achievable in two to three weeks), one medium-term (achievable within two months), and one long-term (achievable within six months). The goals need to be specific and realistic and, most importantly, things that both Amelia and her family want to achieve.

The plan represented in Table 15.3 provides examples of possible goals for Amelia and her family.

Table 15.4 shows further examples of short-, medium- and long-term goals for Amelia.

For further information about quality care plans for community care, go to Chapter 3 of *The Goal Directed Care Planning Toolkit:* https://kpassoc.com.au/resources/gdcp-resources

Table 15.3 *Example of a care plan for Amelia and her family*

Goal	Actions	Person(s) responsible	Time frame	Review date	Outcomes
Short term					
1. Amelia will increase her autonomy in decision making for her own care.	Ask Amelia what decisions she would like to make about her care.	Amelia Kathryn and Jim Healthcare team	2–3 weeks		
2. Amelia will begin to be involved in the management of PEG and enteral nutrition.	Provide Amelia with opportunities to participate in the day-to-day care of her PEG and enteral nutrition.	Amelia Kathryn Community nurse Dietitian	2–3 weeks		
Medium term					
1. Amelia will receive community support to assist with ADLs and socialisation.	Involve Amelia in the process of selecting carers.	Case manager Social worker Community support services	2–3 months		
2. Amelia will develop an identity as an autonomous young adult.	Provide Amelia with opportunities to socialise independently of her family.	Parents Amelia Case manager Friends	2–3 months		
Long term					
1. Amelia will enrol in an online course of her choosing.	Provide Amelia with assistance to research courses and enrol.	Amelia Person of Amelia's choosing	6 months		
2. Amelia will begin the transition to supported accommodation.	Provide Amelia with assistance to research supported accommodation options.	Amelia Case manager/ social worker	6 months		

Source: Based on K. Pascale (2014). *The Goal Directed Care Planning Toolkit: Practical Strategies to Support Effective Goal Setting and Care Planning with HACC Clients.* Melbourne, Victoria: Eastern Metropolitan Region (EMR) HACC Alliance, Outer Eastern Health and Community Services Alliance. Resources available from: https://kpassoc.com.au/resources/gdcp-resources

Table 15.4 *Additional goals to consider for Amelia and her family*

Goal	Actions	Person responsible	Time frame
Short term Family members are discussing the ways in which changing roles is impacting on their relationships within the family.	Family meetings will continue in the community.	• Amelia • Parents and siblings • Community case manager	2–3 weeks
Medium term Amelia has the capability to tell others what is required to maintain enteral nutrition.	Evaluate Amelia's understanding of administration of enteral nutrition.	• Amelia • Community nurse • Dietitian • Medical officer (GP)	2–3 months
Long term Amelia will achieve optimal autonomy and interdependence.	Ensure potential for autonomy and interdependence is realised through regular evaluation of implemented strategies.	• Community case manager	6 months

Source: Based on K. Pascale (2014). *The Goal Directed Care Planning Toolkit: Practical Strategies to Support Effective Goal Setting and Care Planning with HACC Clients.* Melbourne, Victoria: Eastern Metropolitan Region (EMR) HACC Alliance, Outer Eastern Health and Community Services Alliance. Resources available from: https://kpassoc.com.au/resources/gdcp-resources.

7. EVALUATE

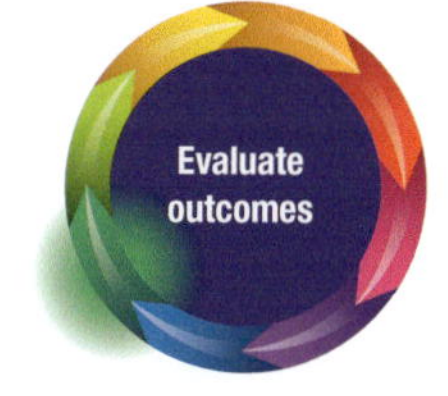

In complex situations such as the one portrayed in this chapter, it can be difficult for members of the interprofessional healthcare team to predict the effectiveness of the planned actions to be put in place. Therefore, it is important at the time of establishing goals to think about how the actions may be evaluated.

Q1 Based on the statements below, evaluate the effectiveness of the planned actions after a period of three months. Label each as *effective* or *ineffective*.

Amelia is . . .	Rating
. . . guiding carers or her siblings on how to administer her enteral nutrition and clean the equipment after use.	
. . . planning her ADLs around a schedule that she has determined, in collaboration with her parents and community support services.	
. . . feeling guilt about her parents refusal to acknowledge her desire to move to supported accommodation.	
. . . meeting new friends through new social groups and activities.	
. . . uncertain about her role in contributing to Sebastian's decision to move out of home.	
. . . engaging in conversation with her family about the new challenges she is encountering through her increasing independence.	
. . . researching online accounting courses through VET and university providers.	

Q2 In this chapter, we have explored issues of delayed transition from adolescence to adulthood for people living with disability. Why do you believe the parents of a child with a disability may contribute to the delayed transition of their child?

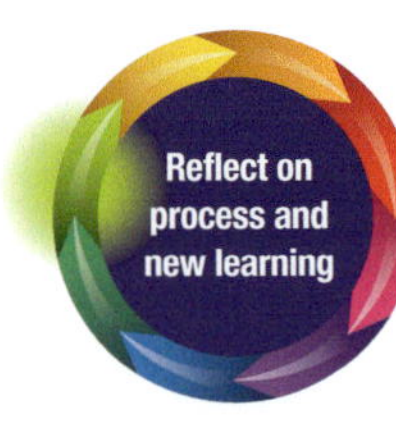

8. REFLECT

In the last stage of the clinical reasoning cycle, it is important to consider what you have learnt and how your learning will inform your future practice.

The Fundamentals of Care Framework (Feo, et al., 2017) outlines three core dimensions for the delivery of high-quality fundamental care:

1. A trusting therapeutic relationship between care recipient and care provider
2. Integrating and meeting a person's physical, psychosocial and relational needs
3. A context of care that is supportive of relationship development and care integration.

Q1 Of the three core dimensions, which do you feel you are capable of delivering in the fundamental care of a young person living with a disability?

Q2 After reflecting on the previous question, and on this chapter, how do you feel your understanding and beliefs of people living with a disability have changed?

Q3 Of the three core dimensions, which do you feel you are *least* prepared for in the planning and delivery of fundamental care for a young person living with a disability?

Q4 What actions will you commit to in order to be better prepared for planning and delivery of fundamental care for a young person living with a disability?

Something to think about . . .

For people who do not live (or have not lived) with disability, understanding the impact of disability on everyday life is difficult to appreciate. In 2020, the Australian Government Department of Social Services commenced a new National Disability Strategy. Consultation reports have been published which highlight the experiences of people with disabilities and their families in Australia. One such report is the Right to Opportunity: Consultation Report to Help Shape the Next Disability Strategy (Commonwealth of Australia, 2019), retrieved from: https://www.dss.gov.au/disability-and-carers-a-new-national-disability-strategy/reports

This report provides stark insights into the worlds of people living with disability.

EPILOGUE

Amelia continues to live with her family. She feels she has a better 'relationship' with her PEG tube and, while she cannot administer the enteral nutrition herself, she can direct people to administer the enteral nutrition and time her 'feeds' to the mealtimes of her family or friends. Amelia has also developed the confidence to tell people her preferences for positioning the PEG tube and setting up her feeding equipment in a way that is inconspicuous.

Strategies developed through regular community-care meetings, coordinated by her community case manager, have enabled Amelia to select and manage her personal carers (of her own age), manage her finances and begin navigation of the social services available to her. For the first time in her life, Amelia has been going out at night with friends, independent of her parents. Amelia still plans to move to supported accommodation in the future, but she understands that this transition will take time.

FURTHER READING

Agency for Clinical Innovation. (2014). *Key Principles for Transition of Young People from Paediatric to Adult Health Care.* Retrieved from: https://aci.health.nsw.gov.au/resources/transition-care/priniciples

Baron, S., Ross, H., Greenwood, E., Warren, A., Dupres, F. & Pretty, K. (2018). *Empathic Care of a Person with Cerebral Palsy: E-simulation Toolkit.* Bournemouth University, England, UK. Retrieved from: https://www.virtualempathymuseum.com.au/wp-content/uploads/2018/10/PERSON-WITH-CEREBRAL-PALSY-TOOLKIT-IN-TEMPLATE.pdf

Gaskin, C. J., Imms, C., Dagly, G., Msail, M. E. & Reddihough, D. (2021). Successfully negotiating life challenges: Learnings from adults with cerebral palsy. *Qualitative Health Research*, *31*(12), 2176–93. doi: 0.1177/10497323211023449

Helen's Story: Insights into the Healthcare Experiences of a Woman With Cerebral Palsy. Retrieved from: https://bournemouth.cloud.panopto.eu/Panopto/Pages/Viewer.aspx?id=506a71f8-657e-42e5-9ec0-a96500ac7b2c

REFERENCES

Agency for Clinical Innovation and Trapeze, The Sydney Children's Hospitals Network. (2014). *Key Principles for Transition of Young People from Paediatric to Adult Health Care.*

Australian Cerebral Palsy Register Group. (2018). *Australian Cerebral Palsy Register: Report 2018.* Retrieved from: https://cpregister.com/wp-content/uploads/2019/02/report-of-the-australian-cerebral-palsy-register-birth-years-1995-2012.pdf

Australian Commission on Safety and Quality in Health Care. (2021*). National Safety and Quality Health Service Standards* (2nd edn). Sydney: ACSQHC.

Baranello, G., Signorini, S., Tinelli, F., Guzzetta, A., Pagliano, E., Rossi, A., … Ricci, D. (2019). Visual Function Classification System for children with cerebral palsy: Development and validation. *Developmental Medicine and Child Neurology*, *62*(1), 104–10. doi: 10.1111/dmcn.14270

Brown, M., Higgins, A. & MacArthur, J. (2019). Transition from child to adult health services: A qualitative study of the views and experiences of families of young adults with intellectual disabilities. *Journal of Clinical Nursing, 29*(1–2), 195–207. doi: 10.1111/jocn.15077.

Commonwealth of Australia (2019). *Right to Opportunity: Consultation Report to Help Shape the Next Disability Strategy.* Australian Government Department of Social Services. Retrieved from: https://www.dss.gov.au/disability-and-carers-a-new-national-disability-strategy/reports

Courtney-Pratt, H. (2021). Documenting and reporting. In A. Berman, S. J. Snyder, B. Kozier, G. L. Erb, T. Levett-Jones, T. Dwyer, … D. Stanley (Eds), *Kozier and Erb's Fundamentals of Nursing* (4th edn). Melbourne: Pearson.

Deloitte Access Economics. (2020). *The Cost of Cerebral Palsy in Australia in 2018.* Sydney, Australia: Report prepared for Cerebral Palsy Australia, Cerebral Palsy Alliance and The Australasian Academy of Cerebral Palsy and Developmental Medicine, 1–67.

Eliasson, A. C., Krumlinde-Sundholm, L., Rosblad, B., Beckung, E., Arner, M., Ohrvall, A. & Rosenbaum, P. (2006). The Manual Ability Classification System (MACS) for children with cerebral palsy: Scale development and evidence of validity and reliability. *Developmental Medicine & Child Neurology*, *48*(7), 549–54.

Feo, R., Conroy, T., Jangland. E., Muntlin Athlin, Å., Brovall, M., Parr, J., Blomberg, K. & Kitson, A. (2017). Towards a standardised definition for fundamental care: A modified Delphi study. *Journal of Clinical Nursing*, *27*, 2285–99. doi: 10.1111/jocn.14247

Furlong, A. (2009). Introduction. In *Handbook of Youth and Young Adulthood: New Perspectives and Agendas*. Milton Park; New York: Routledge.

Hidecker, M. J. C., Paneth, N., Rosenbaum, P. L., Kent, R. D., Lillie, J., Eulenberg, J. B., … Taylor, K. (2011). Developing and validating the Communication Function Classification System for individuals with cerebral palsy. *Developmental Medicine & Child Neurology, 55*(8), 704–10.

Levett-Jones, T., Dwyer, T., Reid-Searl, K., Heaton, L., Flenady, T., Applegarth, J., Guinea, S. & Andersen, P. (2017). *The Patient Safety Competency Framework (PSCF) for Nursing Students*. Retrieved from: https://www.cqu.edu.au/__data/assets/pdf_file/0026/65780/PatientSafetyCompetencyFrameworkFINAL.pdf

Myers, L. L., Nerminathan, A., Fitzgerald, D. A., Chien, J., Middleton, A., Waugh, M. C. & Paget, S. P. (2020). Transition to adult care for young people with cerebral palsy. *Paediatric Respiratory Reviews*, *33*, 16–23. doi: 10.1016/j.prrv.2019.12.002

Nursing and Midwifery Board of Australia (NMBA). (2016). *Registered Nurse Standards for Practice.* Retrieved from: www.nursingmidwiferyboard.gov.au/Codes-Guidelines-Statements/Professional-standards.aspx

Palisano, R. J., Rosenbaum, P. L., Bartlett, D. & Livingston, M. H. (2008). Content validity of the expanded and revised gross motor function classification system. *Developmental Medicine Child Neurology*, *50*(10), 744–50.

Rosenbaum, P. L. & Rosenbloom, L. (2012). *Cerebral Palsy: From Diagnosis to Adult Life*. London, UK: Mac Keith Press.

Sellers, D., Mandy, A., Pennington, L., Hankins, M. & Morris, C. (2014). Development and reliability of a system to classify the eating and drinking ability of people with cerebral palsy. *Developmental Medicine & Child Neurology*, *56*(3), 245–51.

The Royal Children's Hospital Melbourne. (2016). *Clinical Practice Guidelines: Engaging With and Assessing the Adolescent Patient*. Retrieved from: www.rch.org.au/clinicalguide/guideline_index/Engaging_with_and_assessing_the_adolescent_patient

Wimalasundera, N. & Stevenson, V. L. (2016). Cerebral palsy. *Practical Neurology*, *16*(3), 184–94.

Chapter 16

Caring for a person requiring palliative care

JOANNE LEWIS and DEBORAH PARKER

LEARNING OUTCOMES

Completion of the activities in this chapter will enable you to:

- explain why an understanding of palliative care is required for competent care of a person with a terminal illness and their family (**recall** and **application**)
- identify some of the main symptoms experienced by a patient requiring palliative care that will guide the collection and interpretation of cues (**gather, review, interpret, discriminate, relate** and **infer**)
- review clinical information to identify the main nursing diagnoses for a person requiring palliative and end-of-life care (**synthesise**)
- describe the priorities of care for a person requiring palliative and end-of-life care, taking into account their physical, psychological, social and spiritual needs (**goal setting** and **taking action**)
- discuss the role and responsibilities of the palliative care team (**taking action**)
- identify factors that impact on the quality of end-of-life care
- identify clinical criteria for determining the effectiveness of nursing actions taken to manage common symptoms (**evaluate**)
- apply what you have learnt about palliative care to new situations (**reflection** and **translation**).

INTRODUCTION

This chapter focuses on the care of a 37-year-old woman with metastatic breast cancer. You will be introduced to Sally Abraham and follow her journey through palliative care.

The World Health Organization (WHO, 2021) defines palliative care as an approach that improves the quality of life for people who face life-threatening illness and their families, by providing pain and symptom relief, and spiritual and psychosocial support from diagnosis to the end of life and bereavement. Palliative care enables people facing death to be as free as possible from unnecessary suffering, to maintain their dignity and independence throughout the experience, to be cared for in an environment of their choice, to have their grief needs recognised and responded to, and to be assured that their family's needs are being met (Palliative Care Australia, 2018a).

Caring for a person undergoing palliative care not only requires effective clinical reasoning skills but also requires the nurse to practise in a way that is holistic, person-centred and respectful. Holistic healthcare emphasises the importance of the individual as a whole being within a social, cultural, spiritual and environmental context, rather than a person with isolated impairment of a particular system or organ (Kittelson, Eli & Pennypacker, 2015; Murray et al., 2017). Dying with dignity involves physical comfort, autonomy, meaningfulness, usefulness, preparedness and interpersonal connection, and is a critical principle of palliative care (Anderson, 2020, pp. 399–407; Oechsle et al., 2014; Proulx & Jacelon, 2004).

Dying is influenced by the patient's beliefs, values, history, emotions and culture (Ferrell et al., 2018). Although this can be challenging for novice nurses, the clinical reasoning cycle provides a coherent framework for working confidently through the complexities inherent in palliative care.

KEY CONCEPTS

palliative care
holistic care
symptom management
dying with dignity

SUGGESTED READINGS

P. LeMone, G. Bauldoff, P. Gubrud-Howe, M.-A. Carno, T. Levett-Jones, … D. Stanley (Eds). (2020). LeMone and Burke's Medical-Surgical Nursing: Critical Thinking for Person-Centred Care (4th edn). Pearson Australia.

Chapter 4: Nursing care of clients experiencing loss, grief and death

SCENARIO 16.1 The palliative care journey begins

SETTING THE SCENE

To find out more about the investigations used to identify breast cancer, see: https://canceraustralia.gov.au/publications-and-resources/position-statements/early-detection-breast-cancer

Sally Abraham is a 37-year-old single mother who was recently referred to the palliative care outreach team with metastatic breast cancer. When asked about her experiences by the palliative care nurse, Sally recounted her story as follows:

I was 25 when I was diagnosed ... I found a lump in my breast and I went to my GP. My daughter was 2 years old and I thought it was probably a blocked milk duct. The GP wasn't worried. I had a mammogram but it didn't show anything. So I had an ultrasound because the GP could feel the lump. The ultrasound found that there were three lumps in my breast.

Patients benefit from referral to palliative care as soon as possible after a diagnosis of a terminal illness. Often patients and families are fearful of referral to palliative care, but clear communication about the benefits of this referral can often overcome concerns that palliative care is for the imminent dying (Sarradon-Eck et al., 2019).

So I went into hospital to have a biopsy done and found out it was breast cancer. I had a partial mastectomy and two months of radiotherapy. Everything was clear for two and a half years, but then two lumps came up in the initial site and one under my arm. So I had a full mastectomy, followed by six months of chemotherapy. Six weeks later, another lump came up in the scar. For the next few years I developed secondary cancers in my bones and had further radiotherapy and chemotherapy which I was told was palliative not curative. I also started on hormone therapy which I was told would only slow the growth of the cancer. Then last month I developed some abdominal pain and had an abnormal blood test, a PET scan and a biopsy which diagnosed secondary spread to my liver and bones.

My oncologist said that it was unlikely that there would be further benefit from chemotherapy and it would likely make me feel more unwell. When I asked how long I might live for he said it was likely 6 to 12 months. I was completely devastated by this news and asked what else I could do. My oncologist suggested a referral to palliative care to manage my symptoms, and also to support me, my daughter and family.

Mindfulness meditation has many benefits, including reduced stress (Bower et al., 2015; Yazdanimehr et al., 2016), enhanced personal wellbeing (Sears et al., 2011), reduced cortisol levels and improved immune response (Pascoe, Thompson & Ski, 2020). Palliative care patients often find that the practice of mindfulness improves their physical, emotional and spiritual needs (Poletti et al., 2019).

I cried all the way home from the hospital. When I pulled up in the driveway, I was thinking, 'How do I tell my daughter Olivia that I am not going to live long enough to raise her? She's only 11 years old and I'm a single mum.' I couldn't work out a way to do it. So I called my family and said, 'This is what the doctor said and I am going to do all I can to live the best life while I can.' My family were devastated by the news and wanted me to get another specialist opinion, and they said that they thought a referral to palliative care was too soon. My family were angry that I was still using complementary therapies and the relationship became very difficult.

At first, I cried and cried for weeks, thinking, 'Oh ... I am dying ... This is really going to happen. I am really going to die.' Because of these fears I was initially reluctant to meet with the palliative care doctors and nurses but, when I did, I found that they were there to support me to live better, manage my symptoms and to understand what was important to me and what my goals were for my life. I was not expecting them to focus so much on living. I discussed with them my preference for complementary therapies in addition to other medications they thought might help. We also discussed the value of mindfulness and meditation.

Advance care planning is a process or discussion that reflects a person's goals, values, beliefs or preferences, related to future wishes for how their health and care can be managed or prioritised. An advance care plan may include an Advance Care Directive which is a legal document outlining health and care preferences, and can only be enacted when the person it pertains to no longer has capacity to make decisions or communicate those decisions (Advance Care Planning Australia, 2021).

So the palliative care team spoke to me about advance care planning and I understood that it was important for my family to understand my preferences for care and living.

I told Olivia that I loved her every day.

The epidemiology of breast cancer

In Australia, breast cancer is the cancer with the highest incidence for women (Australian Institute of Health and Welfare [AIHW], 2019). It can occur at any age, but it is more common in women over the age of 60. Men can also develop breast cancer, although this is quite rare. Breast cancer is underscored by the impact of genomic instability. In about 5 per cent of women, pathogenic variants, known as BRCA1 and BRCA2, increase the lifetime risk of breast cancer by 40 to 90 per cent (Pietrasik et al., 2020) There have been many risk factors identified in the literature, which include being older, reproduction history, socioeconomic status, exogenous hormones, lifestyle risk factors (alcohol, stress, diet, obesity and physical activity), familial history of breast cancer, having a chronic degenerative disorder, mammographic density and history of benign breast disease (Iacoviello et al., 2021).

Access *Cancer in Australia* (AIHW, 2019) to find out more about the incidence, mortality, death rate and survival rate for breast cancer.

Complementary therapies in palliative care

There is a growing body of evidence indicating that a significant proportion of palliative care patients access complementary medicine physicians for advice and use of medicines for symptom management (Steel et al., 2020). With the increased interest in complementary therapies, there is a need to ensure that these practices are safe, cause no harm and are used to enhance wellbeing (McCabe, 2005; van der Riet, Francis & Levett-Jones, 2011). Integrative healthcare models consider the interface between traditional and complementary therapies and do not force consumers to consider one or the other. Additionally, they manage the risks posed when people don't declare their usage of traditional medicines (Hunter et al., 2020).

Access the Cancer Council NSW website to learn more about the use of complementary therapies in cancer.

National Safety and Quality Health Service (NSQH) Standards

Medication safety standard

The NSQHS Standards specify that in order to promote medication safety, healthcare professionals must partner with consumers, actively involving them in their care and ensuring they have the information required to make appropriate treatment decisions (ACSQHC, 2021).

Many complementary therapies include a combination of pharmacological and non-pharmacological components, such as the oils used in aromatherapy, herbal therapies or 'medicines' prepared by Chinese traditional healers. It is common for people to believe that, because complementary medicines are 'natural' products, they must be good for you. However, like all medicines, there are potential risks associated with some complementary medicines (Sheppard-Hanger & Hanger, 2015; van der Riet, Francis & Levett-Jones, 2011). An understanding of the limits of monitoring and regulation of complementary alternative medicine practice is required along with the necessary professional regulatory guidance to ensure safety and quality measures are addressed (Pokladnikova & Telec, 2020). The use of complementary therapies in palliative care is common in oncology patients and has been increasing over the last decade. However, their use should be reviewed by practitioners as they can interact with chemotherapy agents and other medications (Michalczyk et al., 2021). Many of these therapies are indeed complementary to traditional medicine and support symptom management. In particular, massage (Candy et al., 2020; Corpora, Liggett & Leone, 2021), music therapy (Brungardt et al., 2021; Potvin, Hicks & Kronk, 2021), meditation (Pascoe, Thompson & Ski, 2020) and aromatherapy (Candy et al., 2020) contribute to a reduction in anxiety and improved quality of life for this group of patients. However, safety should always be an important consideration. For example, people who have had chemotherapy may have a reduction in their platelets and a vigorous massage could cause bleeding. This is not to say that massage should not be used; however, nurses should use this modality with care and carefully assess the patient's condition first.

Who are the members of the palliative care team? What are their roles? See www.caresearch.com.au/caresearch/ProfessionalGroups/tabid/55/Default.aspx

Patient Safety Competency Framework (PSCF)

Domain 4—Teamwork and collaborative practice

The PSCF specifies that nurses must have the skills required to collaborate and communicate effectively with members of the healthcare team in ways that facilitate mutual respect and shared decision making.

Source: *The Patient Safety Competency Framework for Nursing Students*, https://patientsafetyfornursingstudents.org

Models of palliative care

1. Generalist palliative care (primary model of care)

All health professionals should have core competencies to provide palliative care, as the majority of people with life-limiting illnesses will be cared for by generalist providers where symptoms are able to be managed without specialist palliative input (Palliative Care Australia, 2018b).

2. Specialist palliative care provision (tertiary)

In this model, care is provided for patients and their families with moderate to high palliative care needs where patients and their symptoms require extra attention. Symptoms may involve pain, breathlessness, nausea and/or vomiting. Referral to the interprofessional palliative care team is required. The goal is one of assessment and management of complex symptoms.

3. End-of-life care (terminal care)

This usually involves the final days or weeks of life. Here, the focus is very much on physical, emotional and spiritual comfort, as well as support for the family. It can be delivered by either generalist providers or specialist palliative care providers or both (Palliative Care Curriculum for Undergraduates [PCC4U], 2020).

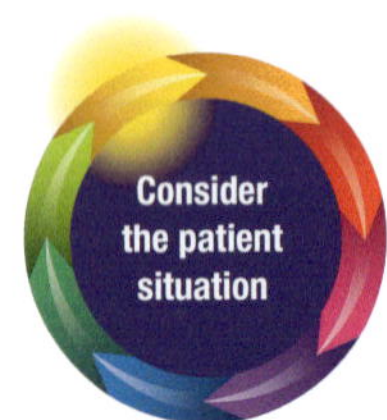

1. CONSIDER THE PATIENT SITUATION

Morning handover for the outreach palliative care team

Sally Abraham is a 37-year-old woman recently referred to the Outreach Community Palliative Care Service with a primary diagnosis of breast cancer with liver and bone secondaries. Her initial visit was last week. She called last night with increasing generalised pain, nausea and vomiting. She is on MS Contin 120 mg BD and morphine (Ordine) elixir 40 mg PRN for breakthrough pain. Sally said she is also using complementary therapies; I'm not sure which ones. She is not keen to be admitted to the hospice for symptom management and wants to stay at home as long as she can. But she lives in a caravan with her 14-year-old daughter.

National Safety and Quality Health Service (NSQH) Standards

Communicating for safety standard

The NSQHS Standards highlight the importance of coordinated delivery as an integral part of caring for an individual at the end of life (ACSQHC, 2021). Coordinated delivery of care involves collaboration, partnership and communication between all team members, with compassionate care the central tenet.

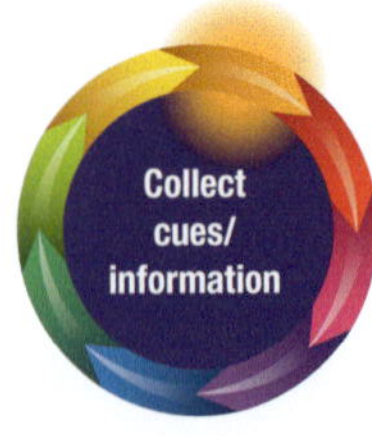

2. COLLECT CUES/INFORMATION

(a) Review current information

You are one of the nurses from the palliative care service. When you visit Sally, she tells you that her pain is worse and that she hasn't been getting around much. Olivia tells you that her mum has been nauseated; she made her ginger tea but she hasn't been able to eat anything solid for a few days.

Something to think about ...

People requiring palliative care may experience a range of symptoms depending on the underlying pathology of the disease, co-morbidities and other psychological, social and environmental factors. Preventing, minimising and treating these symptoms is an important part of the nurse's role. Some of the most common physical symptoms include fatigue, pain, dyspnoea, anorexia and constipation. Each of these, alone or in combination, causes suffering. The onset or exacerbation of symptoms can signal disease progression and this can cause additional emotional distress, anxiety and depression. A person's symptoms don't always follow a predictable pattern; they are experienced differently by each person and have multiple contributing factors and effects (PCC4U, 2020).

(b) Gather new information

Effective and accurate clinical assessment skills are imperative for the nurse working in palliative care. The comprehensive Symptom Assessment Scale (SAS) (Palliative Care Outcomes Collaboration, 2020) is one of the clinical assessment tools recommended by the Australian Palliative Care Outcomes Collaboration.

For more information about the analgesic ladder see: https://professionals.wrha.mb.ca/old/professionals/files/PDTip_AnalgesicLadder.pdf

A comprehensive symptom assessment typically includes:

- an evaluation of contributing factors
- characteristics of the symptoms (such as intensity, location, quality, temporal nature, frequency and associated pattern of disability)
- the meaning of the symptom(s) to the person (including beliefs about the symptom(s) and the effect on the person's physical, psychological and social wellbeing)
- behavioural responses to the symptom(s) (such as, the actions that the person is taking to manage or cope) (PCC4U, 2021).

Q You begin your physical assessment of Sally. Place the following assessments into the correct order based on their level of importance.

a Vital signs
b Mobility assessment
c Falls assessment
d Pain assessment
e Abdominal distention and bowel (elimination) assessments
f Assessment of nausea/vomiting
g Medication history
h Assessment of fatigue
i Assessment of breathlessness/dyspnoea
j Family/carer/social supports

There are seven main principles of pain management in palliative care:

1. Listen to the patient; involve the family.
2. Determine the cause of the pain and treat where possible.
3. Anticipate pain and anticipate side effects of drugs.
4. Start using the least invasive route and follow the WHO analgesic ladder.
5. Give medication regularly 'by the clock' and give PRN doses; use a combination of drugs.
6. Give the right drug and dose to treat the type of pain without unpleasant side effects.
7. Conduct regular reassessment of pain.

You review Sally's medication regime and note that she has been taking MS Contin 120 mg BD and morphine (Ordine) elixir 40 mg for breakthrough pain. She has needed morphine for breakthrough three times in the past 24 hours. She tells you that this is 'just not holding her pain though'.

Review the World Health Organization's pain ladder at www.who.int/cancer/palliative/painladder/en

(c) Recall knowledge

How confident are you about your knowledge of palliative care nursing?

Quick Quiz!

Q1 Individuals with which life-limiting illnesses may access palliative care services?

a Breast cancer
b Motor neuron disease
c Leukemia
d Melanoma
e Chronic obstructive pulmonary disease
f All of these options

Q2 Your own values and beliefs about death and dying may impact on your interactions with a dying person, which is why self-awareness is such an important strategy for the palliative care nurse. *True* or *false*?

Q3 Fill in the missing word: _________ is the most common strong opioid used to treat cancer-related pain.

Q4 Fill in the missing word: _________ are found within opioids (morphine, oxycodone and hydromorphone) and have the potential to accumulate in patients, with renal impairment causing tremors and delirium.

Q5 For MS Contin, which of the following statements are *true* and which are *false*?

a MS Contin is an opioid drug.
b MS Contin is a non-opioid drug.
c MS Contin is used for breakthrough pain.
d MS Contin is a slow-release drug.
e MS Contin can be crushed for easier administration.
f MS Contin should never be cut or crushed.

Q6 Which of the following is the reason that pethidine is rarely used for pain relief in palliative care?

a It has a strong odour.
b There is the potential for accumulation of toxic metabolite.
c It is rarely prescribed so availability is limited.
d It is too long acting.

Q7 What are the potential side effects of opioids? (Select the six correct answers.)

a Tachycardia
b Nausea
c Polydipsia
d Drowsiness
e Hypertension
f Constipation
g Confusion
h Hallucinations
i Vivid dreams
j Anxiety

Sally uses a number of complementary therapies, including:

- Vitamin D
- Ginger tea
- Juices (carrot, beetroot and celery) three times a day
- Slippery elm powder, bovine powder and lavender oil made into a paste for skin irritation on her chest wall
- Echinacea

Although you are not expected to have an extensive knowledge of all complementary therapies, it is important that you have a general understanding of their use.

Something to think about . . .

People seek complementary therapies for a number of reasons; for example, to maintain control, provide hope and retain an active part in their treatment process. To gain an understanding of information you might provide to a person seeking advice about complementary therapies, access the Cancer Council's site:

https://www.cancer.org.au/assets/pdf/understanding-complementary-therapies-booklet

Q8 Sally thinks about visiting another complementary therapy provider and asks you what questions she should ask. What would be the appropriate reply?

a What side effects could there be?
b What is the evidence for the success of the therapy?
c They are only after your money, so I wouldn't waste your time.
d How much will the therapy cost?
e a, b and d.

Patient Safety Competency Framework (PSCF)

Domain 6–Evidence-based practice

The PSCF specifies that nurses must demonstrate the ability to provide care that takes into account best available evidence, clinical expertise and patients' individual needs, values and preferences.

Source: *The Patient Safety Competency Framework for Nursing Students*, https://patientsafetyfornursingstudents.org

Q9 The action of Vitamin D is to:

a Reduce fatigue and pain
b Assist in the prevention of cold and influenza
c Cure breast cancer
d Treat nausea and vomiting

Q10 The action of echinacea is to:

a Reduce inflammation and pain in the joints and lower back
b Boost the immune system and help the body fight infections such as the common cold
c Promote gastric emptying
d Manage pain

A major concern for Sally is her current lack of social support. She tells you that her family became very dismissive when she wanted to talk about her use of complementary therapies and told her she was just giving herself and her daughter false hope. Sally also tells you that she has not talked to her GP (general practitioner) about her complementary therapy use as she is sure he does not believe in their effectiveness.

Conflict between patients and their families and caregivers in palliative care occurs reasonably frequently. It is important to recognise and, where possible, respond to these needs when caring for someone with a terminal illness who needs family support. All members of a multidisciplinary team in palliative care can enable conversations aimed at understanding complex and conflicted family relationships and, where possible, create a space for people where the work of reconciliation can occur. The impacts of family conflict at the end of life are far reaching and may result in poor outcomes for the dying person and all involved. These may include: the reduced likelihood of the person receiving care and dying in their place of preference; distress and anxiety for the family, including poorer outcomes in grief; and distress for staff who are providing care for the person and their family (Wilson et al., 2020).The particular needs for family support at the end of life are especially important when the dying person is the sole parent for children (Hanna et al., 2021), where the focus is on the welfare of the child and preparation for their care in the future.

When caring for an individual with a life-limiting illness, you also need to care for the caregivers. Consider the experience of Sally's family and how their distress at their daughter's terminal diagnosis is impacting them. Although they have had limited contact with Sally, they still have a close relationship with their granddaughter and would like to restore their relationship with Sally.

See CareSearch for further information regarding children with grief and loss: https://www.caresearch.com.au/tabid/6131/Default.aspx?q=children

3. PROCESS INFORMATION

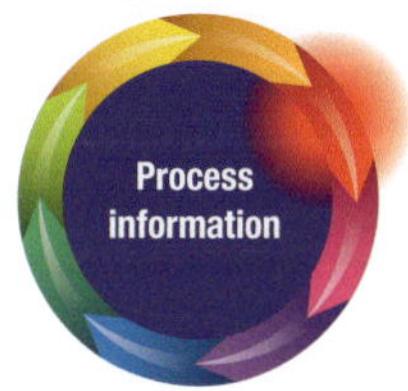

(a) Interpret

Q1 Within palliative care, you may find that a full set of vital signs are attended on an irregular basis and, in home visits, taking a full set of vital signs is rare. Select the vital signs that would be the most important for Sally at this time.

- a Temperature, pulse, blood pressure
- b Pain assessment, bowel assessment, respiration rate
- c Oxygen saturation, respiration, temperature
- d Bowel assessment, blood pressure, temperature

Q2 To assist you with understanding Sally's condition, her vital signs are provided below, along with those assessments that are a priority in palliative care. Which one of these is considered to be within normal parameters for Sally?

- a Temperature: 37.3°C
- b Pulse rate: 120
- c Respiratory rate: 30
- d Blood pressure: 140/95
- e Oxygen saturation level: 95%
- f Abdominal sounds: high-pitched tinkling sounds
- g Skin condition: dry skin
- h Oral mucosa condition: dry with tongue furrowed
- i Abdominal distension: evident on visual inspection

Q3 Sally tells you she feels bloated; she has pain near her rectum and has been passing small amounts of liquid diarrhoea that she can't always control. She also feels nauseated and has vomited small amounts. For a person with metastatic breast cancer, these symptoms are:

- a Unpleasant but expected
- b Typical of bone pain
- c A potential side effect of medications
- d A potential side effect of complementary therapies

(b) Discriminate

Q From the list below, select cues that you believe are *most relevant* to Sally's situation at this time.

- a Respiratory rate
- b Pulse

c Skin irritation
d Oxygen saturation
e Nausea and vomiting
f Lack of appetite
g Urine output
h Pain
i Frequency of bowel movements

See the following CareSearch site to gain a further understanding of constipation: https://www.caresearch.com.au/tabid/6222/Default.aspx

It is important at this stage of the clinical reasoning cycle to recognise *any gaps* in the cues you have collected. From the information you have collected, you begin to think that Sally may be constipated. She cannot remember the last time she had her bowels opened, although she does admit she is never regular. You palpate Sally's abdomen, which reveals an easily palpable colon with a soft and mobile faecal mass. Digital examination of the rectum reveals hard stools.

Clinical reasoning errors: Sally's diagnosis of metastatic breast cancer and her referral to palliative care may limit cue collection. Anchoring could lead you to focus on the pain related to metastatic breast cancer and overlook assessment of the potential side effects of medications.

(c) Relate

Q It is important to cluster the cues together and to identify relationships between them (based on the information you have collected so far). Which two of the following statements are *not* true?

a Sally could be in pain because she has metastatic breast cancer.
b Sally could be in pain as a result of her skin irritation.
c Sally could have nausea and vomiting as a side effect of the MS Contin and oral morphine that she is taking.
d Sally could be hypertensive because she is anxious about dying and leaving her daughter.
e Sally could have nausea and vomiting because she is constipated.
f Sally could be hypertensive as a result of her pain.
g Sally could be tachycardic as a result of her vomiting and pain.
h Sally is probably constipated as a side effect of the MS Contin and oral morphine that she is taking.

(d) Infer

Q It is time to think about the cues that you have collected and clustered about Sally's condition, and to make inferences based on your interpretation of those cues. From what you know about Sally's history, signs and symptoms, as well as your knowledge about palliative care, identify which of the following inferences are correct. (Select the one correct answer.)

Hint: Think about the side effects of morphine.

a Sally is septic.
b Sally is constipated.
c Sally is in shock.
d Sally has metastatic spread.
e Sally is suffering from anorexia nervosa.

(e) Predict

Q1 Predict what might happen if Sally's pain, nausea and vomiting are not corrected. (Select the four correct responses.)

a Sally could go into shock from an electrolyte imbalance.
b Sally's condition will gradually deteriorate over the next few days.
c Sally could go into acute renal failure (acute tubular necrosis).
d Sally could develop pulmonary oedema.
e Sally could die.
f Sally could become hypoxic.

Q2 Predict what might happen if Sally's constipation is not treated. (Select the four correct responses.)

a Sally could become hypotensive.
b Sally could develop a bowel obstruction.

c Sally could have a seizure.
d Sally could become hypoxic.
e Sally could develop toxic megacolon.
f Sally could become confused.
g Sally could become agitated.

Despite the prevalence of constipation in palliative care patients, it is often underdiagnosed and undertreated (Coluzzi et al., 2021).

4. IDENTIFY THE PROBLEM/ISSUE

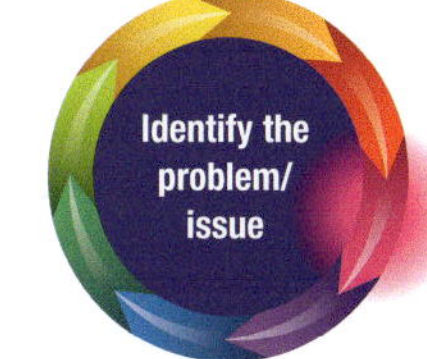

Q Sally is currently experiencing a number of problems. From the following list, select the most appropriate nursing diagnosis at this stage.
a Acute pain related to metastatic spread of cancer, evidenced by high pain score
b Constipation related to opioid use, reduced oral intake and limited mobility, as evidenced by pain, nausea and vomiting
c Metastatic spread of cancer related to abdominal distension, evidenced by high-pitched tinkling sounds
d Sally is experiencing 'typical' cancer pain

Nursing and Midwifery Board of Australia (NMBA) *Registered Nurse Standards for Practice* The NMBA's *Registered Nurse Standards for Practice* (2016) state that RNs must provide care that is person-centred and evidence-based with preventative, curative, formative, supportive, restorative and palliative elements.

5. ESTABLISH GOALS

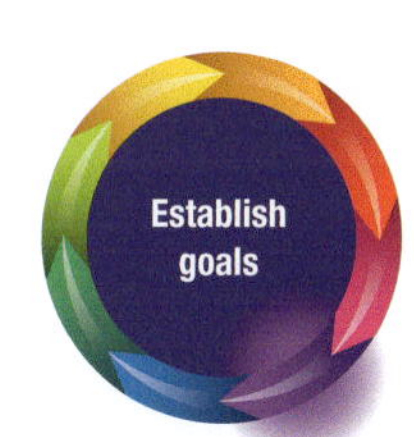

Q1 From the list below, choose the two most important *short-term* goals for Sally at this time.
a For Sally to be free of pain, nausea and vomiting
b For Sally to resume a normal diet
c For Sally's faecal impaction to be cleared
d For Sally to be admitted to a hospice

You are aware that Sally's accommodation could be contributing to her constipation, as she explains that walking to the public toilets is becoming more and more difficult. You are also concerned about how she will manage as her condition deteriorates and there is a lack of social support for her and her daughter.

Q2 Once Sally's immediate physical needs are addressed, it is important for you to do which of the following? (Select the two correct answers.)
a Contact Sally's parents.
b Organise alternative accommodation for Sally and Olivia.
c Plan where Olivia will go when Sally's condition deteriorates.
d Spend time talking with Sally so that you understand her wishes and needs for herself and Olivia.
e Contact anyone that Sally wants to speak to.
f Refer Sally to the social worker for help with possible accommodation.

6. TAKE ACTION

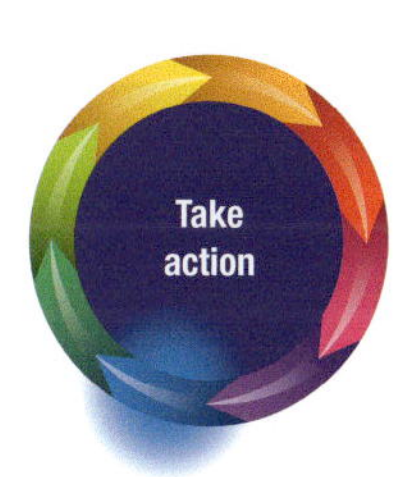

Q At this stage of the clinical reasoning cycle, you need to decide on the most important course of action. Place the following nursing actions into the correct order of priority:
a Negotiate an action plan in case of further episodes of constipation.
b Administer two glycerine suppositories to soften hard rectal stools.
c Ensure the glycerine suppositories are against the wall of the bowel.
d Administer an enema to clear the faecal impaction.
e Educate Sally about the importance of adequate fluids, mobility and use of aperients.
f Contact Sally's doctor to discuss her condition, and for an order for an enema as well as oral aperients or laxatives.

Something to think about ...

Although rectal enemas are sometimes necessary for treating faecal impaction, they should not be part of the regular treatment of every cancer patient with constipation. They are undignified and inconvenient, and may have a considerable negative effect on quality of life.

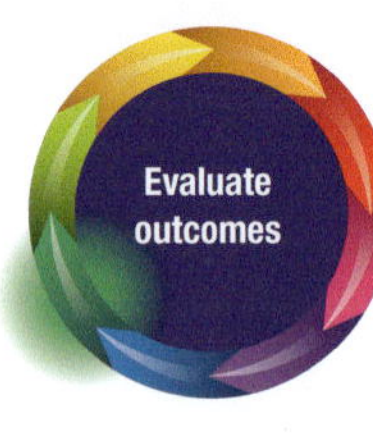

7. EVALUATE

It is now two hours since Sally was given a rectal examination and two microlax enemas.

Q1 Rate each of the following signs and symptoms as *unchanged, improving* or *deteriorating*.

Cognitive status	Patient restless and anxious
Pulse	90
Bowels	Good result but firm stools
Oral mucosa	Mouth is dry and tongue furrowed
Oral intake	Tolerating sips of water
BP	110/70
Colour	Pale
Pain	On scale of 10, Sally reports 2
Nausea	Slight nausea
Vomiting	Nil

Q2 You now need to synthesise these parameters to decide whether Sally's status has improved overall. Which of the following statements is most correct?

- a Sally's pain, nausea and vomiting have improved significantly.
- b Sally's pain, nausea and vomiting have not improved and you need to contact the doctor again.
- c Sally's pain, nausea and vomiting have improved significantly but still require careful monitoring and will require oral aperients.
- d Sally's status has not improved but you will monitor her condition carefully for the next four hours.

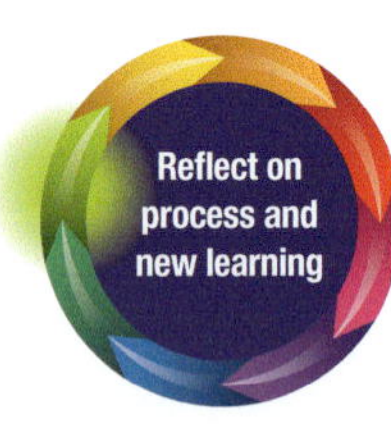

8. REFLECT

Reflect on your learning from this scenario and consider the following questions.

Q1 What actions will you take in clinical practice as a result of your learning from this scenario?

Q2 Why is therapeutic communication and holistic care important when caring for someone requiring palliative care?

Q3 Why is interprofessional communication imperative to the care of the person needing palliative care?

Q4 The *National Palliative Care Standards* (Palliative Care Australia, 2018c) specify that: 'Palliative care should be strongly responsive to the needs, preferences and values of people, their families and carers. A person- and family-centred approach to palliative care is based on effective communication, shared decision making and personal autonomy.' (p. 5). What strategies will you use in your clinical practice to meet this standard when caring for people requiring palliative care?

Q5 What advice would you give if a patient or a friend asked you about the use of complementary therapies for the treatment of cancer or the management of symptoms?

SCENARIO 16.2 The palliative care journey comes to an end

CHANGING THE SCENE

Since referral to palliative care, Sally has continued working with the Outreach Palliative Care Team, including nurses, doctors, allied health, pastoral care, social work and complementary therapists. With their help, she has been able to reconnect with her family who are now more accepting and supportive. Sally shares her story with the palliative care nurse:

> *The housing commission organised this house for me, and my family now support my use of complementary therapies. So now when I get stressed Mum says, 'Come and I'll put a meditation tape on for you'; and Dad says, 'You're running out of vitamin C. I'll go up the road and get you some.'*
>
> *I've also been connected to the support group through palliative care and it's been great. When you're at home and you're doing everything that you can, your family is as supportive as they can be and so are your friends—but it's the same old stuff … they just don't know what it is like. And you go along to a support group and you are not a minority anymore; you're part of the majority. Everybody in the room is going through a similar journey, so you don't feel isolated and lonely.*

Support groups can be another valuable resource for patients and carers. For more information, access: https://www.caresearch.com.au/tabid/6913/Default.aspx

Although referral to palliative care has had a positive effect on Sally's psychosocial wellbeing, her breast cancer has continued to progress. She explains to the palliative care nurse how she responded when she learnt how the disease had spread:

> *I remember when the cancer first spread to my bones … my ribs were hurting a bit. I had a bone scan straightaway … the radiotherapist had written down on the report, there could be signs of metastatic disease. Then everything was going along fine but I started to get aches and pains all over; it was hard to lift my leg up to get dressed, get in and out of bed, just basic things … I thought I had just been bashing myself a bit too much. I didn't think too much about it but I had an appointment a week and a half later with the oncologist. So I thought, I will leave it till then … I went and had another bone scan done and it was everywhere … all through my hips, in the top of my femur in one of my legs, in about eight vertebrae in my spine and six ribs. It has gone into my shoulder, and I think … it's getting worse; I can feel more pains and aches; it has gone into my neck as well, um … and I am kind of in shock that this is it …*

It has now been six months since Sally was first referred to palliative care and in the last month she has noted a decline in her mobility and her independence, as well as an increase in her pain. Sally and her daughter moved in with her parents as she required more care and support. However, over the last week her parents have found it increasingly difficult to manage her pain, discomfort and restlessness, and Sally has agreed to be admitted to the hospice.

1. CONSIDER THE PATIENT SITUATION

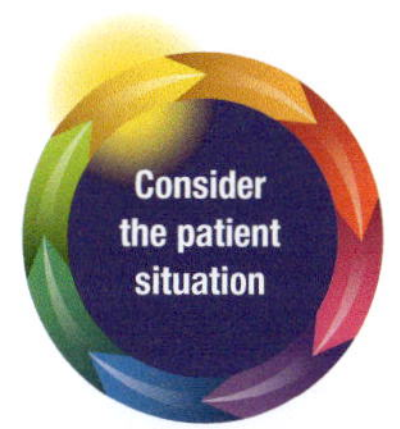

Morning handover at hospice

> *Sally Abraham is a 37-year-old woman with metastatic breast cancer; secondary sites include multiple bone metastases and metastatic spread to the liver. The outreach team commenced analgesia via a syringe driver the day prior to her admission but Sally's pain was not covered and she became increasingly restless. Her family stated that she has been eating only a spoonful of food a couple of times a day and having occasional sips of water. Sally was limited to her bed because of pain and weakness; previously she was walking short distances around the house. Sally was admitted to the hospice yesterday with increasing pain and decreasing consciousness. She has been moved to a single room.*
>
> *Since admission, Sally has commenced on a morphine/midazolam infusion and, although she is sleeping most of the time, she is easily roused. Her mother approached me before I came into handover asking if we are going to commence intravenous fluids because Sally is no longer taking anything orally.*

What does the literature say about medical hydration for dying patients? If unsure, access these articles: Oehme & Sheehan (2018) and Lokker et al. (2019).

Her parents (Nancy and Brendan) and Sally's daughter, Olivia, are staying in the room. Although they are all aware that Sally is dying, her parents are becoming distressed with Sally's agitation and the fact that she is not drinking and eating.

Quick Quiz!

Review the medications being delivered via the syringe driver.

Q1 A syringe driver in palliative care delivers a continuous infusion of medication over a 24-hour period, thus providing continuous dosing and avoiding the 'peak and trough' effect of four-hourly dosing. *True* or *false*?

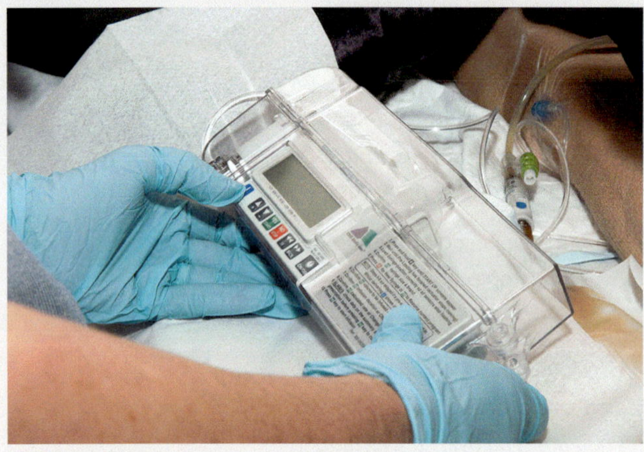

Syringe driver

Dr P. Marazzi/Science Photo Library/Alamy Stock Photo

Q2 A syringe driver is helpful for:

- a Post-operative pain
- b Intractable vomiting
- c Providing hydration and nutrition
- d When a patient is too weak to swallow
- e b and d

Q3 Circle the *true* statements concerning midazolam.

- a It is a benzodiazepine drug.
- b It is a non-benzodiazepine drug.
- c It is used for its anxiolytic and muscle relaxing effects.
- d It is used for pain relief.

Q4 Fill in the missing word: For palliative care patients, _________ delivery of medication is the preferred route (subcutaneous, intravenous, intramuscular)

Q5 Fill in the missing word: Increased agitation, twitching, restlessness and groaning are a form of ________, which may be present in the terminal phase of illness. (psychosis, dementia, terminal restlessness)

2. COLLECT CUES/INFORMATION

Access CareSearch; Syringe drivers https://www.caresearch.com.au/caresearch/tabid/3426/Default.aspx

(a) Review current information

Sally's condition has deteriorated and her family are aware that she is close to death. Bereavement support of carers often commences prior to a patient's death. Therapeutic communication skills make a significant impact on the experience of carers in the terminal phase of their loved one's life.

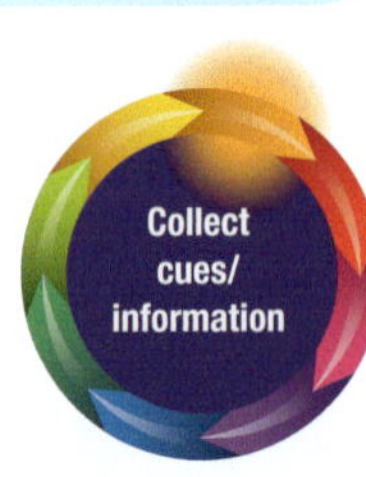

Q What current information might you consider prior to entering Sally's room?

- a Age of Sally
- b Relationships of bereaved to Sally
- c Gender of bereaved
- d Your own self-care strategies when dealing with grief reactions
- e Age of the bereaved
- f All of these options

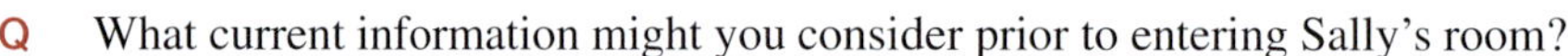

(b) Gather new information

The terminal phase of an illness describes the final days of a person's life. The focus during this stage is to provide symptom management for the patient to ensure that suffering is minimised, but supporting the carers or family is also a focus.

It is important to explain to the family the signs that will indicate Sally is in the terminal phase of her illness.

Hint: Being aware of signs of imminent death are essential for palliative care nurses so that they can fully support the carers or family.

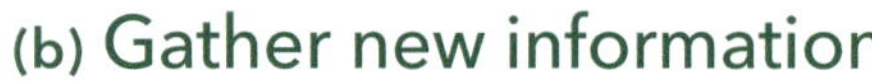

Q1 Indications that Sally is dying may include:

- a Thirst, fatigue and increased pain
- b Mainly asleep, bedbound and little oral intake
- c No bowel movements and increased pain
- d Increased confusion

Q2 Sally's parents and daughter have expressed a need to be with Sally when she dies; however, they are extremely tired. What actions could you recommend for them based on your knowledge of the terminal phase?

a Encourage them to go home and shower and have some rest.

b Encourage them to walk in the garden outside the room for 15 minutes while you sit with Sally.

c Encourage them to go to the cafeteria for a break.

Ascertainment bias

The transition and assessment during this phase can be difficult. The clinical reasoning error of ascertainment bias may occur when a nurse bases his or her judgment of the terminal phase on assumptions rather than on a full assessment of the client and the carer or family's needs.

(c) Recall knowledge

The provision of physical, psychological and spiritual care for patients during the terminal phase is essential.

Spirituality

For the palliative care patient, spirituality is often likened to a search for inner meaning. Complementary therapies can sometimes assist in this process, particularly meditation as it provides a space for contemplation. Many of these therapies, as previously stated, reduce anxiety and this then opens up the space for self-reflection.

Spirituality is an important component of professional nursing (Zumstein-Shaha, Ferrell & Economou, 2020); however, it is also an elusive term with no clear definition (Jastrzębski, 2020) that can mean different things to different people. Amoah (2011) points out that spirituality helps the dying person make sense of their life and that it is an integral component of palliative care. Smyth and Allen's research into nurses' experiences in assessing dying patients found that 'spirituality forms a significant component of the wellbeing of patients and, as such, is integral to delivering nursing care in any setting' (2011, p. 342). Importantly, this study reported that nurses implement 'spiritual care through listening, observing and communicating' (p. 341). For Wright, spirituality is 'what gives people balance when finding meaning in the existential challenges of life' (2005).

Hint: A spiritual assessment tool may assist you. Access: doi.org/10.1016/j.jpainsymman.2009.12.019

How would you communicate with Sally to ensure that you deliver spiritual care that acknowledges her individual needs and wishes?

Q1 When exploring spirituality, which aspects do you need to consider?

a The patient's perspectives

b The views of the interdisciplinary team

c The patient's own thoughts or concepts of spirituality

d Your own perceptions of spirituality and how they might impact on discussions with the patient

e All of the options

Now that Sally is dying, your nursing priorities include:

- promotion of comfort and relief of suffering
- careful assessment and management of symptoms
- pain assessment and management
- consideration of existential issues: spiritual issues, affirmation of life, meaning, unfinished business, reconciliation, culturally appropriate care
- the needs of family and carers: anticipatory grief, emotional support.

Advanced care planning is a strategy that can assist individuals with life-limiting illness to ensure that their wishes are respected when they are no longer able to verbalise them. Sally's parents and daughter have a clear understanding of Sally's wishes in relation to the terminal phase of her illness.

Q2 Advanced care planning is best discussed with the patient in the later stages of their illness.

True or *false*?

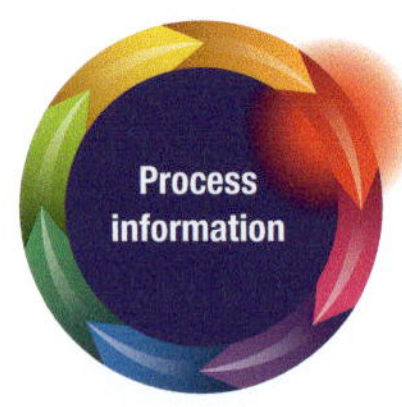

3. PROCESS INFORMATION

(a) Interpret

Sally's mother has approached you as she is upset that intravenous fluids have not been commenced. You have been doing regular mouth care for Sally and are aware that she is not complaining of thirst or hunger.

Quick Quiz!

Q1 Artificial or medical hydration should be considered in the palliative approach where dehydration results from potentially correctable causes. Identify which of the following are correctable.

- a Over-treatment of diuretics and sedation
- b Recurrent vomiting
- c Diarrhoea
- d Hypercalcaemia
- e All of these options

Q2 Medical provision of hydration (intravenous fluids) can make a difference to a dying patient's thirst. *True* or *false*?

Q3 Intravenous fluids in the dying patient can cause burdensome and distressing symptoms. *True* or *false*?

Q4 Terminal dehydration stimulates the production of endorphins. *True* or *false*?

Q5 A decrease in endorphins can cause some degree of analgesia. *True* or *false*?

Q6 Anorexia in the dying person results in ketoacidosis and this removes a feeling of hunger, resulting in analgesia. *True* or *false*?

Q7 Medical provision of hydration (IV fluids) can produce distressing and life-threatening symptoms for patients with end-stage illness and multi-organ failure. *True* or *false*?

Q8 Medical provision of hydration (IV fluids) can produce distressing symptoms because the physiological and metabolic processes of the body are no longer efficient. *True* or *false*?

(b) Discriminate

Q From the cues and information you now have, you need to narrow down the information to what is most important. From the list below, select four cues that you believe are *most relevant* to Sally's situation at this time.

- a Blood pressure
- b Dyspnoea
- c Sally's agitation
- d Oxygen saturation
- e Condition of oral mucosa
- f Level of consciousness
- g Sally is not eating or drinking
- h Urine output
- i Pain
- j Family distress

(c) Relate

Q It is important to cluster the cues together and identify relationships between them (based on the information you have collected so far). Which of the following are *true* statements?

- a Sally is restless because she has terminal restlessness.
- b Sally is restless because she may be frightened of dying.
- c Sally's family are worried about her not eating and drinking.
- d Sally's family feel helpless that Sally is not eating.
- e Sally's family feel that she is suffering because she is not eating and drinking.

(d) Infer

It is time to think about all the cues that you have collected about this situation and to make inferences based on your analysis and interpretation of those cues.

Q From what you know about Sally not eating and drinking, as well as your knowledge about palliative care, identify which of the following inferences is *most* correct.

a Sally is experiencing terminal dehydration.
b Sally is not experiencing terminal dehydration.

(e) Predict

Now is the time to consider the consequences of your actions or inaction by predicting potential outcomes for your patient.

Q1 What could happen if Sally is given intravenous fluids? (Select the four that apply.)

a Sally's family would be more relaxed.
b Sally's breathing would become noisy from the excessive respiratory secretions.
c Sally's peripheral oedema will increase.
d Sally could develop pulmonary oedema.
e Sally could become hypoxic.

Q2 What could happen if Sally is not given intravenous fluids? (Select the three that apply.)

a Sally's condition will gradually deteriorate over the next few days.
b Sally's breathing will be easier and she will not require any hyoscine hydrobromide and glycopyrrolate to dry up her secretions.
c Sally's urinary incontinence will be less.
d Sally will be less oedematous.
e Sally could become hypoxic.

4. IDENTIFY THE PROBLEM/ISSUE

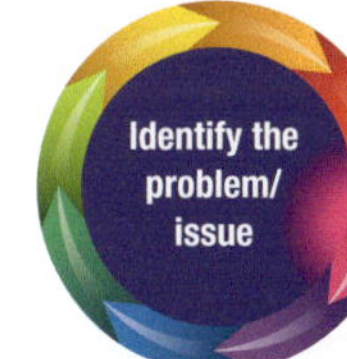

At this stage, you bring together (synthesise) all of the facts you've collected and inferences you've made to identify definitive risk diagnoses for Sally.

Q Select from the following the *incorrect* nursing diagnoses for Sally at this time.

a Risk of aspiration related to oropharyngeal secretions and the provision of oral fluids
b Risk of abdominal discomfort related to accumulation of gas and fluids in the gastrointestinal tract and decreased peristalsis
c Risk of distress and discomfort associated with withholding fluids
d Risk of oral discomfort related to limited oral intake and poor oral care
e Risk of peripheral, cerebral or pulmonary oedema related to excess fluid intake

5. ESTABLISH GOALS

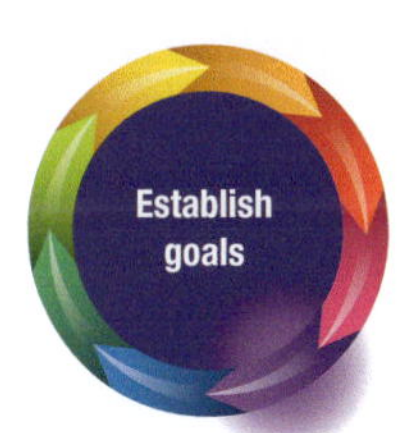

Before implementing any actions to improve this situation, it is important to clearly specify what you want to happen and when.

Q From the list below, choose the two most important *short-term* goals for Sally's management at this time.

a For Sally to be comfortable and treated with dignity
b For Sally to be hydrated with IV fluids
c To prevent dry mucous membranes and oral discomfort

Hint: Read Hemberg and Bergdahl (2020) for more information.

6. TAKE ACTION

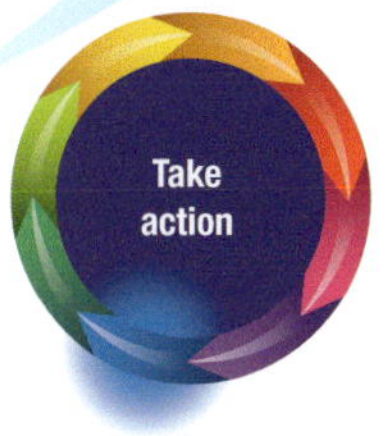

At this stage of the clinical reasoning cycle, you need to decide on your course of action to improve this situation. You should be alert to your role as patient advocate.

Q From the list below, choose the three *most immediate* actions you should take at this stage.

a Call the doctor and set up for the insertion of IV fluids.
b Explain to the family that IV fluids will not promote comfort for Sally. Her body has shut down and will not absorb intravenous fluids.

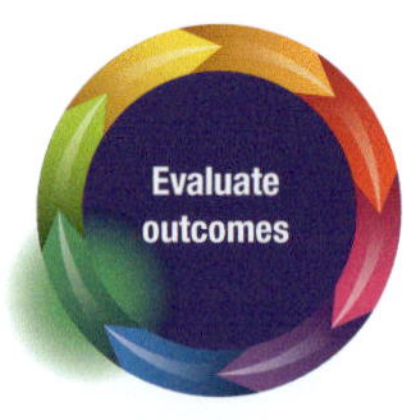

c Provide regular oral care, using moistening swabs with water (not glycerine swabs, as they dry mucous membranes), an oral gel or an oral spray.

d Explain to the family there has been a gradual decrease in food and fluid and that, provided regular mouth care is given, Sally will not suffer the ill effects of terminal dehydration.

7. EVALUATE

In person-centred care, you should refer to the patient and their family regarding their preferences for the use of music and aromatherapy. It is important that nurses do not push their own agenda and preferences.

It is now 24 hours later. Sally's family have been keeping a bedside vigil. Her terminal restlessness has settled. You have been giving her gentle massages when you turn and sponge her. The use of aromatherapy (lavender) in a vaporiser, along with low-level lighting and relaxation music, created a peaceful environment which has helped to calm both Sally and her family.

Sally died peacefully two days after being admitted to the hospice. She was very calm and pain-free in the last two days of her life. Sally's parents and her daughter Olivia were with her when she died and stayed with Sally for an hour longer to say their final farewells. They cried a lot and said how much they loved her. Sally's parents and Olivia chose not to assist in the final bathing of her but they selected a dress they wanted Sally to wear. You sat with them for a while and gently held Olivia's hand.

For the palliative care nurse, the death is not the completion of care. In many palliative care services, nurses will provide a bereavement service to the carers, the provision of support—supporting the expression of grief—and referral to bereavement counsellors or support networks if required.

8. REFLECT

Caring for people who require palliative care can often be stressful and emotionally distressing. Your own fear of death and dying, and feelings of inadequacy in relation to the person's suffering, can add to feelings of distress. When caring for people who are dying, it is important that you have realistic expectations about the degree of support you can provide. It is also important that you know who you can access for support and advice.

Q1 What actions will you take in clinical practice as a result of your learning from this scenario?

Q2 Why are self-care strategies so important in palliative care nursing?

Q3 Who would you talk to if you felt distressed about a dying patient you have been caring for?

Q4 What self-care strategies could you use to assist you in caring for a dying patient?

Q5 What advice or support could you provide for a colleague who is caring for a dying patient?

To find more information about the importance of self-care for your nursing career, go to Palliative Care Australia, Self Care Matters: https://palliativecare.org.au/resources/self-care-matters

EPILOGUE

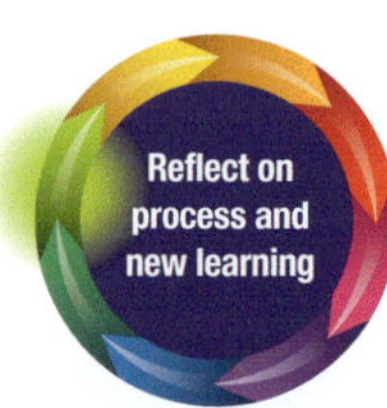

Several months after Sally died, the hospice received a card from her mother to say how much they appreciated the care given to Sally. She spoke of the gentle massages given to Sally when she was restless, and how the time taken to communicate with and comfort the family will always be remembered. Sally's mother said that Olivia is living with them and, although she misses her mother very much, love and care from family and friends and attendance at an adolescent bereavement support group have been very helpful.

FURTHER READING

Cancer Council NSW. Retrieved from: www.cancercouncil.com.au.

CareSearch (2011). *CareSearch: Palliative Care Knowledge Network*. Retrieved from: www.caresearch.com.au/tabid/6129/Default.aspx

Palliative Care Curriculum for Undergraduates (PCC4U). (2021). *Teaching and Learning Hub: Palliative Care Learning Modules*. Retrieved from: https://pcc4u.org.au

REFERENCES

Advance Care Planning Australia. (2021). Retrieved from: https://www.advancecareplanning.org.au

Amoah, C. (2011). The central importance of spirituality in palliative care. *International Journal of Palliative Care*, *17*(9), 353–58.

Anderson, P. L. (2020). Family Involvement: What Does a Loved One Want at the End of Life? In *Surgical Decision Making in Geriatrics*. Denmark: Springer Cham.

Australian Commission on Safety and Quality in Health Care (ACSQHC). (2021). *National Safety and Quality Health Service Standards* (2nd edn). Sydney, Australia.

Australian Institute of Health and Welfare. (2019). *Cancer in Australia 2019*. Cancer series no.119. Cat. no. CAN 123. Canberra: AIHW.

Bower, J. E., Crosswell, A. D., Stanton, A. L., Crespi, C. M., Winston, D., Arevalo, J., … Patricia, A. (2015). Mindfulness meditation for younger breast cancer survivors: A randomized controlled trial. *Cancer*, *121*(8), 1231–40. doi: 10.1002/cncr.29194

Brungardt, A., Wibben, A., Tompkins, A. F., Shanbhag, P., Coats, H., LaGasse, A. B., … & Lum, H. D. (2021). virtual reality-based music therapy in palliative care: A pilot implementation trial. *Journal of Palliative Medicine*, *24*(5), 736–42.

Candy, B., Armstrong, M., Flemming, K., Kupeli, N., Stone, P., Vickerstaff, V. & Wilkinson, S. (2020). The effectiveness of aromatherapy, massage and reflexology in people with palliative care needs: A systematic review. *Palliative Medicine*, *34*(2), 179–94.

Coluzzi, F., Alvaro, D., Caraceni, A. T., Gianni, W., Marinangeli, F., Massazza, G., … & Lugoboni, F. (2021). Common clinical practice for opioid-induced constipation: A physician survey. *Journal of Pain Research*, *14*, 2255.

Corpora, M., Liggett, E. & Leone, A. F. (2021). The effects of guided imagery and hand massage on wellbeing and pain in palliative care: Evaluation of a pilot study. *Complementary Therapies in Clinical Practice*, *42*, 101303.

Ferrell, B. R., Twaddle, M. L., Melnick, A. & Meier, D. E. (2018). National consensus project clinical practice guidelines for quality palliative care guidelines. *Journal of Palliative Medicine*, *21*(12), 1684–89.

Hanna, J. R., McCaughan, E., Beck, E. R. & Semple, C. J. (2021). Providing care to parents dying from cancer with dependent children: Health and social care professionals' experience. *Psycho-Oncology*, *30*(3), 331–39.

Hemberg, J. & Bergdahl, E. (2020). Dealing with ethical and existential issues at end of life through co-creation. *Nursing Ethics*, 27(4), 1012–31.

Hunter, J., Grant, S., Ee, C. & Templeman, K. (2020). What do medical specialists think about a proposed academic, integrative health centre in Australia? A qualitative study. *Complementary Therapies in Medicine*, *53*, 102530.

Iacoviello, L., Bonaccio, M., de Gaetano, G. & Donati, M. B. (2021, July). Epidemiology of breast cancer, a paradigm of the 'common soil' hypothesis. In *Seminars in Cancer Biology, 72*. 4–10.

Jastrzębski, A. K. (2020). The challenging task of defining spirituality. Journal of Spirituality in Mental Health, 1–19.

Kittelson, S., Eli, M. & Pennypacker, L. (2015). Palliative care symptom management. *Critical Care Nursing Clinics of North America*, *27*, 315–39.

Levett-Jones, T. Dwyer, T., Reid-Searl, K., Heaton, L., Flenady, T., Applegarth, J., Guinea, S. & Andersen, P. (2017). *The Patient Safety Competency Framework (PSCF) for Nursing Students*. Sydney, NSW.

Lokker, M. E., van der Heide, A., Oldenmenger, W. H., van der Rijt, C. C. & van Zuylen, L. (2019). Hydration and symptoms in the last days of life. *BMJ Supportive & Palliative Care, 11*(3), *335–43.*

McCabe, P. (2005). Complementary and alternative medicine in Australia: A contemporary overview. *Complementary Therapies in Clinical Practice*, *11*(1), 28–31.

Michalczyk, K., Pawlik, J., Czekawy, I., Kozłowski, M. & Cymbaluk-Płoska, A. (2021). Complementary methods in cancer treatment—cure or curse? *International Journal of Environmental Research and Public Health*, *18*(1), 356.

Murray, S. A., Kendall, M., Mitchell, G., Moine, S., Amblas-Novellas, J. & Boyd, K. (2017). Palliative care from diagnosis to death. *British Medical Journal*, 356.

Nursing and Midwifery Board of Australia (NMBA). (2016). *Registered Nurse Standards for Practice*. Retrieved from: http://nursingmidwiferyboard.gov.au/Codes-Guidelines-Statements/Professional-standards.aspx

Oechsle, K., Wais, M., Vehling, S., Bokemeyer, C. & Mehnert, A. (2014). Relationship between symptom burden, distress, and sense of dignity in terminally ill cancer patients. *Journal of Pain and Symptom Management*, *48*(3), 313–21.

Oehme, J. & Sheehan, C. (2018). Use of artificial hydration at the end of life: A survey of Australian and New Zealand palliative medicine doctors. *Journal of Palliative Medicine*, *21*(8), 1145–51.

Palliative Care Australia. (2018a). *Palliative Care 2030—Working Towards the Future of Quality Palliative Care for All*. PCA, Canberra.

Palliative Care Australia (2018b). *Palliative Care Service Development Guidelines*. Canberra: PCA. Retrieved from: PalliativeCare-Service-Delivery-2018_web2.pdf

Palliative Care Australia. (2018c). *National Palliative Care Standards*, 5th edn. PCA, Canberra.

Palliative Care Curriculum for Undergraduates (PCC4U). (2020). Project Team, with funding from the Australian Government Department of Health. *Palliative Care Curriculum for Undergraduates (PCC4U)*. Retrieved from: www.pcc4u.org.au

Palliative Care Curriculum for Undergraduates (PCC4U). (2021). *Teaching and Learning Hub: Palliative Care Learning Modules*. Retrieved from: https://pcc4u.org.au

Palliative Care Outcomes Collaboration. (2020). *Symptom Assessment Scale*. Retrieved from: Palliative Care Outcomes Collaboration.

Pascoe, M. C., Thompson, D. R. & Ski, C. F. (2020). Meditation and endocrine health and wellbeing. *Trends in Endocrinology & Metabolism*, *31*(7), 469–77.

Pietrasik, S., Zajac, G., Morawiec, J., Soszynski, M., Fila, M. & Blasiak, J. (2020). Interplay between BRCA1 and GADD45A and its potential for nucleotide excision repair in breast cancer pathogenesis. *International Journal of Molecular Sciences*, *21*(3), 870.

Pokladnikova, J. & Telec, I. (2020). Provision of complementary and alternative medicine: Compliance with the health professional requirements. *Health Policy*, *124*(3), 311–16.

Poletti, S., Razzini, G., Ferrari, R., Ricchieri, M. P., Spedicato, G. A., Pasqualini, A., … Bandieri, E. (2019). Mindfulness-based stress reduction in early palliative care for people with metastatic cancer: A mixed-method study. *Complementary Therapies in Medicine*, *47*, 102218.

Potvin, N., Hicks, M. & Kronk, R. (2021). Music therapy and nursing cotreatment in integrative hospice and palliative care. *Journal of Hospice and Palliative Nursing*, *23*(4), 309.

Proulx, K. & Jacelon, C. (2004). Dying with dignity: The good patient versus the good death. *American Journal Hospice Palliative Care*, *21*(2), 116–20.

Sarradon-Eck, A., Besle, S., Troian, J., Capodano, G. & Mancini, J. (2019). Understanding the barriers to introducing early palliative care for patients with advanced cancer: A qualitative study. *Journal of Palliative Medicine*, *22*(5), 508–16.

Sears, S., Kraus, S., Carlough, K. & Treat, E. (2011). Perceived benefits and doubts of participants in a weekly meditation study. *Mindfulness*, *2*(3), 167–74. doi: 10.1007/s12671-011-0055-4

Sheppard-Hanger, S. & Hanger, N. (2015). The importance of safety when using aromatherapy. *International Journal of Childbirth Education*, *30*(1), 42–47.

Smyth, T. & Allen, S. (2011). Nurses' experiences assessing the spirituality of terminally ill patients in acute clinical practice. *International Journal of Palliative Care, 17*(7), 337–43.

Steel, A., Schloss, J., Diezel, H., Palmgren, P. J., Maret, J. B. & Filbet, M. (2020). Complementary medicine visits by palliative care patients: A cross-sectional survey. *BMJ Supportive & Palliative Care, 12*(e1), e47–e58.

van der Riet, P., Francis, L. & Levett-Jones, T. (2011). Complementary therapies in healthcare: Design, implementation and evaluation of an elective course for undergraduate students. *Nurse Education in Practice*, *11*, 146–52.

Wilson, D. M., Anafi, F., Roh, S. J. & Errasti-Ibarrondo, B. (2020). A scoping research literature review to identify contemporary evidence on the incidence, causes, and impacts of end-of-life intra-family conflict. *Health Communication*, 1–7.

World Health Organization (WHO). (2021). *Palliative Care*. Retrieved from: https://www.who.int/news-room/fact-sheets/detail/palliative-care

Wright, S. G. (2005). *Reflections on Spirituality and Health*. London: Whurr Publishers Ltd.

Yazdanimehr, R., Omidi, A., Sadat, Z. & Akbari, H. (2016). The effect of mindfulness integrated cognitive behaviour therapy on depression and anxiety among pregnant women: A randomised clinical trial. *Journal of Caring Sciences*, *5*(3), 195–204.

Zumstein-Shaha, M., Ferrell, B. & Economou, D. (2020). Nurses' response to spiritual needs of cancer patients. *European Journal of Oncology Nursing*, *48*, 101792.

Chapter 17

Caring for a person who is refusing treatment

LORINDA PALMER

LEARNING OUTCOMES

Completion of the activities in this chapter will enable you to:

- outline the ethical and legal dimensions of clinical reasoning in a refusal-of-treatment context
- relate the concepts of futile and burdensome treatment, quality of life and person-centred care to the process of making a decision to refuse treatment
- describe the process for making a valid advance care directive (ACD) in Australia
- interpret the balance of benefits and harm associated with refusal of cardiopulmonary resuscitation (CPR)
- reflect on personal and professional values relating to refusal of treatment decisions
- identify how experience, emotions and situational contexts can affect clinical reasoning
- investigate relevant areas of legislation, common law, departmental/NSW Health policies and the National Safety and Quality Health Service (NSQHS) standards applicable to the refusal of CPR (and other potentially life-saving treatments) in Australia.

INTRODUCTION

This book would not be complete without a chapter exploring the ethical issues that nurses may encounter when caring for a person who is refusing potentially life-saving treatment; in this case cardio-pulmonary resuscitation (CPR). Mr George McAllister, who you will meet in the following pages, is one such person.

As we have learned, 'failure to rescue' occurs when nurses miss vital cues and do not detect a patient's deterioration early enough to prevent a serious and potentially preventable outcome from occurring. But, what if cues that a patient is trying to refuse treatment are missed, misinterpreted or overlooked? Not all attempts to 'rescue' are appropriate if the treatment being given is futile and burdensome, not in the person's best interests, or not in accordance with their wishes.

However, the process of determining what is in a person's best interests and what accords with their wishes can be fraught with difficulties. Good communication skills are needed in the context of a therapeutic relationship incorporating an ethos of culturally appropriate, person-centred care (Hall, Roland & Grande, 2019).

Another complication is that, while many hospitals have protocols for how to respond when a patient's condition deteriorates, clear procedures do not always exist for when a patient wants to refuse treatment, particularly potentially life-saving treatments such as CPR.

These decisions can be complex as they often involve both technical and ethical elements–that is, discussion of broader issues, such as the limits of technology, the uncertainty of outcomes, eliciting patient's preferences, navigating potential family conflicts, and talking about death and dying (Hayes, 2013). These are difficult conversations to have and there are highly sensitive issues for everyone involved to traverse. There is evidence that, as a result, 'people from ethnic minority groups and people with conditions other than cancer are less likely to receive the care that meets their wishes and needs' (Hall, Roland & Grande, 2019, p. 330).

This situation is compounded by the lack of legal clarity; although this is perhaps less of an issue in jurisdictions such as Victoria, where legislation addressing the refusal of life-saving treatment and making advance care directives has been enacted. New South Wales is not one of those jurisdictions, so the legal situation there relies on common law cases and their interpretation in NSW Health guidelines and hospital policies (Forrester & Griffiths, 2014). Refusal cues may also be overlooked if clinicians feel compelled to do everything possible to try to 'save' someone; and in many ways (in both myth and reality), performing CPR is one of the classic 'rescue' missions.

KEY CONCEPTS

ethical reasoning
ethical dilemma
advance care directive (ACD)
futile and burdensome treatment
CPR decision making
withdrawal of treatment and withholding treatment
end-of-life care

SUGGESTED READINGS

C. Bergland. (2019). *Integrating Law, Ethics and Regulation: A Guide for Nursing and Health Care Students*. Melbourne: Oxford University Press.
Chapter 9: Timeless quandries at the beginning and end of life

K. Forrester & D. Griffiths. (2014). *Essentials of Law for Health Professionals* (4th edn). Sydney: Elsevier.
Chapter 8: Refusal of treatment

I. Kerridge, M. Lowe & C. Stewart. (2013). *Ethics and Law for the Health Professions* (4th edn). Sydney: Federation Press.
Chapter 18: CPR and no-CPR orders

Whatever the reasons, decisions to withhold potentially life-saving treatments—not to rescue—are among the most frequent and difficult moral problems that nurses encounter in practice (Adams et al., 2011). They require excellent clinical reasoning and decision-making capability, combined with person-centred care and therapeutic communication capabilities, and a sound understanding of the relevant legislation and case law.

Patient Safety Competency Framework (PSCF)

Domain 2–Therapeutic communication

The PSCF specifies that nurses must demonstrate the ability to use verbal and non-verbal communication skills to convey respect and empathy, and to encourage the person to express their feelings and needs while at the same time maintaining professional boundaries.

Source: *The Patient Safety Competency Framework for Nursing Students*, https://patientsafetyfornursingstudents.org

This chapter explores how the clinical reasoning cycle can be used to assist in the ethical reasoning process associated with a situation involving the withholding of CPR.

Questions and answers in this chapter

Ethical dilemmas such as the ones explored in this chapter rarely have unequivocally correct answers. For this reason, the answers provided on the Pearson website to the questions asked in this chapter are not intended to be definitive. Instead, they are provided to promote reflection and discussion, and they also suggest avenues for further reading and learning.

SCENARIO 17.1 The night before Christmas ...

SETTING THE SCENE

It is late in the evening on Christmas Eve, on a busy cardiology unit about an hour before handover and change of shift, when notification comes of a new admission. He is Mr George McAllister, a 78-year-old man who had surgery that day at another hospital but is being transferred because he needs specialist cardiac care. He has had a post-surgical myocardial infarction following radical prostatectomy. He has a bladder irrigation in-situ, a history of poorly controlled type 2 diabetes and right-sided hemiplegia from a stroke five years ago. Pathology results on the grading and staging of his prostate cancer are pending.

> Access this AIHW website page Australia's *Health 2020* to find out more about the incidence, prevalence, morbidity and mortality associated with the four health conditions that George has: myocardial infarction, stroke, type 2 diabetes and prostate cancer: https://www.aihw.gov.au/reports-data/australias-health

George arrives just before the shift ends, so there isn't time to do much more than settle him in, ensure he is comfortable and pain free, check whether he has any medications due, assess his vital signs and check that his bladder irrigation is patent.

George feels exhausted by his traumatic day—major surgery for prostate cancer, chest pain, a heart attack, a late-evening transfer to a different hospital, the pain from surgery and the discomfort caused by his urethral catheter.

In just a few hours it will be Christmas Day.

VALUES

Clinical decisions about treatment cannot be separated from the whole person. Up until this point, the healthcare professionals involved in George's care have been focused on diagnosing and treating his medical conditions. But all of these things have a deep impact on George's life and his ability to live it in a way that is satisfying and meaningful to him. That is, George's values and perceptions of his quality of life, which up until now have not been a significant factor in his care, are about to become so.

Thus far, he has accepted, in a fairly unquestioning way, advice about what surgeries, tests and treatments he should have. But things have now reached the point where he wants to reconsider the course he is on.

Review the information on this NSW Health website about advance care planning and how people can make their wishes known: www.health.nsw.gov.au/patients/acp/pages/default.aspx

Thinking about this overnight, George decides that, if something happens and he has another heart attack, he does not want to be 'jumped on' and revived. He has known for quite some time that he doesn't want to be 'kept alive on machines', and he feels that now would be a good time to make that known. He is not sure what to say specifically, or to whom, but he is sure that the nurses will know. He determines to ask someone about it in the morning. The young male nurse who settled him in said he would be back for the morning shift. George thought that he seemed really nice and very assured, and that he would be the right person to talk to.

Something to think about ...

George's personal values underpin his beliefs and guide his decisions. The nurse caring for George is guided by the values and standards of his profession. These are expressed in the International Council of Nurses (ICN) Code of Ethics for Nurses *(2012), the NMBA* Code of Conduct for Nurses *(2016) and the NMBA* Registered Nurse Standards for Practice *(2016): https://www.nursingmidwiferyboard.gov.au/Codes-Guidelines-Statements/Professional-standards.aspx*

Review these professional codes and standards and identify which values and expectations are most relevant to George's situation, as well as how they relate to the clinical decisions and care that George's nurses should be providing for him. Also note the common threads that run across all four of these documents.

PERSON-CENTRED CARE—WHO IS GEORGE?

In order to understand why George might feel this way about his situation, it is necessary to know much more about him than just the results of his tests and scans. In common with many of his generation, who lived through the depression and World War II, George has worked hard all his life and values independence and thrift. He has been married twice—his first wife is now deceased and his second marriage did not work out, resulting in divorce several years ago. He has no contact with his ex-wife and his only daughter died over five years ago from cancer. Apart from his sister and her extended family, George has no close relatives. He tries to keep up an active social life and interests, and up until five years ago when he had the stroke, he was very physically active. But the disability arising from the stroke has been a huge blow from which he has not recovered. He has always been very particular about his appearance and his physical ability, and the loss of these has been steadily eroding his confidence and happiness. He has had counselling and psychological support but none of it has helped much and, for George, life entails a daily struggle to cope, with deep wounds to his psyche that have never healed.

Patient Safety Competency Framework (PSCF)

Domain 1—Person-centred care

The PSCF specifies that nurses must consider the person's rights, preferences, needs and values when planning and providing care, and support the person to make informed choices about their healthcare.

Source: *The Patient Safety Competency Framework for Nursing Students*, https://patientsafetyfornursingstudents.org

More than anything, George fears having another stroke or illness that renders him even more unable to function than he already is. Stroke survivorship has taught him harsh lessons about the nature of quality of life after stroke that perhaps only those who have lived through it—or care for those who do—can fully appreciate. He does not want to end his remaining years in an aged care facility, or be dependent on full-time care. He has seen this happen to some of his relatives and friends, and he is determined that this will not happen to him.

Mostly, what George wants is that, when the time comes for him to die, he retains the same fierce independence, pride and dignity that have been so integral to his character for his entire life. He is not sure whether that time is now but somehow it feels as though it might be. George is not afraid of dying. He has lived a good life and takes great comfort from his memories. What he is terribly afraid of now is losing control over his mind, body and life for whatever remaining time that he has.

> This information about George is mostly unknown to the healthcare professionals who have been caring for him. One reason is that few health assessments entail asking patients about their values, beliefs or wishes regarding the limits to continued treatment, such as CPR. Read *The value of taking an 'ethics history'* by Sayers et al. (2001) for a discussion on this issue: www.jstor.org/stable/27718658

It makes sense that for truly person-centred and compassionate care, George's perspectives on the situation need to be well understood by all those who are providing care for him at this critically important time. Despite the fact that Greg has not had much time to get to know George, the imperative for person-centred care is no less vital. Rather, it is more so, and we are about to find out just how much.

National Safety and Quality Health Service (NSQH) Standards

Partnering with consumers and Communicating for safety standards

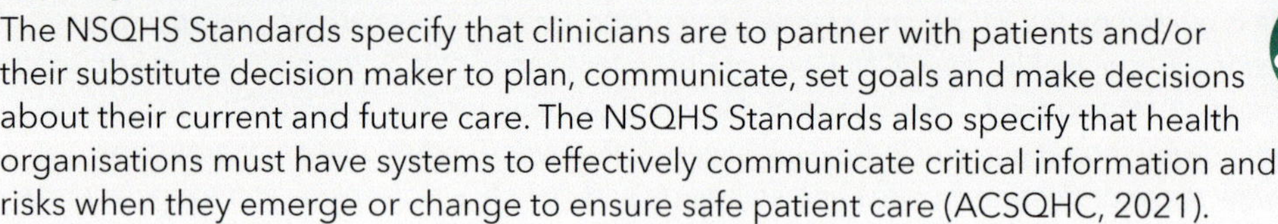

The NSQHS Standards specify that clinicians are to partner with patients and/or their substitute decision maker to plan, communicate, set goals and make decisions about their current and future care. The NSQHS Standards also specify that health organisations must have systems to effectively communicate critical information and risks when they emerge or change to ensure safe patient care (ACSQHC, 2021).

SCENARIO 17.2 Christmas morning

CHANGING THE SCENE

The next morning, George is happy to see Greg, the nurse who looked after him the evening before, walk back into his room and greet him. Today, George will find the right time to tell Greg about the decision he made the night before. Not just yet, though, because breakfast is arriving and there is quite a bit of festive cheer being bandied about. People are coming in and out of the four-bed room and Greg looks a bit busy with other patients in the room; but soon, when the moment is right …

Eventually, the moment does arise and George tells Greg that he 'doesn't want any heroics' if he has another heart attack or stroke. Greg is surprised, because not many patients come out and say things so directly so he wasn't expecting this. But after a short conversation, he tells George that the best thing to do is to wait until a bit later in the morning when Dr Jones, George's cardiologist, does his rounds and the matter can be discussed with him.

It is now 1030 hours and George has been in the unit for just over 14 hours. Dr Jones has come to see him to assess his condition and options for treatment. The bedside visit is quite short and is focused on George's physical problems, particularly the tests and medications relating to his heart attack. George feels a bit intimidated. Dr Jones looks busy and the room is still quite noisy and full of people, so George doesn't raise the issue of not wanting CPR. As Dr Jones leaves the room, George whispers a reminder to Greg to go after him and tell him about his decision. Greg catches up to Dr Jones at the desk as he is writing in George's notes and tells him what George has said to him earlier; how he feels about not having CPR. Dr Jones thinks for a moment and replies, 'We'll talk about that later after his pathology results [tests for the staging and grading of his prostate cancer] come back.' He closes the chart and walks away.

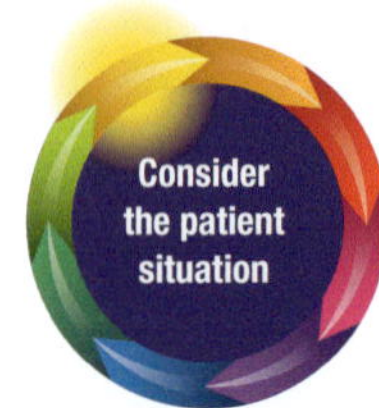

1. CONSIDER THE PATIENT SITUATION

What should Greg do in this situation? He has a number of options, but finding the best—or least worst—will not be easy. He is having a very busy shift and, on top of that, it is Christmas Day. Should he seek advice from someone; if so, from whom? And what should he tell George now? Should he go after Dr Jones immediately and ask him to come back to talk with George? Should he just do as he was told and wait? What if George has a cardiac arrest in the meantime? Should Greg do CPR even though he now knows that George does not want it and has specifically refused it? Is that refusal legally valid?

Greg has spent only a few hours with George and does not know him very well. Could he be depressed? He has had a terribly stressful 24 hours. Is he in the right frame of mind to be making a decision like this? On the other hand, everyone has accepted that his frame of mind is perfectly okay to consent to continuing treatment, so why should it be questioned only when he wants to refuse it?

The dilemma Greg is facing here is not uncommon. There are a number of complex and conflicting issues and, before deciding what to do next, Greg needs to carefully think through the ethical and legal aspects of the situation. This is the process of ethical reasoning and decision making. The aim of this process is to try to identify what could be done, what should be done, what actually will be done, and why.

Jewell (2000, cited in Henderson, 2005, p. 190) poses an interesting question: is a moral person 'one who feels strongly about moral issues, one who understands moral issues or one who acts ethically when dealing with other[s]'?

Let's now work through the clinical reasoning cycle, with a focus on the ethical and legal dimensions of the situation, to see if you can identify what should be done, and what you actually would do if you were the nurse caring for George.

According to the clinical reasoning cycle, the first stage involves carefully considering the patient. Contextual reality may have a considerable impact at this stage. George's late arrival on Christmas Eve has the potential to be a distraction. Matters that are not urgent or life threatening, like advance directives and discussions about no-CPR decisions, can safely be left until after Christmas ... can't they?

Another factor is the sheer complexity and difficulty of the ethical problems that arise in healthcare. Ethical dilemmas, by their very nature, are often difficult and messy, and may involve conflict, taking time to address and resolve. It requires a particular state of mind to 'see' the ethical dimensions of clinical situations, and a deliberate act of will to go beyond the surface 'routine' of clinical practice to address the ethical complexities of the situation. Epstein (2006, p.115) calls the ability to do this 'mindful practice [in] the tacit ethics of the moment'. How the moral agent views these issues will have a significant impact on the way this situation unfolds, and on the outcome.

Therefore, the first stage of the clinical reasoning cycle, 'consider the patient's situation', should ideally focus as much on George as a person as on George having a number of serious and potentially life-threatening medical conditions. Will those caring for George consider his values and perspectives just as important as his diagnosis? Getting that balance right is extremely difficult and requires a high degree of willingness to listen to the points of view of others, as well as insight into one's own.

2. COLLECT CUES/INFORMATION

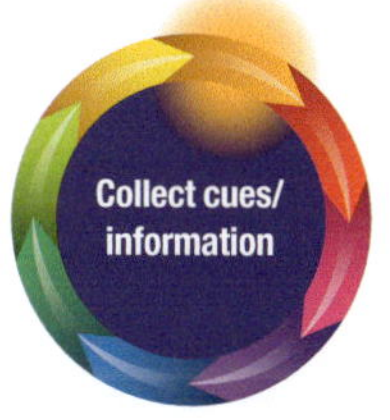

(a) Review current information

There is a great deal that Greg does not know about George, especially the things that lie beneath the reasons for his decision to refuse CPR. One short conversation without privacy was not enough. George did appear to be very certain though, and what was also apparent was his trust in Greg that he would know what to do.

On the other hand, Greg does not feel confident that George's refusal was sufficiently informed and not unduly influenced by his distressing experiences of the previous day. Greg wants to act in George's best interests, but it is not clear at the moment exactly what those are. Greg is very aware of the need for information to inform decisions; however, he is also uncomfortable with Dr Jones' view that George cannot refuse CPR until he has a clearer diagnosis and prognosis for his prostate cancer. Greg needs more information too, not only from George, but also about the wider ethical and legal ramifications of the situation.

(b) Gather new information

Nurses are familiar with conducting health assessments and taking patient histories, but such histories rarely involve deliberately eliciting information about a patient's values and treatment preferences, particularly concerning things like CPR. One of the ways of doing this is through an ethics history, in which information about George's understanding of his current situation, his values and wishes and the reasons for them, family relationships and other crucial but as yet unknown issues could be directly and explicitly explored. Sayers et al. (2001, p. 115) suggest some questions that could be useful in taking an ethics history, for example:

Very occasionally patients have what is called a cardiac arrest. This means their heart stops beating. Usually we try to restart it using artificial respiration, drugs and sometimes an electric shock. Usually doctors decide what to do, but some patients prefer to decide [this] for themselves.

Would you like to make this decision?

Would you like us, or a family member, to decide?

Do you need more information before answering?

Some people make advance directives ... Have you heard of this? If so, are there any such directives that you would want us to know about?

Greg also needs to know what processes should be followed for George's refusal of CPR to be recognised in law. There is variation between the states in regard to legislation and case law as well as different processes for making an advance care directive (ACD). Therefore, nurses need to be aware of the relevant polices and guidelines in their jurisdiction. The NSW Health (2021) document *Making an Advance Care Directive* provides guidance for people to work through the process of making an ACD. If an ACD is valid it must be followed. The ACD includes a section on personal values about dying and a section on directions about medical care, one of which specifically addresses accepting or refusing CPR. One of the things that Greg would need to know is whether George already has an ACD or, if not, whether he would like to make one now.

Consider the following questions:

In Victoria, people can also complete an advance care directive (under the *Medical Treatment Planning and Decisions Act 2016)*: https://www.advancecareplanning.org.au/create-your-plan/create-your-plan-vic Identify what laws, policies and processes for ACDs apply in your state.

Q1 Do you think that nurses should be involved in making CPR decisions, or is this outside their scope of practice? Explain.

Q2 If you are in NSW, download and read the NSW Health *Making an Advance Care Directive* document at the following link: https://www.health.nsw.gov.au/patients/acp/Publications/acd-form-info-book.pdf

In NSW, does an ACD have to be filled out on the form provided in that official document and witnessed?

Q3 The NSW Health *Making an Advance Care Directive* document states (on p. 5) the elements that make an ACD valid in NSW. What are they?

(c) Recall knowledge

The knowledge of ethics and law that each individual nurse has will depend on their education, experience and professional ethos. While most nurses have had ethics content as part of their undergraduate education, one study found that many nurses (74%) feel that they need more continuing ethics education in the workplace (Johnstone, Da Costa & Turale, 2004). One effect that ethics education has been found to have is to make it more likely that the nurse will encounter ethical issues in their practice. This is believed to be because they become increasingly likely to 'see' the ethical dimensions of practice—in other words, their perceptions fundamentally change as a result of such education. But being more attuned and aware of the ethical dimensions of practice is just the first step. To practice effectively, nurses also need to be able to correctly apply that knowledge to the situation at hand. This can be difficult because the details of each case are frequently quite distinctive in their nuances and content, and clinicians have to make inferences to determine how the generalities of codes or the specifics of different law cases apply.

Go to: https://www.advancecareplanning.org.au/understand-advance-care-planning/advance-care-planning-for-aboriginal-and-torres-strait-islander-peoples and scroll down to 'Access culturally appropriate resources' and 'Take control of your health journey'.

The *ICN Code of Ethics for Nurses* (2012) should be well known to all nurses practising in Australia. Greg is aware that the Code values respect for human rights, choice and dignity, and to be treated with respect. However, these value statements are quite broad, and Greg has to translate them into the specifics of this situation. For example, this might entail:

- knowing what the benefits and risks of CPR actually are for George in this situation
- knowing how to assess whether George has made an informed refusal
- knowing how to ensure that George's values, beliefs and wishes are both elicited and respected
- knowing which actions are consistent with these value statements and which are not.

Greg is also aware that the NMBA's *Code of Conduct for Nurses* (2016) requires him to practise in accordance with current laws. Some of the specific aspects of law that apply to this situation, and that Greg will need to know about, include:

- knowing what George's legal rights are in relation to refusing CPR
- knowing how best to inform George of these rights
- knowing his own legal responsibilities in either instigating or withholding CPR in the absence of a clearly documented no-CPR decision.

Consider the following questions.

Q1 Assuming that George does have decision-specific capacity, does he have the legal right to refuse CPR?

Q2 What might the potential legal consequences be of instigating CPR in the current situation (i.e., knowing George has refused it, but in the absence of any documentation)?

The epidemiology of in-hospital cardiac arrest

Studies of the morbidity and mortality of in-hospital cardiac arrests show some interesting findings, some of which may surprise you. For example, we know that older people with chronic illnesses (such as George has) are much less likely to survive to discharge, are less likely to be discharged to their home and have significantly worse outcomes than those who do not have chronic illnesses (Stapleton et al., 2014). Conversely, patients and the general public considerably overestimate their chances of surviving a cardiac arrest. A study by Kaldjian et al. (2009) found that patients think the probability of surviving a cardiac arrest is 60 per cent, whereas actual rates are closer to 12–19 per cent (van Gijn et al., 2014). This figure may be even lower, depending on factors such as age, co-morbidities and peri-arrest variables (such as time taken to initiate CPR). There are also other risks that many people may not consider, such as surviving with permanent neurological damage, and/or needing nursing home care rather than being able to be discharged home.

A famous study of the depiction of CPR in movies and television found that it was shown to be successful over 75 per cent of the time, many times greater than happens in reality (Diem et al., 1996; Portnova et al., 2015). For more details on the epidemiology of CPR, go to: doi.org/10.1016/j.resuscitation.2013.02.021

This doesn't mean that we should not be doing CPR. What it does mean is that the potential benefits and risks should be carefully and realistically considered for each patient's situation. In George's case, since he was so fearful of losing any more of his physical and mental capability, the risks are particularly applicable.

Q How does this information affect your assessment of whether CPR is in George's best interests?

3. PROCESS INFORMATION

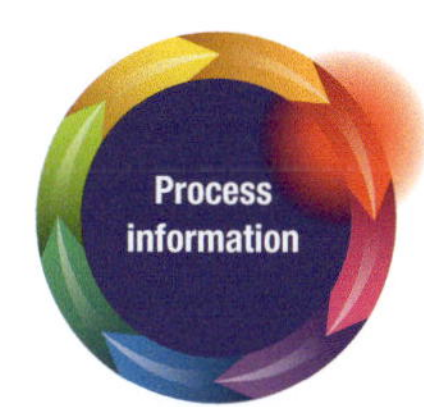

The third stage of the clinical reasoning cycle relates to the processing of information.

(a) Interpret

Interpretation can be difficult when the information that you are working with is subjective and not in the form of quantifiable and objective data, such as that derived from physiological signs and symptoms.

This stage of interpretation will also be filtered through the person doing the interpreting, and we know that human beings are not value-neutral when they make interpretations. Each person has had past experiences, both personal and professional, of situations such as this. Each person has personal beliefs and opinions about such matters, perhaps informed by a religion or perhaps not. These past experiences and personal values will affect how Greg feels about what George is requesting. Some nurses may interpret what George is requesting as irrational, a product of fear or stress or depression, and call into question his capacity to make such a decision. Others may interpret his refusal of treatment as synonymous with a wish to die. Greg's interpretation of these complex factors will have a significant impact on the outcome. Another nurse may interpret things differently and come to quite a different conclusion. This is yet one more way in which George is vulnerable in this situation. He is, to a considerable extent, dependent not only on the way others see him but also on their preparedness to act (or not) based on their interpretations.

According to the moral psychologist Jonathan Haidt (2000), human beings do not make moral judgments judicially and reasonably; rather, they do so quickly and instinctively, relying on innate intuitions, emotions, and socially and culturally derived perceptions and values. For Haidt, reason comes into play only after we have already made a judgment, and it is used mainly to rationalise or justify the judgment to ourselves and to others. Haidt's challenging ideas provide a fascinating insight into the ways in which a reasoning process may be far less rational than we realise.

Consider the following questions.

Q1 This situation potentially involves a clash of differing values and moral views. We are now well aware of George's values, but those of Greg and Dr Jones are much less visible. How might they affect the situation?

Q2 What values do you hold that would influence your interpretation of the information that you have about this situation?

Read about some of the debates on how humans came to be moral, the sources of our moral views and differences, and how we make moral judgments at The Situationist website: http://thesituationist.wordpress.com/2008/06/17/jonathan-haidt-on-the-situation-of-moral-reasoning

(b) Discriminate, (c) Relate, (d) Infer and (e) Match

These elements of the clinical reasoning cycle might involve Greg being able to:

- distinguish what is more important from that which is less so
- identify what is most relevant from that which is least relevant
- identify which aspects of his past experiences with similar situations might be helpful in this one
- identify how his emotions and feelings about what has happened might be influencing his reasoning.

All of these elements require careful consideration of nuanced and detailed information. Is it more important for George's wishes to be respected or more important that his carers are sure that those wishes are informed? Is following the 'correct' process of refusing CPR more or less important than the outcome? Is it possible that processes which are intended to give rise to better ethical decisions may not, in fact, do so in some situations? Could this be one of those? These four elements—discriminating, relating, inferring and matching—all require experience and skill to engage in effectively. If this is the first time that Greg has encountered this kind of situation, his thinking, feelings and overall approach at this stage of the clinical reasoning cycle are likely to be very different from his approach if he is used to and comfortable dealing with complexity, nuance and ambiguity.

(f) Predict

Thinking ahead to predict the outcome of each possible option for decisions in this situation is not a straightforward undertaking. There are a bewildering number of possibilities. However, Greg may identify the following options:

a Explain to George what has happened.
b Ask George whether he would like the involvement and support of family and/or friends.
c Undertake a proper ethics history.
d Make a thorough and detailed documentation of the information elicited from the ethics history.
e Explain to George how he can go about making a legally binding advance care directive.
f Call Dr Jones back and ask him to see George again.
g Notify the immediate clinical supervisor about what has happened and ask for advice.
h Do nothing except document George's request and Dr Jones' response.
i Do nothing at all now; not mention anything to George about what has happened, not document anything, and leave it until the next shift or even later.
j Various combinations of these options.

Options (a) to (g) will, to varying degrees, be time consuming. Even though it is Christmas morning, it is still very busy and Greg has four other patients to care for. So it is possible that this will also be a factor in determining what happens next, even though this may not be explicitly acknowledged.

Apart from the time factor, there is also the question of how both Dr Jones and George might respond. Options (a) to (f) all require some degree and form of moral agency or advocacy from Greg, on George's behalf. Seal (2007), in a study of nurses and advocacy in advance care planning, found that up to 49 per cent of nurses felt powerless to advocate for their patients when issues of end-of-life care, or making decisions to withdraw or withhold treatment, were concerned. However, with the involvement of an institutionally supported intervention—the Respecting Patient Choices Program—this dropped to 19 per cent.

This suggests that, even if Greg decides he should pursue options (e) and/or (f), he might feel he does not have the power to do so. Greg may feel that he lacks institutional or collegial support for any decision he might make that involves advocating for George, and his perception of the consequences of doing this may be a significant concern at this point.

4. IDENTIFY THE ETHICAL PROBLEM/ISSUE

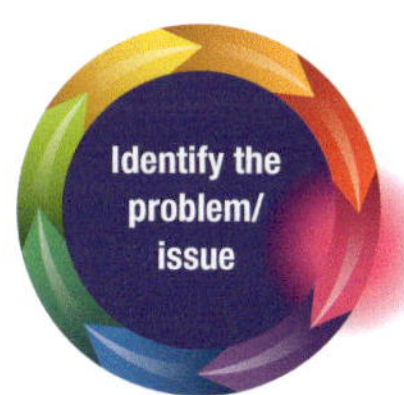

The core problem here is the question of who is responsible for making a no-CPR decision, and how that decision should be discussed, formally recognised and followed through. George thinks it is his decision. Unfortunately, he has little real understanding of the legal and procedural complexity that lies behind his request not to have CPR.

Dr Jones thinks it is his decision. He believes that he has both the expertise and the ultimate authority. The procedural need for formal documentation of some kind makes it unclear what should happen now, and if and how such an authority might legitimately and usefully be challenged.

Greg is caught in the middle but if George has a cardiac arrest, then it will become Greg's decision. The moral problem for Greg is three-fold: First, can he find a way for George's refusal of treatment to be formally acknowledged? Second, can he make it happen in time? And, finally, what will he do if he can't?

5. ESTABLISH GOALS

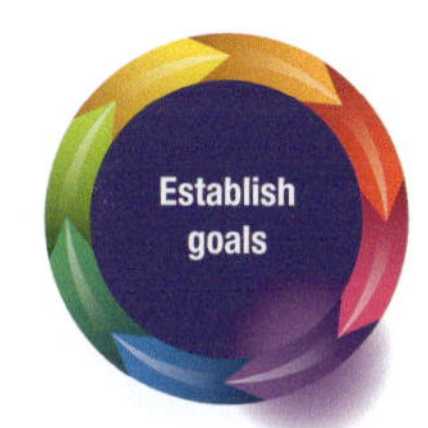

The people involved in this situation have different goals arising from their different values and perspectives about what is most important. Dr Jones values a clear diagnosis and that is his goal. His perception of George's best interests is to make a CPR decision based on having that information. George feels that he doesn't need that information. His decision about CPR isn't predicated on knowing if he has prostate cancer or not; it is about not wanting to live with a quality of life any less than he has now. These positions are fundamentally different.

The question is, whose goals (and values) come first? Nurses and doctors should and do put patients first, but it is possible (as we have seen) to have a different perspective about what that entails. In this situation, Greg's goal might well be to try to bridge the gap between George and Dr Jones, to make each aware of the other's position, and to try to resolve the situation in a collegial way that reflects the principles and goals of a best-practice advance care planning process.

There is something else that might be worth considering here. The Greek philosopher Aristotle wrote a great deal about the human virtues that lead to making good moral decisions. He believed that humans of good character or virtue would act rightly and make correct decisions, and that we should, throughout our lives, work consciously and deliberately to develop these character traits. For Aristotle, 'goodness' included traits such as kindness and generosity. He wrote in *Nichomachean Ethics*, '… we do not act rightly because we have virtue or excellence, but we rather have those because we have acted rightly. We are what we repeatedly do.'

Habits of thought and practice might be highly influential at this stage of the process. They may even determine the outcome. It is also possible that certain decisions and actions may be able to be definitely excluded as being the antithesis of 'goodness' and 'virtue'. Examples of such behaviours would include lying to George (even by omission) or avoiding him until the shift is over, behaviours that arise from self-centred rather than person-centred goals.

6. TAKE ACTION

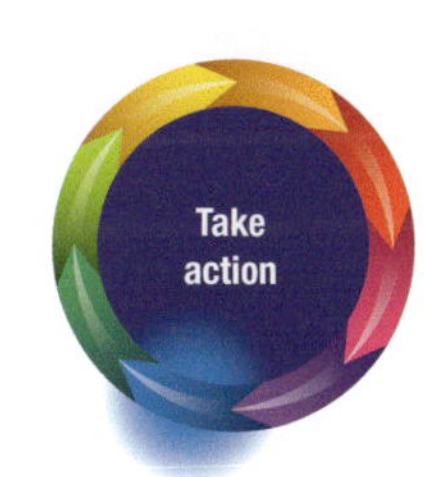

It turns out that Greg's time for thinking about the situation and taking action is cut short. What happens next is something he hasn't really believed could happen, even though he knows it is a possibility.

George's condition has been stable since his transfer and he's had no further chest pain. He begs Greg to allow him to take a shower on a commode chair because he hates bed baths and doesn't want to have one on Christmas Day. So Greg takes him to the shower on a commode chair and is with him when George has a cardiac arrest.

Greg then has to make yet another decision about what to do and this time there is no time for thinking. So he pushes the emergency buzzer, turns off the shower, eases George from the commode to the floor and starts CPR. The team arrives with the crash cart and George is carried naked from the bathroom to the corridor just outside where an attempt to resuscitate him continues in full public view, with just a towel over his groin in a meagre attempt to preserve his modesty.

As someone else takes over doing chest compressions, the realisation hits Greg that what is happening is precisely what George has been trying to avoid.

After a prolonged resuscitation, George is taken to the coronary care unit (CCU) and Greg is left to wonder if he has done the right thing and what, if anything, he could have done differently.

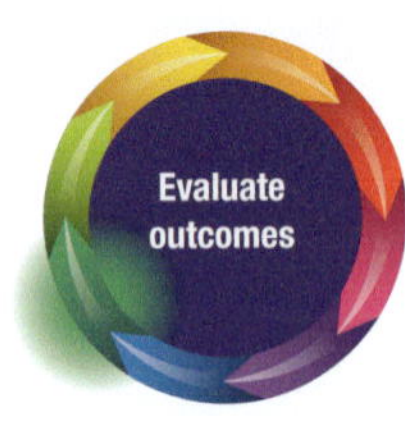

7. EVALUATE

As Greg is thinking about what has happened and wrestling with his feelings of guilt, a call comes from the CCU. George's sister is there and wants to talk to him. Greg is a little apprehensive but it turns out that she wants to talk about the documentation he wrote in the notes earlier, in which he explained in detail the results of his conversations with George. She has found out about it because the CCU staff wanted to confirm the information with her. George's sister tells Greg how thankful she is that Greg has done this and has taken the trouble to get to know George. She tells Greg that George has told her several times that, when his time comes, he wants to go quickly and calmly. George's sister goes on to say that George has not regained consciousness and that his life support is about to be turned off. She then asks if Greg would like to be there when it is.

Greg agrees; so he, the last person to know George, is there with George's sister, who knows him best, to say goodbye at the end.

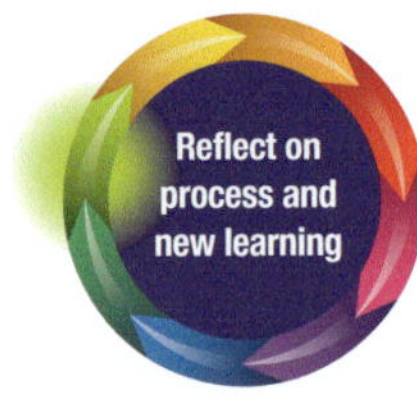

8. REFLECT

Reflecting on the whole situation afterwards, Greg realised that he could have done some things differently. He should have known that George was quite likely to have another cardiac arrest, and he should have factored that eventuality more into his thinking. But he also realised that, even knowing about the possibility, he hadn't really believed the cardiac arrest would happen when it did.

Greg felt sad and conflicted, knowing that George had an awful death, so lacking in the dignity that characterised his life, but also that, without the CPR attempt, his sister would not have had the opportunity to see him and say goodbye. So there had been both good and bad in what had happened. Greg knew, though, that he could never tell George's sister the reality of George's resuscitation, naked on the floor, in full view of almost the whole ward. So instead he gave a silent apology to George for not being able to protect him from that.

He wouldn't ever forget George and, if something like this happened again, Greg knew what he would do differently. He now knew that, whatever the time of day or year, patients' requests for refusing treatment have to be decisively followed up then and there. He knew now that he should have asked Dr Jones to go back and speak to George instead of saying nothing as the doctor walked away. He also realised that the ward needed clearer guidelines on what the nurses should do in situations like this, so that outcomes would be less up to the vagaries of chance.

It is a hopeful signal for change that the need for better end-of-life care planning has been recognised and acted upon by the Australian Commission on Safety and Quality in Health Care. The NSQHS standards now include a *Partnering with consumers* standard which aims to address gaps in quality and safety, such as those that occur when we are not person-centred in our approach to care and fail to determine people's preferences for care (ACSQHC, 2017). The future prospects for comprehensive end-of-life care planning for patients like George are now much improved.

Reflect on your learning from this scenario and consider the following questions.

Q1 What are three of the most important things that you have learnt from this scenario?

Q2 Identify the full range of specific nursing actions that you think may have prevented George from having CPR against his wishes.

Q3 Considering your answer to Q1 and Q2, what would you have done in this situation and why?

Q4 What resources, information and support is available in your state to help people make an advance care plan?

FURTHER READING

Australian Commission on Safety and Quality in Health Care (ACSQHC). (2019). *End-of-Life Care*. Retrieved from: https://www.safetyandquality.gov.au/our-work/end-life-care

Relevant legislation and common law:

Advance Care Planning Australia. (2021). *Advance Care Planning and the Law*: https://www.advancecareplanning.org.au/law-and-ethics/advance-care-planning-and-the-law

Brightwater Care Group Inc. v Rossiter [2009] WASC 229. Read the decision via eCourts Portal of Western Australia at: https://ecourts.justice.wa.gov.au

Hunter and New England Area Health Service v A [2009] NSWSC 761. Read the decision via NSW Caselaw at: https://www.caselaw.nsw.gov.au/decision/549ffbac3004262463c78daf

Medical Treatment Act 1988 (VIC) (Repealed Act): https://www.legislation.vic.gov.au/repealed-revoked/acts/medical-treatment-act-1988/051

Medical Treatment Planning and Decisions Act 2016 (V): https://www.legislation.vic.gov.au/in-force/acts/medical-treatment-planning-and-decisions-act-2016/009

NSW Health. (2021). *Making an Advance Care Directive*: https://www.health.nsw.gov.au/patients/acp/Pages/acd-form-info-book.aspx

REFERENCES

Adams, J. A., Bailey, D. E., Anderson, R. A. & Docherty, S. L. (2011). Nursing roles and strategies in end-of-life decision making in acute care: A systematic review of the literature. *Nursing Research and Practice*. doi: 10.1155/2011/527834

Aristotle. (n.d.). *Nichomachean Ethics*. Retrieved from: http://classics.mit.edu/Aristotle/nicomachaen.html

Australian Commission on Safety and Quality in Health Care (2021). *National Safety and Quality Health Service Standards,* (2nd edn). Sydney: ACSQHC. https://www.safetyandquality.gov.au/standards/nsqhs-standards

Diem, S. J., Lanton, J. D. & Tulsky, J. A. (1996). Cardiopulmonary resuscitation on television—Miracles and misinformation. *New England Journal of Medicine*, *334*, 1578–82. doi: 10.1056/NEJM199606133342406

Epstein, R. M. (2006). Mindful practice and the tacit ethics of the moment. In W. Shelton (Ed.), *Advances in Bioethics*. New York: Emerald.

Forrester, K. & Griffiths, D. (2014). *Essentials of Law for Health Professionals* (4th edn). Sydney: Elsevier.

Haidt, J. (2000). The emotional dog and its rational tail: A social intuitionist approach to moral judgment. *Psychological Review*, *108*, 814–34. doi: 10.1037/0033-295x.108.4.814

Hall, A., Rowland, C. & Grande, G. (2019). How should end-of-life advance care planning discussions be implemented according to patients and informal carers? A qualitative review of reviews. *Journal of Pain and Symptom Management*, *28*(2), 311–35. doi.org/10.1016/j.jpainsymman.2019.04.013

Hayes, B. (2013). Clinical model for ethical cardiopulmonary resuscitation decision-making. *Internal Medicine Journal*, *43*(1), 77–83. doi: 10.1111/j.1445-5994.2012.02841.x

Henderson, L. (2005). Combining moral philosophy and moral reasoning: The PAVE moral reasoning strategy. *International Education Journal*, *6*(2), 184–93.

International Council of Nurses. (2012). *Code of Ethics for Nurses*. https://www.icn.ch/sites/default/files/inline-files/2012_ICN_Codeofethicsfornurses_%20eng.pdf

Johnstone, M., Da Costa, C. & Turale, S. (2004). Registered and enrolled nurses' experiences of ethical issues in nursing practice. *Australian Journal of Advanced Nursing*, *22*(1), 24–30.

Kaldjian, L. C., Erekson, Z. D., Haberle, T. H., Curtis, A. E., Shinkunas, L. A., Cannon, K. T. & Forman-Hoffman, V. L. (2009). Code status discussions and goals of care among hospitalised adults. *Journal of Medical Ethics*, *35*(6), 338–42. doi: 10.1136/jme.2008.027854

Levett-Jones, T. Dwyer, T., Reid-Searl, K., Heaton, L., Flenady, T., Applegarth, J., Guinea, S. & Andersen, P. (2017*). The Patient Safety Competency Framework (PSCF) for Nursing Students*. Sydney, NSW.

Nursing and Midwifery Board of Australia (NMBA). (2016). *Code of Conduct for Nurses*. www.nursingmidwiferyboard.gov.au/Codes-Guidelines-Statements/Codes-Guidelines.aspx#competencystandards

Nursing and Midwifery Board of Australia (NMBA). (2016). *Registered Nurse Standards for Practice*. www.nursingmidwiferyboard.gov.au/Codes-Guidelines-Statements/Professional-standards.aspx

NSW Health. (2021). *Making an Advance Care Directive*. https://www.health.nsw.gov.au/patients/acp/Pages/acd-form-info-book.aspx

Portnova, J., Irvine, K., Yi, J. Y. & Enguidanos, S. (2015). It isn't like this on TV: Revisiting CPR survival rates depicted on popular TV shows. *Resuscitation*, *96*, 148–50. doi: 10.1016/j.resuscitation.2015.08.002

Sayers, G. M., Barratt, D., Gothard, C., Onnie, C., Perera, S. & Schulman, D. (2001). The value of taking an 'ethics history'. *Journal of Medical Ethics*, *27*, 114–17. dx.doi.org/10.1136/jme.27.2.114

Seal, M. (2007). Patient advocacy and advance care planning in the acute hospital setting. *Australian Journal of Advanced Nursing*, *24*(4), 29–36.

Stapleton, R. D., Ehlenbach, W. J., Deyo, R. A. & Curtis., J. R. (2014). Long-term outcomes after in-hospital CPR in older adults with chronic illness. *Chest*, *146*(5), 1214–25. doi: 10.1378/chest.13-2110

van Gijn, M. S., Frijns, D., van de Glind, E. M. M., van Munster, B. C, & Hamaker, M. E. (2014). The chance of survival and the functional outcome after in-hospital cardiopulmonary resuscitation in older people: A systematic review. *Age and Ageing*, *43*(4), 456–65. doi.org/10.1093/ageing/afu035

GLOSSARY

acquired brain injury Any injury or damage that occurs to the brain after birth.

acute pain A severe pain episode lasting from a few seconds to six months duration that may occur due to trauma, surgery or a medical condition.

advance care directive (ACD) A document by which a person makes provision for healthcare decisions in the event that, in the future, he or she becomes unable to make those decisions.

adverse drug event A harmful or unintended reaction or symptom from an administered medication.

aetiology The cause or origin of a disease or abnormal condition.

altered level of consciousness Any level of consciousness other than normal rousability and responsiveness.

analyse Separation into components: the breaking down of the whole into its parts (deductive reasoning).

anchoring The tendency to lock onto salient features in the patient's presentation too early in the clinical reasoning process, and failing to adjust this initial impression in light of later information.

anxiety Feelings of apprehension, uneasiness, tension and restlessness, often precipitated by different or unfamiliar experiences.

arrhythmias Abnormal heart rhythms or beats.

ascertainment bias When a nurse's thinking is shaped by prior assumptions and preconceptions, e.g. ageism, stigmatism and stereotyping.

asthma A respiratory condition that causes airways to become inflamed, swell and narrow; along with extra production of mucus, breathing becomes difficult.

autoimmune disease A condition where the immune system responds abnormally and attacks healthy cells within the body.

blood component therapy Transfusion of one or a number of components of whole blood, e.g. packed red cells or platelets.

cardiac arrest An emergency situation where a person's cardiac output and effective circulation suddenly ceases.

caregiver burden The level of multifaceted strain perceived by the caregiver from caring for a family member and/or loved one over time.

cerebral palsy A group of permanent disorders of development, movement and posture caused by non-progressive disturbances to the developing brain during pregnancy or soon after birth.

cerebrovascular accident Damage to the brain caused by interruption to its blood supply; characterised by the rapid onset of neurologic symptoms that generally last more than 24 hours.

chest pain A physical symptom requiring immediate evaluation, diagnosis and treatment. May be symptomatic of a cardiac complication, or could be musculoskeletal, gastrointestinal or psychogenic.

chronic Persisting for a long time, either recurring frequently or continuing for the rest of a person's life.

clinical reasoning The process by which nurses (and other clinicians) collect cues, process the information, come to an understanding of a patient problem or situation, plan and implement interventions, evaluate outcomes, and reflect on and learn from the process.

cognitive decline A gradual reduction in the speed at which individuals acquire information as they age.

community-acquired pneumonia Pneumonia (acute infection of the lungs) that has developed in the community, outside of a healthcare setting.

co-morbidity Two or more diseases experienced at the one time that are connected with each other via pathogenetic mechanisms.

complementary therapies A group of diverse medical and healthcare systems, practices and products that are not generally considered to be part of conventional medicine.

complex post-traumatic stress disorder A mental health condition that can occur after prolonged and repeated trauma. It can cause problems with memory and disrupt the development of a person's identity and their ability to form meaningful relationships.

complexity Sometimes referred to as multi-morbidity, a person with more than one chronic condition.

confirmation bias The tendency to look for confirming evidence to support a nursing diagnosis rather than look for disconfirming evidence to refute it.

CPR decision making The decision about whether to initiate CPR in the event of cardiac arrest.

critical thinking A complex collection of cognitive skills and affective habits of the mind.

cues Identifiable physiological or psychosocial changes experienced by the patient, perceived through history or assessment and understood in relation to a specific body of knowledge and philosophical beliefs. Cues also include the context of care and the surrounding clinical situation.

cultural safety Effective person-centred healthcare of an individual and/or their family as determined by their cultural background and traditional wishes.

data A piece or pieces of information about health status.

dehydration Extreme loss of fluid from cellular tissues in the body as a result of illness or lack of fluid intake.

delirium An acute reversible clinical syndrome of cognitive function, characterised by an acute decline that impairs cognitive and physical function.

dementia An umbrella term that is used to describe a gradual, progressive, irreversible deterioration of cerebral function, which results in disturbance of many higher cortical functions, including memory, thinking and judgment.

depression A mood disorder that causes a persistent feeling of sadness and loss of interest, and that can affect how a person feels, thinks and behaves.

deterioration Gradual decline or worsening of a condition.

diabetes A term covering a complex group of dangerous diseases that result in an imbalance of blood glucose levels. The three key types of diabetes include type 1 (insulin in pancreas is destroyed by the immune system); type 2 (pancreas does not produce enough insulin, or the insulin produced is not effective); and gestational diabetes (occurs during pregnancy, usually disappearing after birth of baby).

diabetic ketoacidosis A highly dangerous complication of diabetes that may occur when the body is profoundly deficient in insulin with symptoms of hyperglycaemia, ketosis, acidosis and dehydration.

diagnostic momentum When a label attached to a patient starts as a possibility but gathers increasing momentum until it is seen as definite and other possibilities are excluded.

disability A physical or mental condition that limits a person's movements, senses or activities.

discharge planning Activities that facilitate continuity of care during a person's transfer from one healthcare setting to another, or to home. It is a multi-disciplinary process involving doctors, nurses, social workers and possibly other healthcare professionals.

discriminate To use good judgment, note or observe a difference accurately, distinguish relevant from irrelevant information, recognise inconsistencies, narrow down information to what is most important and recognise gaps in cues collected.

dying with dignity Death that occurs in accordance with the wishes and values of a patient.

electrolyte imbalance An imbalance of electrolytes in the body, such as sodium, potassium, magnesium or calcium.

end-of-life care Physical, emotional, social and spiritual care for patients who are near the end of life and have stopped treatment to cure or control their disease.

ethical dilemma Situations in which there is a choice to be made between two options, neither of which resolves the situation in an ethically acceptable fashion.

ethical reasoning The ability to identify, assess and develop ethical arguments from a variety of ethical positions.

evaluate To make a judgment about the worth or value of something.

'failure to rescue' Mortality of patients who experience a hospital-acquired complication.

family-centred care Healthcare delivery centred around a partnership with a child's family and/or significant others.

fundamental attribution error The tendency to be judgmental and blame patients for their illnesses rather than examine the circumstances that may have been responsible.

futile and burdensome treatment Treatment that is of no benefit or is not in the person's best interests.

goals A desired outcome and a guidepost to the selection of nursing interventions.

haemotological diseases Diseases or disorders affecting the blood.

harm reduction Policies, programs and practices that aim to minimise negative health, and social and legal impacts associated with drug use.

healthcare transition The coordination and continuity of healthcare during a movement from one healthcare setting to another or to home, and/or between healthcare providers during the course of a chronic or acute illness.

heart failure When the heart is not able to effectively maintain blood flow to ensure sufficient circulation. Sometimes referred to as chronic or congestive heart failure.

holistic care Comprehensive healthcare that takes into consideration a person's physical, emotional, social, economic and spiritual needs.

hyperglycaemia An abnormally high blood glucose level.

hypervolaemia An abnormally high level of fluid in the circulating blood volume—or fluid volume deficit.

hypoglycaemia An abnormally low blood glucose level.

hypovolaemia An abnormally low level of fluid in the circulating blood volume.

hypoxia When an inadequate amount of oxygen is reaching tissues in parts of the body.

inconsistency Something that contradicts something else or that is not in keeping with it; not regular or predictable.

infer To make deductions or form opinions that follow logically by interpreting subjective and objective data; to consider alternatives and consequences.

interpret Analyse data to come to an understanding; to explain or tell the meaning of; to present in understandable terms.

interprofessional healthcare team Team members from two or more different healthcare professions who learn with, from and about each other to enable effective collaboration and improve health outcomes.

ischaemia A restriction or lack of blood supply to tissues in the body causing inadequate oxygen levels, sometimes leading to tissue necrosis.

kidney disease A disease where renal function is impaired, either acutely or chronically, sometimes requiring dialysis.

lactate An organic molecule produced by most tissues in the human body, with the highest production found in muscle.

match Information or cues that correspond to each other or cluster together naturally.

medication error A preventable incident where an incorrect medication is administered which may lead to patient harm or inappropriate use.

medication safety A model that aims to prevent medication errors occurring.

mental state examination A clinical assessment tool used in mental health assessment that provides a methodical way to observe and record an individual's thoughts, emotions, behaviour and demeanour.

mild cognitive impairment A syndrome characterised by cognitive decline that is different from normal ageing and does not meet the criteria for mild dementia.

motor symptoms Symptoms that affect movement, such as tremor, stiffness and slowness of movement.

multi-disciplinary healthcare team When healthcare professionals from a range of disciplines with different but complementary skills, knowledge and experience work together to deliver comprehensive care aimed at providing the best possible outcome for the physical and psychosocial needs of a patient and their carers.

multimodal pain management A combination of two or more analgesic medications or techniques acting on different mechanisms to provide optimal pain relief whilst using less opioids.

multimorbidity Two or more diseases appearing randomly without any connection to each other through pathogenetic mechanisms.

multisystem autoimmune disease An autoimmune disease that impacts multiple organs.

neurodegenerative condition Occurs when nerve cells in the brain or peripheral nervous system lose function over time and ultimately die.

neurological deterioration Gradual decline or worsening of the neurological state, which may appear as a decline in sensory and motor responses.

non-motor symptoms Symptoms that are not associated with movement, such as pain, anxiety, depression, orthostatic hypotension, disordered sleep, fatigue, bladder and bowel problems, sexual difficulties and swallowing problems.

nursing diagnosis A patient problem that becomes apparent following a thorough and systematic interpretation of subjective and objective data.

outcome A measurable change in a client's status in response to nursing care.

overconfidence bias Believing we know more than we do, reflecting a tendency to act on incomplete information, intuition or hunches.

oxygenation The process of oxygen diffusing from the alveolus to the pulmonary capillary.

pain management plan An agreement made between the medical officer and patient to use medication and/or alternative therapies in an effort to meet pain management goals.

pain myths A well-known but false idea or belief about pain and/or pain management.

palliative care An approach that improves the quality of life of people facing a life-limiting illness, through the prevention and relief of suffering by identification, assessment and treatment of pain and other physical, psychosocial and spiritual problems.

persistent (chronic) pain Pain that continues past a 'normal' healing time of around three months.

person-centred care A holistic approach to the planning and delivery of healthcare that is grounded in a philosophy of personhood. It is a way of practising that acknowledges and respects each individual's autonomy, personal beliefs, values, needs and desires.

predict To envisage or foresee something that may happen.

pre-emptive pain management Analgesia that is initiated before surgery in order to prevent the establishment of central sensitisation evoked by the incisional and inflammatory injuries occurring during surgery and in the early post-operative period. Also refers to all analgesic strategies that aim to prevent rather than treat pain after it has manifested.

premature closure The tendency to accept a nursing diagnosis without sufficient evidence and before it has been fully verified.

primary healthcare Generally the first contact a person has with Australia's health system. It relates to treatment of patients that can be provided in the home or in community-based settings.

psychological wellbeing A person's level of psychological happiness/health, encompassing life satisfaction, and feelings of accomplishment.

psychosis A state of mind where there is a disconnect with reality.

psych-out error When clinical reasoning errors occur in people with mental illness, and co-morbid conditions are overlooked or minimalised. A variant is when medical conditions (e.g. hypoxia, delirium, electrolyte imbalance or head injuries) are misdiagnosed as psychiatric conditions.

raised intracranial pressure A rise in pressure of the cerebrospinal fluid surrounding the brain and spinal cord, due to either an increase in fluid volume or swelling of the brain.

rapid response A system whereby a team of healthcare professionals (sometimes referred to as a medical emergency team) immediately responds to a call for a patient who is exhibiting signs of serious clinical deterioration.

recall To remember or recollect a past situation or piece of knowledge.

recovery model A model that supports an individual's recovery from mental illness.

reflection A critical review of practice with a view to refinement, improvement or change; the process of looking back and the careful consideration of an experience; to explore the understanding of what one did and why and the impact it has on oneself and others.

rehabilitation The process of restoring an individual's health and mental or physical abilities to the pre-operative or pre-injury level through guided therapy.

relate To connect or link; to discover new relationships or patterns; to cluster cues together to identify relationships between them.

'rescue' The ability to recognise deteriorating patients and to intervene appropriately.

respiratory distress A life-threatening condition involving breathing difficulties due to narrowed airways or when alveoli fill with fluid.

risk nursing diagnosis A clinical judgment about a potential problem where the presence of risk factors indicates that a problem may develop unless nurses intervene appropriately.

sepsis A potentially life-threatening infection—often of the blood.

septic shock A serious medical condition that occurs when sepsis, which is organ injury or damage in response to infection, leads to dangerously low blood pressure and abnormalities in cellular metabolism. It can cause multiple organ failure and death.

stigma A mark, blemish or sign of disgrace, shame or dishonour.

stroke Brain damage from an interruption to the blood supply. Two types of stroke include haemorrhagic (bleeding in the brain) and ischaemic (blocked artery). A transient ischaemic attack (TIA) may also occur, which is when the blood supply is interrupted, but for a short time only.

substance use dependence A condition in which the use of one or more substances leads to a clinically significant impairment or distress. It refers to a cluster of cognitive, behavioural and physiological symptoms indicating that the individual continues using the substance despite significant substance-related problems.

symptom management To prevent or treat as early as possible the symptoms of a disease, side effects caused by treatment of a disease, and psychological, social, and spiritual problems related to a disease or its treatment.

synthesis The putting together of parts into the whole (inductive reasoning); the integration of new knowledge with previous knowledge, to form a 'new whole'.

terminal dehydration A type of isotonic fluid imbalance that occurs at the end of life, which can lead to feelings of euphoria and an increasing level of comfort during the dying process.

terminal restlessness A particularly distressing form of delirium that sometimes occurs in dying patients characterised by spiritual, emotional or physical restlessness, anxiety, agitation and cognitive failure.

time-critical medications Medications where early or delayed administration of maintenance doses, more than 30 minutes before or after the scheduled time, may cause harm or result in substantial sub-optimal therapy or pharmacological effect.

transfusion reactions Adverse signs or symptoms that appear or occur during, or up to 24 hours after, infusion of transfused product.

transient ischaemic attack A brief episode of neurological dysfunction resulting from an interruption in the blood supply to the brain or eye, sometimes as a precursor to stroke.

trauma-informed care A framework for healthcare delivery that is based on knowledge and understanding of how trauma affects people's lives.

unpacking principle Failure to collect and unpack all relevant cues, and consider differential diagnoses, resulting in significant possibilities being missed.

withdrawal of treatment The removal of a therapy that has been started in an attempt to sustain life but is not, or is no longer, effective.

withholding treatment The decision not to make further therapeutic interventions.

INDEX

D

E

P